KETAMINE

The Story of Modern Psychiatry's Most Fascinating Molecule

By

Keith G. Rasmussen, M.D.

Professor of Psychiatry, Mayo Clinic, Rochester, Minnesota

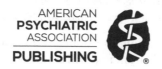

AMERICAN
PSYCHIATRIC
ASSOCIATION
PUBLISHING

Copyright © 2024 American Psychiatric Association Publishing

ALL RIGHTS RESERVED

First Edition

Manufactured in the United States of America on acid-free paper
27 26 25 24 23   5 4 3 2 1

American Psychiatric Association Publishing
800 Maine Avenue SW, Suite 900
Washington, DC 20024–2812
www.appi.org

Library of Congress Cataloging-in-Publication Data

Names: Rasmussen, Keith G., author. | American Psychiatric Association
  Publishing, issuing body.
Title: Ketamine : the story of modern psychiatry's most fascinating
  molecule / by Keith G. Rasmussen.
Description: Washington, DC : American Psychiatric Association Publishing,
  [2024] | Includes bibliographical references and index.
Identifiers: LCCN 2024003272 (print) | LCCN 2024003273 (ebook) | ISBN
  9781615375448 (paperback ; alk. paper) | ISBN 9781615375455 (ebook)
Subjects: MESH: Ketamine | Phencyclidine | Mental Disorders--drug therapy |
  Phencyclidine Abuse
Classification: LCC RD86.K4 (print) | LCC RD86.K4 (ebook) | NLM QV 81 |
  DDC 615.7/81--dc23/eng/20240228
LC record available at https://lccn.loc.gov/2024003272
LC ebook record available at https://lccn.loc.gov/2024003273

British Library Cataloguing in Publication Data
A CIP record is available from the British Library.

For Gemma and Sigrid – Salamat

Contents

About the Author

Keith G. Rasmussen, M.D., is Professor of Psychiatry at the Mayo Clinic, Rochester, Minnesota.

Disclosure

Dr. Rasmussen stated that he had no competing interests during the year preceding manuscript submission.

Chapter 1

Ketamine's Precursor: The Discovery of PCP

KEY POINTS IN THIS CHAPTER:

- PCP was synthesized in 1956 by Harold Maddox.
- PCP was developed as an anesthetic drug, but it caused emergence agitation.
- Most eventual uses of ketamine were presaged by PCP.

What is ketamine? To Calvin L. Stevens, Wayne State University chemistry professor and consultant to the Parke-Davis pharmaceutical company, it was one of the compounds he synthesized in his laboratory in 1962. To his bosses, the Parke-Davis executives, it was a potentially profitable medication. To Edward Domino, a University of Michigan pharmacologist, it was a drug with interesting psychological effects. To John Krystal, Yale University psychiatry professor, it is a neuropharmacological probe to study the neurobiology of schizophrenia. To anesthesiologists, it has proved to be an excellent anesthetic that does not suppress respiration or blood pressure. To the field of psychiatry, it is a simple-looking molecule that has breathed new life into a stale and anemic psychopharmacopeia. To modern practicing psychiatrists, it is much-needed relief from the grinding drudgery of prescribing pills that don't work very well. To some entrepreneurial doctors who oversee ketamine clinics, it is a precious commodity with which to enrich themselves. To chronically depressed people, it is hope that they don't have to spend their lives thinking about suicide. To the psychedelic connoisseur, it is a pathway to enlightenment. To the ketamine addict, it is a pathway to hell.

Like no other compound, whether prescribed by doctors or used recreationally, ketamine has a perplexing duality about it. Does it protect the brain or damage it? Does it cause addiction or treat addiction? Does it worsen psychiatric disorders or cure them? Does it lead to philosophical insight or just a fool's drug high? Some people who take this drug love it; others hate it.

Of all the molecules in modern psychiatry, ketamine is the most fascinating. Think about it—what other molecules could be considered more charismatic? Are any of the other drugs we introduce into people, such as antidepressant, antipsychotic, antianxiety, antimanic, stimulant, and hypnotic agents, really that engrossing? Most of them are weakly active at best and barely distinct from placebo. Thus the intense interest in ketamine. And then of course there are all the innumerable molecules inherent in the human brain. Dopamine, serotonin, and norepinephrine captured the imagination of psychiatry for three decades but seem rather tired now, yesterday's news. The old notions that psychosis is caused by "too much dopamine" and depression by "too little serotonin or norepinephrine"— hypotheses that seemed so sophisticated in the 1970s—now seem ludicrously simplistic. All the other neurohormones and neuromodulators have caused but the barest ripples of interest.

No, in modern times it is ketamine that stands head and shoulders above the others in fascination. Just open an internet browser, enter "ketamine," and appreciate the media and scientific interest in this compound.

In this book, the story of ketamine is told. It is the author's wish that, as he has been captivated by this story, so too will the reader. Since its first synthesis in 1962, ketamine has generated a great deal of excitement and has traversed several pathways. These include anesthesiology and pain medicine; psychedelic drug use; the neuropharmacology laboratory to study psychotic processes such as schizophrenia, brain damage, and neuroprotection; and most recently, psychopharmacology to treat depression and other psychiatric disorders. It is on a steep trajectory, and it is not clear where—to a revolution in psychiatry, perhaps? Or a dead end like lobotomy?

In this book, the various ways in which scientists and others have studied and used this drug are reviewed. But first, as a launching point, we cover the backstory—how did this versatile molecule come about? Biographies of people begin with a description of the main character's parents. In like manner, seeing this book as a biography of ketamine, we begin with ketamine's "parent," an interesting, unusual, and even legendary compound: phencyclidine (aka PCP, aka angel dust). Virtually all of the pathways traversed by ketamine over the decades really begin with phencyclidine. So, where did PCP come from?

The Discovery of Phencyclidine

The story begins with a chemist born in 1871 in Cherbourg, France, with the regal-sounding name of François Auguste Victor Grignard (pronounced roughly "greenyar"). Dr. Grignard won the Nobel Prize for chemistry in 1912 for discovery of a type of chemical reaction that now bears his name. The *Grignard reaction* allows the formation of carbon-carbon bonds, which is enormously helpful in the chemical synthesis of thousands of useful compounds. *Grignard reagent* refers to organometallic halides (an organic moiety attached to usually magnesium bromide), which are used to effect a wide variety of chemical syntheses.

In the early part of the twentieth century, Grignard reagents turned out to be critical for the synthesis of a type of compound at the beginning of the pathway that led to PCP and ketamine. This class of compounds, known as the *arylcyclohexylamines*, consist of three parts: an aryl group, a cyclohexyl group, and an amine group. An aryl group is aromatic, a cyclic structure that is planar and very stable. A cyclohexyl group is based on cyclohexane, a six-membered ring of carbon atoms that is not aromatic, meaning the six carbon atoms are not coplanar. An amine group contains a nitrogen atom, which may be part of a ring of carbon atoms, or attached to two hydrogen atoms, or a carbon-based group such as a methyl or ethyl group.

Arylcyclohexylamines have interesting biological activity. In 1956, Dr. Harold Maddox, a chemist working for Parke-Davis in Detroit, Michigan, was looking into this class of compounds as possible analgesics or sedatives (Maddox 1981). Using an old reagent with the barely pronounceable name of piperidinocyclohexanecarbonitrile, he added "phenyl Grignard," otherwise known as phenylmagnesium bromide, a Grignard reagent. After a few more steps, the final product was the arylcyclohexylamine compound now known as phenylcyclohexylpiperidine—or phencyclidine. The aryl group of PCP was a phenyl group, with the amine group being a piperidine ring, of course with the cyclohexyl ring that is always present in an arylcyclohexylamine. The molecular structure of PCP is outlined in Figure 1–1. Note that the phenyl and amine groups are geminal, which in chemistry means they are bonded to the same carbon atom on the cyclohexyl group. Several names for this new compound emerged over the years: CI-395 (as denoted by the drug company before a common name was agreed on), Sernyl, Sernylan, and, on the street, the notorious angel dust.

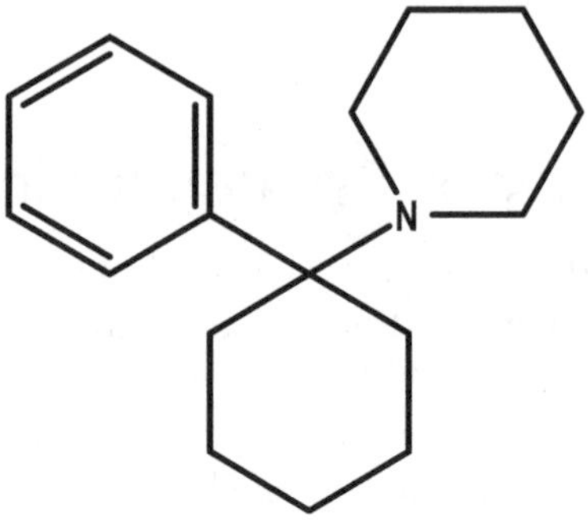

FIGURE 1–1.   The molecular structure of PCP
(phenylcyclohexylpiperidine or phencyclidine)

So the year is 1956, and chemist Maddox, relying on Grignard reactions, has synthesized this new compound, phencyclidine. What next? Maddox of course had no preexisting idea what clinical applicability PCP might have. It was synthesized in the hope of finding a better sedative or analgesic drug, hot chemical commodities in those days. In pharmacological drug development, before a compound can be used in humans, it is first used in animals to test for basic safety and see whether there is a signal for efficacy. Thus, CI-395 was handed over to animal pharmacologists for experimentation.

Animal Testing: The Rise of PCP

The first person to take custody of the newly synthesized PCP was expert animal pharmacologist Dr. Graham Chen, a Parke-Davis employee. When Maddox synthesized PCP, he was looking for a sedative or analgesic. Thus, Chen started experimenting to see whether PCP had such properties in various animal species, and also of course to see whether it was safe (Chen 1981). He and his colleagues published an initial detailed description (Chen et al. 1959). They studied PCP in rats, mice, rabbits, guinea pigs, dogs, cats, hamsters, monkeys, pigeons, frogs, and fish. The investigators noted that PCP caused either behavioral stimulation (usually at high doses) or depression (mainly at low doses), effects that varied by species. For example, rats and mice tended toward excitation, and other species tended toward depression or a *cataleptoid state*, an expression that appears frequently in the PCP and ketamine literature of the 1960s. Derived from the term *catalepsy* (when an organism assumes a fixed posture and does not respond to stimulation, used to describe humans who are catatonic), a cataleptoid state was considered the analogous phenomenon in animals. As described by Chen et al. (1959), PCP commonly caused a cataleptoid state in which the animal would lie still and unresponsive and could be handled and even surgically operated on without becoming agitated. That made PCP attractive as a potential anesthetic drug. From low to high doses, Chen et al. (1959) noted the following general progression of animal behavioral effects of PCP: 1) being able to be handled; 2) cataleptoid state; 3) deep surgical anesthesia; and 4) convulsions. At lower doses, PCP also prevented pharmacologically or electrically induced seizures, thus raising the question of whether it could be an antiepileptic drug. (The latter finding from the late 1950s progressed all the way to the present with PCP's progeny, ketamine, but that story is explored later.)

At PCP doses sufficient to induce anesthesia for surgery in animals, respirations and blood pressure were not suppressed as happened with the anesthetic agents then in use, mostly barbiturates. This finding was enormously important: for some patient populations, it is desirable to perform a procedure without having to give manual respirations or agents to keep blood pressure from falling. Thus, the finding that PCP did not suppress respirations or blood pressure was critical in instilling interest in human trials. Although the Chen et al. (1959) paper focused on animals, the authors did make the cryptic comment that PCP causes humans to react "similarly as monkeys and cats."

In a later publication, Chen and Weston (1960) focused on the effect of PCP in monkeys. The animals would assume a "far-away look" with lack of responsiveness, so that a procedure could be done. Upon awakening from PCP, the animals remained calm. There was no behavioral toxicity with PCP—the animals went into and out of the cataleptoid state without agitation. Thus, to Parke-Davis executives, it appeared as though they may have a blockbuster anesthetic drug on their hands, and they approved it for experiments in humans. Little did they know what was about to be unleashed.

Human Testing: The Fall of PCP

Filled with excitement and enthusiasm about this potential anesthetic, and reassured about safety and efficacy in animals, Parke-Davis executives now ordered human trials. They named the drug *Sernyl*.[1] In those days of rela-

---

[1]According to Edward Domino, the discoverer of the pharmacological effects of ketamine in humans, the name was a portmanteau of *serenity* and *tranquility* (Domino 1980), two descriptors that could hardly have been less apropos to the drug's later reputation. A more suitable name may have been *Ralence*, a combination of *rage* and *violence*.

tively easy Food and Drug Administration (FDA) approval for new drugs, Sernyl was granted approval in 1957, almost before human data were even gathered. The drug company enlisted anesthesiologists at Detroit Receiving Hospital to use PCP for anesthesia. The results were published by Greifenstein et al. (1958). In initial dose-finding work, it was found that 0.5–1.0 mg/kg produced excitation or even convulsions, but doses of 0.25 mg/kg produced good analgesia.

At this point, some definition of anesthesiologic terms is in order. *Analgesia* means lack of pain perception. *Anesthesia* means lack of any sensation, which can be local (such as with lidocaine) or general. There are no general anesthetic agents that do not also cause unconsciousness, or at least a diminution of conscious awareness. Theoretically, in surgical or other procedural work, what is needed is analgesia, so that the procedure can be conducted without the patient having pain. Most true analgesics, such as aspirin, acetaminophen, or even narcotic opioids, are not strong enough for invasive procedures to be done comfortably. Thus, for surgeries, general anesthetic agents are needed, and as noted, all of them cause unconsciousness—or at least all of them until PCP.

What Greifenstein et al. (1958) discovered was that some of the patients undergoing surgery (there were a total of 64) did·obtain enough analgesia with PCP that the procedure could be done, but some of the patients were not completely asleep. The dose of 0.25 mg/kg was enough to cause patients not to respond to auditory or painful stimuli. In about one-fourth of the patients, some degree of excitation occurred during the surgery. Postoperative euphoria, what seemed like an intoxicated state, was common and lasted for many hours. Ten of the 64 patients were frankly agitated and behaviorally unmanageable upon recovery from anesthesia, a phenomenon called *emergence delirium* or *emergence agitation* (in this context, *emergence* referring to emerging from the state of general anesthesia, or regaining consciousness). Some had hallucinations. Interestingly, despite the emergence agitation being quite prolonged (e.g., into the next day), some patients had no memory of it or of the surgery. That was important, because anesthesiologists do not want their patients to recall any aspect of surgery, as such memories are quite traumatic and emotionally distressing. Thus, *amnesia* (a gap in one's memory) is a goal of anesthesia in addition to analgesia.

Besides these behavioral issues, the authors did note that, as with animals, there was no diminution in blood pressure or suppression of respiration with PCP, both very desirable characteristics. Thus, a summary of this first human experience with PCP was that almost all patients achieved good analgesia during the procedure with maintenance of blood pressure and breathing, with amnesia of it later on—but a fairly high percentage experienced unacceptable emergence behavioral reactions.

The study was followed by a more in-depth report by Johnstone et al. (1959), working out of Crumpsall Hospital and Manchester Royal Infirmary, both in Manchester, England. Sernyl was supplied by Parke-Davis. The authors tested the utility of Sernyl in three phases: preoperative sedation (something to help patients relax before surgery), operative anesthesia, and postoperative analgesia. For preoperative sedation, 42 patients were given Sernyl 10 mg intramuscularly 1 hour before surgery. In patients older than 60, the reaction was one of detachment, calmness, even amusement. In those younger than 60, the reactions were more varied and included dissociative states, out-of-body experiences, and hallucinations. Two patients who received their 10-mg dose intravenously experienced behavioral excitement, obviously not a desired reaction in preoperative patients. None of the patients had problems with breathing or blood pressure, and pain seemed to be diminished.

For operative anesthesia, 67 patients were given 10- to 20-mg doses of intravenous Sernyl. Reactions were unanticipated: some went into a catatonic stupor or *akinetic mutism* (lack of movement or speech); some appeared ecstatic; and two believed they were with God. Several patients could not be successfully anesthetized with Sernyl—in other words, they did not reach a deep enough state of unconsciousness to do surgery. Some patients had delirium with rambling speech, obviously too much excitement for surgery (Johnstone et al. 1959, p. x). Of note, when the patients for surgery were pretreated with a combination of thiopental (a barbiturate anesthetic) and halothane (a gaseous, inhaled anesthetic) and then treated with Sernyl, none of the behavioral toxicity occurred, and anesthesia proceeded optimally. Upon emergence from Sernyl anesthesia, the older patients were noted to be a bit euphoric; the young and middle-aged patients were noisy and excited, sometimes violently so, especially the men, and this would go on for hours sometimes, obviously an undesirable situation. However, analgesia and amnesia were good, and blood pressure and breathing were maintained.

For the final usage of Sernyl in the Johnstone et al. (1959) study, postoperative analgesia, the authors used 10 mg intramuscular Sernyl after surgery in 50 patients to control postsurgical pain. They found that Sernyl given in this manner indeed achieved good analgesia (pain control) without behavioral excitement (as long as the thiopental-halothane combination had been used earlier). Thus, in summary, the Johnstone et al. (1959) study confirmed the impressions of the smaller Greifenstein et al. (1958) study. Pertinent findings were that Sernyl was a potent analgesic agent, making patients oblivious to pain without rendering them unconscious, thus allowing some light surgical procedures to be done entirely with Sernyl. Additionally, there was no suppression of respiration or drop in blood pressure, unlike what traditional anesthetic agents caused. Pharyngeal and laryngeal reflexes were maintained, so aspiration of refluxed gastric contents or oral secretions into the lungs did not occur. However, behavioral toxicity as manifested by emergence delirium/agitation occurred in young adults and middle-aged people, and not in the elderly and not in the presence of thiopental-halothane.

In the first report of PCP/Sernyl administered to children (Johnstone 1960), a dose of 20 mg was used for adults, and less for children. A catatonic trance resulted, in which there was a lack of verbal responsivity, and patients could be handled and manipulated without resisting. Excitation and hallucinations occurred in young adult males, but not in the elderly, in children, or in the presence of thiopental-halothane. The authors mentioned that low doses might be useful serially to treat pain syndromes—the first mention of the use of an arylcyclohexylamine to treat pain. This issue never went anywhere for PCP, but ketamine eventually caught on as a treatment for various chronic pain syndromes, a topic to be discussed in more detail in Chapter 6, "Ketamine for Chronic Pain."

Following up on the use of Sernyl in children, an important report from Muir et al. (1961) described the use of Sernyl for burn dressing changes in 50 children from Booth Hall Children's Hospital in Manchester, England. In the children older than 5, about half had troublesome behavioral and emotional reactions: some had restlessness that would last for hours, three had hallucinations, several cried, and one 7-year-old boy was "noisy and abusive" for 2 hours. Complete analgesia was achieved in 78% of Sernyl administrations. Dissociative, out-of-body experiences were described by some of the older children. Interestingly, the children younger than 5 had none of these problems. Taking into account the lack of behavioral/emotional effects in the very young (<5) and elderly (as seen in previous reports), the authors speculated that the brain substrate for this type of reaction to Sernyl was not developed until about age 5 and atrophied in older age.

Attempts were made to mitigate the emergence agitation with Sernyl in humans. Gool and Clarke (1964) tried using either chlorpromazine or haloperidol before Sernyl administration in 735 surgeries (a very large sample size). About 5%–10% of patients developed agitated states, which may be a bit less than reported with Sernyl alone. Like several other groups, Gool and Clarke mentioned that the emergence agitation did not occur in the very young or very old.

By the mid-1960s, it was abundantly clear that PCP/phencyclidine/Sernyl had not lived up to its original promise for anesthesiology use in humans, and it was abandoned for that purpose.

PCP: Epilogue

Although PCP was a nonstarter with regard to human use in anesthesiology, it did enjoy a few years of useful existence in veterinary medicine. For example, Kroll (1962) studied several dozen species of zoo animals and found that Sernyl with proper dosing effectively rendered the animals subdued for handling without suppressing respiration or circulation. No emergence reactions were noted, in marked contrast to the human reactions to this drug. Tavernor (1963) described his experience giving Sernyl to 110 pigs for procedural sedation and extolled the same benefits as in other research, namely good sedation without emergence reactions. Ortega and Otter (1967), in a creative use of Sernyl, found that with a specially constructed Sernyl gun, stray dogs could be handled safely without behavioral excitation. Vondruska (1965) gave Sernyl intramuscularly to 86 baboons for the purpose of buttock tattooing (as identification for behavioral research). No emergence reactions were noted. The animals were observed to stare off into space, something that is seen with humans as well. Barany (1963) studied Sernyl in vervet monkeys (whose Latin name is the regal-sounding *Cercopithecus ethiops*). Sernyl helped the investigators measure ocular pressures in this otherwise highly uncooperative population. In the 109 animals, they noticed a good 45 minutes of the cataleptoid state, and there were no emergence agitation reactions. In a related study, Young (1963) used a variety of anesthetic techniques to sedate 26 monkeys for vision research and concluded that Sernyl was the best, with no emergence reactions.

These are but a few examples of innumerable publications showing how well PCP worked for veterinary medicine. Essentially, it was used to manage procedures for animals in an office (dogs and cats), on the farm (cattle and horses), in a zoo, and in the wild (e.g., managing large game on wildlife reserves). So there was a place for PCP, although its developers had had higher hopes.

Thus PCP had use for animals and was abandoned in humans—or so it was thought, for something very sinister and entirely unexpected was about to happen. An epidemic of pain and tragedy was about to be unleashed. Considering the dysphoric emotional and behavioral reactions described above with PCP in human studies, we may wonder why such a drug would ever be taken recreationally—yet that is exactly what happened. Ultimately, because of thefts from veterinary offices and the horrible PCP epidemic of the 1970s (a topic to be discussed in Chapter 3, "Recreational Use of Ketamine"), PCP was finally taken off the market in 1978. It is a Schedule II drug in the United States, which means it can be used only under experimental conditions with special governmental approval. Given the usefulness of PCP, however, its descendant ketamine piqued the interest of veterinary researchers, and it turned out to be just as good in veterinary medicine as PCP was. In fact, to this day, ketamine is widely used in veterinary medicine, although that usage is not further explored in this book.

In addition to being investigated for anesthesiology in the late 1950s and early 1960s, PCP's interesting psychological effects in humans were pursued. It continues to be used in neuropharmacology laboratories, usually in rodent studies looking at various aspects of brain function. In particular, some investigators believed its effects could help elaborate the neurobiological basis of psychotic states, notably schizophrenia. Thus commenced a pathway of studies that lasted well into the 1970s, looking into the neurobiological effects of PCP as clues to the neurobiological basis of psychiatric illness. That line of investigation also led directly to the use of ketamine for the same purpose (see Chapter 5, "The Ketamine Model of Schizophrenia"). There was even an early hint that PCP might actually treat neurotic states such as anxiety and depression (Bodi et al. 1959). Of course, this notion was prescient considering modern psychiatry's current boom of ketamine for such states. (More on that in Chapter 7, "Ketamine for Depression," and Chapter 8, "Other Uses of Ketamine in Psychiatry.")

Every facet of ketamine (anesthetic agent, abused substance, neuropharmacological probe, antidepressant) was preordained by PCP. PCP was a precursor of almost all aspects of the ketamine story—further reason to call PCP the "parent" of ketamine. Next, we visit the story of ketamine's birth.

Chapter 2

The Birth of Ketamine

KEY POINTS IN THIS CHAPTER:

- The synthesis of ketamine in 1962 by Calvin Stevens culminated from an intense search for a better-tolerated alternative to PCP for anesthesia.

- Ed Domino discovered the fascinating dissociative effects of ketamine in humans.

- Ketamine was approved for anesthesia in 1970 in the United States.

So phencyclidine was a bust. Now what? The Parke-Davis scientists and executives who developed it had two general options: either give up on that class of medications, or keep trying to find similar compounds that might have a better efficacy/side effect profile. They chose to keep going. Recall that phencyclidine belongs to the class of medications called *arylcyclohexylamines*. Scores of aryl, cyclohexyl, and amine groups are available to chemists, so a furious effort was undertaken in the laboratory to synthesize new arylcyclohexylamines and test them for the benefits of phencyclidine without the emergence agitation. Dr. Duncan McCarthy, who was a Parke-Davis scientist at the time, later described the frenzied pace to find a replacement for phencyclidine (McCarthy 1981). McCarthy indicated that some 300 total compounds were evaluated at various stages of testing during the late 1950s and early 1960s, but alas, none of them seemed to fit the bill.

As McCarthy (1981) tells the tale, a new chemist joined the group in the early 1960s, Dr. Calvin Stevens, a chemistry professor at nearby Wayne State University in Detroit, who also had consulted with Parke-Davis. Ste-

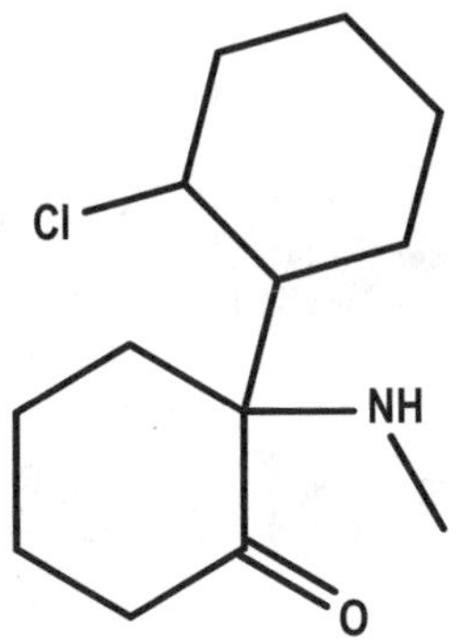

FIGURE 2–1. **The molecular structure of ketamine (2-(2-chlorophenyl)-2-(methylamino) cyclohexanone)**

vens, who was asked to contribute to the search for a better arylcyclohexylamine, fine-tuned his molecular syntheses, and in April 1962 developed the following molecule: 2-(2-chlorophenyl)-2-(methylamino) cyclohexanone (see Figure 2–1). This newly synthesized molecule was assigned the code CL-369 and tested on animals. It was recognized as outstanding (McCarthy 1981), and further study ensued. As shown in Figure 2–1, the cyclohexyl component of this molecule has a carbon-oxygen double bond, with two other single carbon-carbon bonds on the carbon atom bonded to the oxygen. Such an arrangement in chemistry is called a *ketone*; combining that word with *cyclohexyl* yields *cyclohexanone*. A phenyl group with a chloride ion attached at the number 2 position is itself attached to the number 2 position of the cyclohexanone moiety, and a methylamino group is also attached to the number 2 position on that moiety. Thus, all three elements required of an arylcyclohexylamine are present: the cyclohexanone core (cyclohexyl group), the amino group (in this case methylamino), and the aromatic phenyl group (which also has a chloride ion attached to it). The reader is encouraged to read the name of this new molecule and look at the figure closely so as to attain some lasting familiarity with it, because it is none other than the protagonist of this book: ketamine.

Of course, the name *ketamine* is much easier to remember. It was coined by Parke-Davis chemists as a portmanteau of *ketone* and *amine*. As ketamine's potential began to be appreciated by Parke-Davis scientists, the code name was changed from CL-369 to CI-581 (McCarthy 1981), which predominates as an identifier for this compound in the early literature. (In fact, no published papers use CL-369.) Eventually, as human use took off, the common name ketamine proliferated in the literature. Occasionally, some variation of the chemical name has been used, but not often.

Now we take a closer look at the first animal and human experience with this most fascinating drug. First we will cover the animal literature.

Ketamine Captures the Interest of Animal Pharmacologists

The year 1965 was a banner year for ketamine. Many publications came out in that year, including the first animal report and the first human report. One of the first papers was a study by Parke-Davis animal pharmacologist Chen (1965), who, as the reader will recall, also studied PCP in animals. Several anesthetic compounds with ketamine were tested to see whether they resulted in *catalepsy*, a state of muscular rigidity, posturing, and lack of response to manipulation (in animals) or verbal stimulation (in humans).[1]

In humans, catalepsy is often seen as a sign of *catatonia*, a syndrome consisting of mutism, stupor, posturing, waxy flexibility (*cerea flexibilitas*), echolalia, echopraxia, automatic obedience, rigidity (*gegenhalten*), and other signs. In modern psychiatric parlance, the term catalepsy has been replaced by the terms *posturing* and *waxy flexibility*. In the 1960s, the term catalepsy was quite popular in the animal pharmacology literature, thanks to its pronounced appearance after animals were given drugs such as PCP and later ketamine.

Catalepsy captured the fascination of early animal pharmacologists such as Chen because it allowed animals to be manipulated or even operated on without loss of respiration or drop in blood pressure, as discussed in Chapter 1. Chen (1965) explored this phenomenon with PCP as well as three other arylcyclohexylamines, one of which was ketamine. All four compounds caused catalepsy in pigeons (an animal easy to obtain and in whom a characteristic cataleptic reaction occurs), and he detailed the reaction and the dose-response relationship of the compounds. Beyond this, nothing in this early paper distinguishes PCP from ketamine or the other agents used. It is largely a technical report.

In another study published that year (McCarthy et al. 1965), a group of rhesus monkeys was given phencyclidine, CI-581 (aka ketamine), or the barbiturates thiamylal or pentobarbital. Both barbiturates were commonly used at the time and reliably induced anesthesia, but at the cost of suppressing breathing and lowering blood pressure. The study assessed the ability of the four agents to anesthetize the monkeys and noted any adverse reactions. Intrave-

---

[1]Note that *catalepsy* is not to be confused with the similar-sounding *cataplexy*, which is a state of muscular weakness, loss of muscle tone, and in severe cases, drop attacks whereby the patient suddenly falls to the floor. In humans, cataplexy is a symptom of narcolepsy, a condition of excessive sleepiness.

nous injections were given over a 1-minute period. Outcomes were the minimum dose to achieve anesthesia (anesthetic threshold dose [ATD]), duration of anesthesia, minimum dose to cause adverse effects (undesirable effects dose [UED]), and minimum lethal dose (MLD). The MLD/ATD ratio, a reflection of how much higher the lethal dose is relative to the dose needed to achieve anesthesia, was 26 for PCP, 16 for CI-581, 6.5 for thiamylal, and 3.3 for pentobarbital. Thus, one would have to give 26 times the minimal anesthetic dose of PCP to cause death, and 16 times for ketamine. The barbiturates obviously had much lower ranges of safety, and the arylcyclohexylamines emerged as safer anesthetics, at least for rhesus monkeys, than barbiturates.

The main undesirable side effect with PCP was convulsions, which did not occur with CI-581. The UED/ATD ratio, a reflection of how much higher a dose causing undesirable side effects is relative to the minimal anesthetic dose, was 8 for PCP, 15 for CI-581, 6 for thiamylal, and 3 for pentobarbital. Thus, one had to give a much higher dose of CI-581 to get undesirable side effects (respiratory depression) than of PCP (convulsions). Again, the barbiturates had a much lower range of safety. CI-581 had the shortest duration of action, followed by thiamylal, PCP, and pentobarbital. Thus, as far as inducing anesthesia in monkeys, CI-581 seemed superior to PCP.

Chen and colleagues at Parke-Davis published a thorough neuropharmacological animal study of CI-581 in mice, pigeons, and monkeys (Chen et al. 1966). Early studies showed that CI-581, like PCP, was a behavioral stimulant in these animals at low doses, a depressant at higher doses, and a cataleptic, albeit with a shorter duration than PCP. Also unlike PCP, CI-581 did not produce convulsions in pigeons, mice, or monkeys at high dosages. Thus, it was investigated as a possible anticonvulsant drug as well as an anesthetic in these species. Decades later, this possibility would become clinically relevant to humans (see Chapter 9, "Is Ketamine a Neuroprotectant or a Neurotoxin?").

Clearly, CI-581 looked better than barbiturates in the animal studies. It also looked somewhat better than PCP, having a shorter duration of action and not causing convulsions at high doses. The issue of interest, though, was whether CI-581 caused less emergence agitation in humans. Thus, human studies were undertaken, and the results opened up a wellspring of curiosity that continues to this day.

Initial Experience Giving Ketamine to Humans

After the animal pharmacology staff at Parke-Davis in Ann Arbor, Michigan, were essentially finished with their studies establishing the safety and efficacy of CI-581 in a variety of animal species, the drug was handed off to human pharmacology investigators. The first-ever human trials were entrusted to Dr. Edward Domino, a pharmacology specialist physician, and Drs. Guenter Corssen and Peter Chodoff, anesthesiologists, all associated with the University of Michigan Medical Center in Ann Arbor. The reason anesthesiologists were involved in these studies was simple: Parke-Davis was pursuing it as an anesthetic.

For their first study, to assess basic safety and pharmacological response in humans, the investigators administered CI-581 to 20 prison inmate volunteers (such practices, which are now considered unethical, were widespread in those days) (Domino et al. 1965). CI-581 was infused intravenously (IV) to each participant over 1 minute in doses of 0.1–2.0 mg/kg. Several variables were assessed: laboratory blood work, analgesic and anesthetic effects, hemodynamics (i.e., heart rate and blood pressure), respiration, electroencephalography (EEG), and visual and somatosensory evoked responses. Laboratory studies indicated no effect of CI-581 on various blood chemistries. The effects on the other parameters were more complex.

The primary outcomes were quality of analgesia and anesthesia. The Domino et al. (1965) group wanted to know whether CI-581 caused analgesia (diminution of pain sensation) and anesthesia (unconsciousness), and if so, whether it did so safely. To study the analgesic effects of CI-581, the investigators administered relatively small doses (because analgesia can be tested only if the patient is conscious), and while the participant was still able to respond, strongly pinched skin over the chest area (which is normally very painful) and asked about pain. To test for anesthesia, or loss of consciousness, such an effect was inferred when the participant stopped responding to questions. Duration of anesthesia was taken as the time it took from onset of unconsciousness until verbal response resumed.

At doses of 0.1 mg/kg, none of the patients lost consciousness. At 0.5 mg/kg, half the patients lost consciousness for 3–4 minutes, and the other half remained conscious. At doses of 1.0, 1.5, and 2.0 mg/kg, all patients lost consciousness, usually for 3–12 minutes, without much of an increase in duration from 1.5 to 2.0 mg/kg. At the onset of losing consciousness, patients' eyes often remained open, an unusual finding. Before losing consciousness, patients often said they felt numb all over even though sensation was intact. Lack of response to pain stimuli was noted—CI-581 was a good analgesic. Upon recovering consciousness, some subjects showed a variety of emotional responses, and some were completely calm. Almost all felt numb at this stage, and some even felt as if they lacked limbs or were dead. Sensation was intact, however (thus, there was a dissociation between sensation being intact and emotional response to the sensation). Dreamlike states or visual hallucinations were described by some participants. Some thought they were in outer space. Most described their CI-581 experiences as not unpleasant or even pleasant, although two patients refused further infusions because of frightening experiences. During infusions in which unconsciousness was avoided, complete analgesia was noted. This was in sharp contrast to traditional barbiturate anesthetic drugs, in which no analgesia occurs without loss of consciousness (and breathing as well). Thus, the advantages of this drug for use in a variety of procedures were readily appreciated.

Cardiovascular responses generally consisted of increases in heart rate and blood pressure, another advantage vis-à-vis barbiturates, which cause decreases in these parameters. As mentioned, breathing was generally sustained without the need for airway assistance except at higher doses beyond what was minimally needed for analgesia. EEG showed replacement of the awake state alpha rhythm (8- to 12-Hz frequencies) by theta rhythms (4- to 7-Hz frequencies), not a surprising finding. Evoked responses (EEG responses to visual or somatosensory stimuli) showed diminution in concert with the deeper states of anesthesia.

In summarizing the effects of CI-581 in humans, the investigators called it qualitatively similar to phencyclidine but of shorter duration. It did not cause convulsions at high doses, unlike phencyclidine. The frightening or dysphoric emotional and mental side effects of phencyclidine were seen in lesser intensity and of shorter duration with CI-581, although it was rightly pointed out that experience in clinical anesthesia was needed. The investigators considered the drug possibly useful for short procedures, based on the profound analgesia seen at doses that did not cause respiratory depression. The term *dissociative anesthesia* was coined to describe this class of medications, although no rationale for the use of the term was given. The Domino et al. (1965) paper contains all the elements that would later fascinate ketamine enthusiasts: the dreamlike states, the trips to outer space, and the feelings of disembodied consciousness and near-death experiences.

Drs. Corssen and Domino followed up this initial experience giving CI-581 to prisoner volunteers with a second study, giving it to more volunteers; importantly, they tried it out in clinical anesthetic procedures at the University of Michigan Medical Center at Ann Arbor (Corssen and Domino 1966). The first part of this second study involved 10 prisoners and basically confirmed the original findings: doses of ~1.0 mg/kg resulted in anesthesia with mild increases in heart rate and blood pressure and only slight respiratory suppression. Serial doses did not seem to cause any particular problems. They concluded that it was time to use this new drug clinically.

In the clinical part of the study, CI-581 was given to 130 patients undergoing 133 procedures. The average duration of the procedures was ~10 minutes—thus, these were fairly simple, short procedures such as dressing burns, setting bone fractures (orthopedic), stricture repair (urologic), ophthalmologic, head and neck, and miscellaneous others. In 93 of the 133 procedures, one injection of CI-581 was sufficient for the entire procedure. Patient ages ranged from 6 weeks to 86 years (in very small children, intramuscular administration was used). Protective reflexes (pharyngeal, laryngeal, corneal, eyelid) remained intact. No endotracheal tubes were needed. Ventilation was fairly easy, as respirations for the most part were sustained by the patient without support. Average time to recovery of orientation to person, place, and time was ~11 minutes from completion of the procedure. Full recovery took 30–60 minutes.

Vivid dreams and hallucinations were experienced by some patients, described by some as pleasant and others as unpleasant, reflecting the fascinating dual nature of this compound. The dreams often were experienced as a trip to outer space and lasted 5–15 minutes. Two patients thought they had died and were going to hell during this state. One patient displayed 40 minutes of postprocedural agitation, which is clearly a problem. Regarding the cases of postprocedural emergence agitation, the authors commented that it was less frequent than with PCP and less intense as well, but clearly it happened. They suggested that sensory isolation, rather than stimulating the patient with questions, was an appropriate strategy. Also, they speculated that use of sedatives may help prevent the emergence agitation, anticipating the standard strategy years later of using benzodiazepines along with ketamine.

Amnesia was noted for the procedure itself—in other words, patients did not recall being operated on—but there was vivid recall of the emergence time period, the awakening phase. The authors made the following conclusions:

1. In clinical anesthesia practice, at least for short procedures, CI-581 was a powerful analgesic and anesthetic.
2. The state produced by CI-581 was different from the sedation/sleepiness produced by traditional anesthetics; they referred to this state as catalepsy—lack of verbal responding, lack of spontaneous motor behavior, and increased muscle tone, but awakeness at lower doses.
3. CI-581 altered reactivity of the central nervous system to sensation without blocking sensation itself. They theorized that sensory input to primary cortical areas was intact but that further input to the association areas, where information from multiple sensory modalities is in-

tegrated, was blocked. Thus, the term *dissociative* was used in this
context to refer to the presumed dissociation of cortical areas from one
another.[2]

4. Emergence reactions did occur with CI-581 but were not as frequent,
   as severe, or as prolonged as with phencyclidine.
5. It was proposed that sensory destimulation in the recovery period, as
   opposed to stimulating patients with questions, would help mitigate
   emergence reactions.
6. It was proposed that premedication with some type of sedative may
   prevent emergence reactions.
7. Patients had amnesia for the procedure but not for the unpleasant
   emergence reactions.
8. Analgesia was good for relatively superficial procedures, but it was not
   known whether it would be good for deep visceral surgeries.
9. Emergence reactions did not occur in infants or small children, similar
   to what was noticed with phencyclidine earlier.
10. Blood pressure elevations were a drawback, but fortunately blood
    pressure drops did not occur.

Ketamine Goes Prime Time: Approval for Use in the United States and Elsewhere

These initial reports were encouraging, but to gain regulatory approval to
market ketamine, more data were needed to establish safety and efficacy. In
the late 1960s, multiple studies in several countries were commissioned by
Parke-Davis. Studies emanated from Italy, Germany, and Japan, in addition
to the United States. Clearly there was a lot of interest in ketamine at this
time: a Medline search of terms such as CI-581 and ketamine for the years
1966–1970 returns many dozens of hits. A few are reviewed here to show
what anesthesiologists were looking at with ketamine.

Pannacciulli et al. (1966), in a report from Italy, gave ketamine anesthesia to 200 individuals during surgery. Emergence phenomena were described, but ketamine proved a good anesthetic agent. Virtue et al. (1967),
working at the University of Colorado Medical Center, had similar results

---

[2]Of note, in another part of the paper, and indeed in a later paper from Domino
(2010), the origin of the word *dissociative* in relation to the state produced by CI-581
referred to the psychological state of being dissociated from the environment, in a
dreamlike trance. It appears that that is the true origin of the term *dissociative anesthesia*, and the theory about dissociation of cortical areas from one another came
later, as a neurophysiologic explanation for the psychological state.

in 150 cases in which ketamine was used to induce anesthesia for surgery. Dreaming was noted upon emergence. Corssen, introduced earlier as one of the first anesthesiologists to study ketamine (Corssen 1966), indicated that in his opinion, ketamine was contraindicated in adults due to the "psychotic reactions" but not in those younger than 15, in whom such effects were not noted. Falls et al. (1966), from Germany, described the use of ketamine for ophthalmologic procedures and noted emergence dreams and visual hallucinations in adults but not in children or infants. In another report from Germany, Langrehr et al. (1967) detailed ketamine use in 500 cases, a large sample size. Emergence dreaming was noted as in other reports. Podlesh and Zindler (1967) reported favorably on a series of 239 patients, mostly children, who received ketamine anesthesia. Iwatsuki et al. (1967) used ketamine for anesthesia in Japan. In the most comprehensive and largest report from that era, Corssen et al. (1968) used ketamine in approximately 900 anesthesia inductions in Ann Arbor. Children and infants were noted, as above, not to experience emergence agitation or dreams. Emergence reactions were noted to be diminished if patients were free from verbal or tactile stimulation during recovery. Rates of various emergence reactions were provided: vivid dreaming 2.8%, emergence delirium 3.3%, hallucinations 0.2%, euphoria 0.4%, disturbance of body image 0.4%, and feelings of numbness 0.33%.

Based on these and similar anesthesia-related reports, ketamine was approved for use in multiple countries, including Great Britain and the United States in 1970. Ketamine had gone prime time: any hospital or clinic could now purchase the drug for use in anesthesia settings. Over the decades since, many thousands of reports on ketamine in anesthesiology have been published. Collier (1972), reporting experiences of patients anesthetized with ketamine, indicated that 29 of 50 patients in one sample said they would not want ketamine again due to unpleasant dreaming, out-of-body experiences, floating in space, and the perception of being dead. Of 84 patients in the series anesthetized with ketamine, 31 accepted it, meaning that 53 did not. Emergence agitation, although clearly not as bad as with PCP, still happened, and some patients hated ketamine. To mitigate this side effect, a benzodiazepine such as diazepam was used, as described in the classic paper, "The Taming of Ketamine" (Coppel et al. 1973). The authors used 0.17 mg/kg diazepam at the end of the procedure, which mitigated the unpleasant dreamlike states and greatly reduced emergence delirium. End-of-procedure diazepam with ketamine for anesthesia induction is still used today (Longnecker et al. 2018).

Decades later in 2010, Edward Domino, the scientist most responsible for discovering ketamine's fascinating psychological effects, mused that the drug was a "tiger," and that those who chose to take it or administer it (as the field of psychiatry was beginning to do) should beware and not be complacent (Domino 2010). Many have not heeded Domino's advice and have paid a price for messing with the ketamine tiger.

Epilogue: Ketamine in Modern Anesthesiology

Ketamine is now a standard drug in modern anesthesiology practice (Longnecker et al. 2018), and the World Health Organization includes ketamine on its list of essential medicines (World Health Organization 2024). Thus, the effort to find a substitute for phencyclidine worked fabulously for anesthesiology. In modern anesthesiology practice, ketamine is used judiciously to induce general anesthesia (usually cardiac cases), and diazepam is given at the end of the procedure to mitigate emergence dysphoria. Patients are (or should be) prepared in advance for emergence phenomena, and during the recovery phase, care is taken to avoid overstimulation.

The uses of ketamine in modern anesthesiology can be divided into four types:

1. Induction and maintenance of general anesthesia (FDA approved);
2. Procedural sedation and analgesia (FDA approved);
3. Postoperative analgesia and other acute pain syndromes; and
4. Chronic pain management.

IV doses of ketamine used to induce general anesthesia are usually ~1–3 mg/kg; intramuscular doses are higher. Two particularly important applications of ketamine for general anesthesia are on the battlefield and in developing countries, where sophisticated monitoring equipment needed for other anesthetic drugs is not available and ketamine is indispensable (Bonanno 2002). Further elaboration of the techniques and indications of ketamine for general anesthesia are beyond the scope of this book.

Procedural sedation and analgesia (PSA) refers to the use of a drug to induce not unconsciousness, but rather a state of light sedation and pain control (analgesia), to perform procedures such as setting a bone, suturing a laceration, draining a large abscess, inserting an arterial line, dressing a burn, and many others. Usual doses of ketamine for PSA are much lower than for anesthesia, ~10–30 mg IV (more if administered intramuscularly). Of note, ketamine for PSA is quite often used in emergency department settings, especially for children (see Green et al. 2011 for guidelines), by emergency medicine physicians. Elsewhere in the hospital setting, anesthesiologists usually administer ketamine for PSA.

Ketamine is also used by anesthesiologists in the intra- and postoperative setting for patients awakening from anesthesia who need pain control without suppressing respiration (see Brinck et al. 2018 for a review of this topic). Even though ketamine is not specifically approved by the FDA for this purpose, it is used because it decreases the use of opioid medications, which do suppress respiration. Occasionally, ketamine is used for in-hospital analgesia of acute pain syndromes not related to a procedure or surgery, such as in sickle cell anemia patients experiencing a pain crisis.

Thus, circa 1970, ketamine made its way into the field of anesthesiology. Patients tolerated it but sometimes hated it. Those familiar with the drug—the scientists who first studied it and the clinical anesthesiologists who used it—assumed the story of ketamine would end there.

They were wrong.

Chapter 3

Recreational Use of Ketamine: The World Discovers the K-Hole

> At no time did it seem possible that I or anyone else could
> become a "ketamine junkie." As far as I can tell the substance is
> both physically and psychologically nonaddictive.
>
> —Marcia Moore, *Journeys Into the Bright World* (p. 38)

KEY POINTS IN THIS CHAPTER:

- The dissociative effects of ketamine have fascinated recreational users for decades.

- Ketamine abuse has become a major problem in Asian regions such as China, Taiwan, and Hong Kong.

- Long-term heavy use of ketamine causes urinary bladder failure, called ulcerative cystitis.

The above assertion by Marcia Moore could not have been more incorrect. Many people have been seduced into the illusion that ketamine is harmless, and by the time they realized they were addicted, ketamine had taken over their lives. We will meet Moore later in the chapter—her story is one that illustrates the allure and danger of ketamine.

What led to the recreational use of ketamine? In the early 1970s, ketamine was freshly approved for clinical use in anesthesiology, which would ordinarily mean that an insular, small group of doctors would be using it.

Somehow it migrated to street use, rapidly becoming a drug of recreational use and addiction. And as usual for ketamine, it followed a trail first blazed by PCP.

Phencyclidine Recreational Use and Abuse

When human use of PCP began in the 1950s, it caused highly agitated psychotic states. Why would anybody want to use such a drug recreationally? Edward Domino (the discoverer of the pharmacological effects of ketamine in humans) was perplexed, even downright stunned, that PCP would be taken recreationally (Domino 1980).

In a review of the PCP problem of the late 1970s, Cohen (1977) indicated that pleasant "drug trips" with PCP could include mild dissociation and euphoria and that some people enjoyed the frank psychedelic aspects, like "going off into outer space." Dr. Solomon Snyder, the renowned neuroscientist at Johns Hopkins University, broached the issue of why people would take PCP (Snyder 1980): he supposed it was due to the dreamy, hallucinatory state that resulted.

Alternatively, analogy to a roller coaster seems fitting. People flock to amusement parks and wait in long lines to experience rides that routinely cause nausea and fear, yet also a thrill—perhaps a similar experience to taking PCP. After all, the dysphoric effects of alcohol, the most abused drug in the world, are well known. A depressant, alcohol routinely causes users to feel sad, suicidal, angry, and belligerent, yet drinkers keep drinking. Some people want to feel different from their usual, baseline emotional state, and any drug that delivers will serve.

The first report of recreational or street use of PCP was in a then-new publication called the *Journal of Psychedelic Drugs*, founded by one of the co-authors, Dr. David E. Smith, who also founded San Francisco's Haight Ashbury Free Clinic, which provides care to drug users and others. In their esoteric report, Meyers et al. (1967) described a drug the pushers called the "peace pill," apparently after the initials PCP. (The word *peace* betrays a bit of snake oil salesmanship in the name as well.) Not many details were provided about the drug's circumstances or effects. In a later publication, Smith and Wesson (1980) clarified that the peace pill was purchased at a rock concert in San Francisco and that 25–30 people high on the drug ended up at the Haight Ashbury Free Clinic because of toxic reactions including hypertension, *nystagmus* (uncontrolled eye movements), *ataxia* (lack of coordination), and alterations in cognition and behavior. The authors reported that because of those unpleasant reactions, PCP failed to become popular in subsequent years among the recreational drug crowd in the San Francisco area: they knew the peace pill wasn't so peaceful.

The Source of PCP

Where did the street PCP come from? As it happens, the synthesis of PCP is not complicated, and the basic ingredients are easy to come by (Allen et al. 1993). Thus, "kitchen chemists," or people synthesizing the drug in clandestine labs or their own homes, became a big source of illicit PCP. For example, one report in a journal called *Drug Enforcement* (Anonymous 1974) describes in some detail the raid by law enforcement officials of two clandestine PCP labs of shockingly large scale. One was a Maryland warehouse purportedly making electronics parts, wherein the ringleader of the operation became ill one day. Somebody called first responders, and that led to an investigation revealing elaborate chemical equipment and the ingredients to synthesize PCP. The other operation was in the attic of a home in Michigan, under investigation because authorities had been tipped off by chemical supply companies alarmed at the enormous quantities of reagents ordered to a residential address. Astonishingly, that operation was said to be capable of making up to a million PCP pills per week.

In addition to clandestine PCP synthesis, the drug was diverted from legitimate pharmaceutical supply chains. Rainey and Crowder (1974a, 1974b), in two letters to prestigious American journals, pointed out that PCP was discovered in a lot of samples of other street drugs, such as marijuana and LSD. Thus, some ingestion that led to PCP-induced agitation or psychosis was unintentional. Hart et al. (1972) also found that street drug samples containing PCP were billed and sold as something else. As news reports spread of this phenomenon, parents became terrified that their children would be exposed to it accidentally.

The Effects of PCP

The reactions to PCP are complex: after first ingesting it, the user may feel calm and euphoric; however, with time depending on dose, violent psychosis may supervene. Fauman and Fauman (in Domino 1980, chapter 19) described a series of PCP abusers from the 1970s. Typically, phencyclidine was used along with multiple other drugs, such as alcohol, marijuana, opiates, and stimulants. Users at first enjoyed the mild dissociative effects and may have felt some euphoria. With continued use, however, they needed to take ever-increasing amounts to obtain the same effects (an effect known as *tolerance*). Additionally, pleasurable dissociative states tended to be replaced by uncomfortable, dysphoric states with the development of irritability and even violence. Some users became persistently psychotic. A compulsive need to keep using was common, even though by that time a lot of users experienced nothing but unpleasurable effects. It became known as "angel dust" on the street.

Burns et al. (1975) studied 55 patients experiencing PCP intoxication. PCP was available on the street as a powder; it was sprinkled on herbs and smoked or just snorted outright. Pills were sometimes available. Clinical features included nystagmus, hypertension, agitation, coma, ataxia, blank stares, or catatonic posturing (reminiscent of the cataleptoid states in animals at Parke-Davis in the 1950s). The authors noted that some young users would try it looking for something new and then hate it; alternatively, some did not know what it was. Some users were attracted to the drug and went on to use it regularly.

In their study, Burns et al. (1975) noted 15 deaths presumably due to PCP in California from 1970 to 1975, mostly accidents or suicides. Two features noted about PCP in animals and humans distinguish it from ketamine: the presence of behavioral stimulation at relatively low dosages (ketamine does not cause stimulation in animals or humans except mildly at low doses) and convulsions at high doses.

Luisada (1978), working at an inpatient psychiatric facility in the Washington, DC, area in the mid-1970s, described 11 patients admitted with symptoms that seemed indistinguishable from schizophrenia: profound psychosis, agitation to the point of violence, disorganized thinking, occasional catatonia, blunted affect, and unpredictability. As the patients improved while taking antipsychotic medication, a history of PCP use was revealed. The patients had no prior psychotic episodes and had been functioning normally (in contrast, typical schizophrenia has a prodromal stage). The patients seemed to go through three phases: first, a phase of extreme paranoia, uncooperativeness, and propensity toward unpredictable violence; second, a phase of continued psychosis but more cooperative behavior; and third, a phase of rapid reintegration to baseline functioning. The author postulated that some people may have a predisposition to schizophrenia and that use of PCP essentially unmasks it by causing a psychosis more prolonged than is usually seen in others who take it (in whom the psychosis, if it happens, lasts at most a few hours). On the other end of the spectrum are those with frank schizophrenia in whom PCP precipitates prolonged psychotic episodes. In support of the theory, some of the patients in the Luisada series presented with psychotic episodes at later times without any PCP use, indicating a probable predisposition.

Smith and Wesson (1980) and Smith (1980), reporting from the Haight Ashbury Free Clinic in the late 1960s and 1970s, indicated that 32% of patients having toxic reactions did not know they were using PCP—it had been sold as something else, usually marijuana (sold as a premade joint to hide the PCP powder). The authors divided PCP toxic reactions into four types:

- Type I was acute toxicity, whereby the effects lasted only as long as the drug was in the body. Usually, nystagmus, hypertension, and agitation or psychotic symptoms occurred and lasted up to a few hours. Also seen were combativeness, catatonia, convulsions, or coma (the 4 C's, as the authors put it).
- Type II PCP reactions consisted of a more prolonged psychosis that lasted beyond the drug's presence in the body, maybe a few days or so. These reactions occurred in people with premorbid normal function.
- Type III reactions consisted of a full-blown psychotic episode, up to a month or more, precipitated by a single dose of PCP. The authors believed that Type III reactions occurred in people with underlying predispositions to psychotic disorders, such as schizophrenia.
- Type IV PCP reactions consisted of depression resulting from chronic use and could occur either alone or after any one of the other types of reaction.

The Public Scourge of PCP

During the 1970s, recreational use of PCP became a big problem because of the agitated, violent, psychotic states induced by the drug. Emergency departments in urban centers became stressed with the high volume of PCP-induced psychotic patients, who were typically brought in by law enforcement.

Morgan and Kagan (1980) presented an interesting review of media portrayals of the PCP epidemic of the late 1970s. They rounded up 323 newspaper articles on the subject between 1958 and 1979. Fifty-nine of them portrayed violent or "shocking" themes (e.g., a case of self-inflicted enucleation of the eyes). Among the 23 magazine articles on PCP in 1977–1979 alone, 10 involved "PCP horror stories," again of shocking violence committed while somebody was under the influence of PCP. Numerous television news broadcasts covered these stories, and PCP-induced violence was dramatized in TV shows. In particular, 1978 was a year of intense media and cultural attention to PCP abuse, at least in the United States.

Dogoloff (1980), representing the Domestic Policy Office at the White House, summarized the response to the PCP epidemic at the federal level. He estimated that at that time, 7,000,000 Americans had used PCP, and that in 1978 alone, 310 people died from it and 14,000 emergency department admissions resulted from it. His article outlined government agency, legislative, and law enforcement initiatives designed to attack the PCP problem.

It reads as one would expect from a politically motivated bureaucrat: on paper, it sounded like a lot of progress had been made, but in reality, PCP was wreaking havoc in America.

The Range and Consequences of PCP

In a residential format in Illinois called Crossroads, a determined married couple ran a program that, among other things, treated PCP users (Fauman and Fauman 1979; 1980a, 1980b). They pointed out the commonality of intravenous use of PCP and the cognitive problems chronic users complained of, which seemed to last for months. Also, they described in some detail the violent acts associated with PCP.

Aniline et al. (1980), using a then-new ultra-sensitive blood assay for PCP, found in a survey of 135 consecutive admissions to a Los Angeles urban hospital psychiatric ward that 106 were positive for PCP, an enormously high number indicating the drug's widespread use during that era. East and central Los Angeles, where the hospital was located, were known to be an epicenter of PCP trafficking at the time.

An excellent data set was provided by Feldman and Waldorf (1980), funded by the U.S. National Institute on Drug Abuse, describing PCP use in four American cities: Seattle, Philadelphia, Miami, and Chicago. One hundred PCP users were interviewed. Its street use appeared in all four cities in 1968. Violence was rare; use was mostly among adolescents. "Burning out" was reported, consisting of blunted emotionality and cognition. Most used once or twice a week. It was cheap, easy to obtain, and had a reputation as tough to handle, thus giving its users bragging rights.

One interesting observation about PCP is that, unlike other psychedelics and ketamine, there have been no "celebrity" PCP users who wrote about their experiences as mystical, spiritual journeys. Nobody extols the profound insights to be gained by PCP. Nobody shows up in emergency departments just having taken PCP and wanting to tell the staff there about a new religious insight or a meeting with God. It would seem that PCP use is relegated to the street user, the young, alienated, troubled drug-purchaser looking for anything that will numb feelings.

Treatment programs were developed for PCP addiction. Eventually, because of widespread illicit and dangerous phencyclidine use, it was moved to Schedule II from Schedule III, signaling a higher level of abuse risk and dictating more stringent regulation. PCP eventually was replaced in veterinary medicine with ketamine and now is made pharmaceutically only for laboratory research involving animals.

Over the years, the use of PCP declined but did not disappear. For example, Peters et al. (2005) described interviews with 38 young people in the

Houston, Texas, area using a mixture called "fry," in which tobacco or marijuana cigarettes were laced with embalming fluid and PCP and smoked. The respondents did perceive this experience to be fraught with negative outcomes such as hallucinations and addictive potential. In a review from the New York City Medical Examiner's Office, an autopsy series was presented of 138 cases in which PCP was found in the blood (deRoux et al. 2011). Dominici et al. (2015), from the Department of Emergency Medicine at Duke University, recorded 184 visits featuring PCP use from June 2011 to March 2013. The mean age was 32.5 years, 65.2% were male, and 83.2% had smoked the PCP. Urine was positive for PCP in 82.1% of samples. Nystagmus, hypertension, and agitation were common. A few needed admission to a medical or psychiatric floor; most could be discharged from the emergency department in a few hours. PCP abuse continues to be a problem, albeit not the center of attention that opiates and stimulants are.

Ketamine Recreational Use and Abuse

Early in clinical and scientific investigations, it became clear that, like PCP, ketamine did more than induce typical analgesia or anesthesia. For example, Sadove et al. (1971), reporting on the potent analgesic effects of ketamine for medical procedures, wrote:

> It was the distinct impression of the observer that most of the patients who had received ketamine experienced a sense of well-being which supplemented the analgesic effect of the drug in such a way as to give increased relief from postoperative pain. This observation, coupled with the comments of the volunteers that they had experienced a pleasant psychic experience, tends to suggest that this drug has a definite potential for being abused. (p. 457)

This was a prescient observation by the investigators. The addictive qualities of ketamine were distinguishable early, beginning with animal experiments. The data in animals are outside the scope of this book, but it is well documented that animals will do anything they can to get ketamine (Liu et al. 2016).

To examine ketamine's pathway to recreational use in humans, some background on psychedelic drugs is in order.

Use of Psychedelic Substances

In 1956, Dr. Humphry Osmond, a psychiatrist from Regina, Saskatchewan, Canada, coined the term *psychedelic* from the Latin roots *psych* (mind) and *delein* (to reveal). Thus, psychedelic drugs are said to be "mind revealing," although it is not clear whether the effects of these drugs actually reveal anything. The assertion relates to the belief that psychedelic states, rather than being merely random perceptual distortions induced by pharmacological substances, actually impart important information about a person's subconscious mind that might enhance spiritual growth or mental health.

For instance, in psychedelic-assisted or -facilitated psychotherapy, a person being treated by a mental health professional receives a drug resulting in a non-ordinary state of consciousness (NOSC) to assist in psychotherapy sessions. (See more in Chapter 8, "Other Uses of Ketamine in Psychiatry.") Similarly, psilocybin (aka magic mushrooms) and methylenedioxymethamphetamine (MDMA; aka *ecstasy* or *molly*) are being investigated for depression and PTSD, respectively.

As a neuropharmacological probe, studies of the effects of psychedelics on brain processes can lead to important information about normal and abnormal brain function. Much of this research has been in animals, the utility of which is somewhat suspect, but human research using modern methods of brain imaging is proving to be informative. *Model psychoses* refer to drug-induced states that are thought to mimic schizophrenia and may be informative regarding pathophysiology and the search for new drug targets. Early on after the discovery of the effects of LSD, psychiatrists wondered whether its perceptual distortions mimicked in some way the psychotic process in schizophrenia. If *psychedelic psychosis* was a pharmacological model for schizophrenia, it would provide an excellent and easily available laboratory model to study the neurobiology of schizophrenia and test putative new treatments. This interesting line of research is covered in Chapter 5, "The Ketamine Model of Schizophrenia."

Mind control, brainwashing, and forced interrogation constitute an ugly application of psychedelic drugs, although not involving ketamine (at least as far as is publicly known). Governmental agencies and other groups have used LSD and other agents for nefarious purposes, such as extracting information from captives, trying to control people's behavior, or brainwashing people into political ideologies. In the United States, this happened predominantly in the 1950s and 1960s under a project secretly known as MK-ULTRA. A fascinating book, *The Search for the "Manchurian Candidate"* (Marks 1991), reviews these clandestine activities. One can only hope nothing similar is happening these days.

Outside of those uses, why would people experiment with psychedelic drugs? Recreationally, some use psychedelic drugs simply for fun, often in a social context (parties, raves), as a way to stave off boredom or enhance communion with others. Spiritual, religious, and mystical rituals are apropos to the use of psychedelic plants by various cultures around the world. To some, use in modernized, industrialized cultures may lend a sense of transcendent meaning in a busy life filled with responsibilities and materialism.

As far as this chapter is concerned, namely the nonmedical or recreational use of ketamine, the main reasons people take this drug in this manner are essentially for a joy ride or for some kind of deeper spiritual or psychological growth.

Ketamine Sources

Early on, no countries regulated ketamine, so the amount and location of supplies in surgical units and pharmacies was not recorded. When supplies were distributed to hospitals and clinics around the world, first for research purposes and later as part of approved medical care, virtually anybody working in such environments could take it without being detected. Furthermore, licensed physicians could simply purchase ketamine from Parke-Davis and then use it any way they pleased (!)—take it themselves or give it to others.

The chemical synthesis of ketamine, unlike that of PCP, requires difficult-to-obtain reagents that must react with one another in a precise sequence, requiring meticulous conditions and equipment. Thus, nonindustrial synthesis of ketamine has never been a significant source of recreational supplies. There probably have been a few kitchen chemists over the years, those with sophisticated knowledge of organic chemistry coupled with access to the reagents and equipment, who have made small supplies of their own. Indeed, entering "how to synthesize ketamine" in Google leads to many sites claiming to know the answer. Nonetheless, the vast majority of ketamine is synthesized in pharmaceutical factories. Diversion from this process, starting in the factory itself and sometimes from later steps in the supply chain, accounts for illicit ketamine supplies. Theft from veterinary clinics was also a big source of recreational ketamine.

Recreational Ketamine: Higher Consciousness or Just Getting High?

The first appearance of ketamine in recreational use is obscure. What appears to be the first mention in the literature comes from Reier (1971), reporting from Ohio State University Hospital. The author mentioned that people were using ketamine recreationally but provided no specifics or references. A landmark paper of sorts was published by Siegel (1978), an addictions specialist, who described states of intoxication with both PCP and ketamine. He described a phenomenon called *meditatio mortis*, wherein somebody taking PCP had an unusual preoccupation with death; this probably represented the near-death-like experiences that later became a fascination for some ketamine users. Siegel described two cohorts: ~400 PCP users and

23 ketamine users. PCP was used for experimentation, for social recreation, and for certain contexts (e.g., a concert, a bout of depression); some people were intensive, compulsive PCP users. Siegel mentioned that, to his knowledge, the first street use of ketamine was in Los Angeles and San Francisco, in liquid form in 1971 and in powder form or tablets in 1974. Of the cohort of 23 ketamine users, 10 inhaled it and 13 injected it intramuscularly. Anecdotally, it was noted (as elsewhere over the decades) that some of the early users were Vietnam War veterans exposed to ketamine on the battlefield, where it was used to safely stabilize injured soldiers. The psychedelic aspects of the ketamine trips were said to be more vivid than those with PCP.

This first generation of ketamine users were among the *psychonauts* (from the Greek words for "mental" and "sailor"; thus a voyager of the mind) interested in the transcendent quality of ketamine trips and the out-of-body experiences as sources of new insights or spiritual development. Psychonauts would contemplate their ketamine trips after the fact to extract something of value to enhance their lives of consensus reality. Of course, some became addicted to ketamine and descended into compulsive, uncontrolled use.

From first-person narratives of ketamine trips (Jansen 2001), there seem to be two fundamental dissociative qualities of ketamine attractive to regular users: out-of-body experiences and transcendence. In the former, a person has no sensation of having a body, essentially resembling a disembodied consciousness (i.e., a dreamlike state). Transcendence refers to a feeling of being in an alternate reality or outer space. Often the user experiences a meeting with an archetypal religious figure, deity, or ineffable, nonhuman being. In addition, ketamine users have emotional reactions, visual illusions, and hallucinations.

Elements of ketamine trips have similarities with other drugs of abuse: perceptual distortions like other psychedelics; euphoria like stimulants; mellow feelings like marijuana; and emotional disinhibition and inebriation like alcohol, with attendant sadness or anger. The ketamine trip as a whole, however, is much more than a sum of these things. Ketamine is unique; experienced drug users insist there is nothing like it.

Bremner et al. (1998), researching dissociative experiences of people with PTSD, developed a scale that is useful for cataloguing the dissociative effects of ketamine. The Clinician-Administered Dissociative States Scale (CADSS) consists of 27 items, each scored as present or absent (possible score of 0–27). Eight of the items are observer-rated, beginning with the phrase, *Did the subject...*

- Seem eerie or strange or make you uncomfortable?
- Blank out, space out, or lose track?

- Seem detached?
- Say something bizarre or unexpected?
- Behave bizarrely?
- Have to be put back on track?
- Show facial grimacing or twitching?
- Have rolling of the eyes?

The other 19 items are subject-rated, beginning with the phrase, *Do you feel…* or *Do things seem…*, and pertain to experiences of slow motion; derealization; feeling detached; experiencing disembodied consciousness; altered sounds, colors, or time passage; feeling motionless; altered body perception; tunnel vision; and amnestic periods. CADSS has been used quite extensively to study the relationship of ketamine experiences to schizophrenia and to document side effects when ketamine is used therapeutically in psychiatry or pain medicine.

In September 1979, the FDA warned American medical practitioners of the then-growing problem of ketamine recreational use (FDA 1979), which was particularly prevalent at that time on the West Coast. (By that time, PCP had been put into Schedule II, which meant it was highly regulated.) The FDA cited the Fine and Finestone (1973) and Johnson (1971) papers warning about persisting psychosis and delayed onset psychosis from ketamine. Upon close inspection of those reports, however, the evidence they provided was rather weak, leftover from the LSD panic that swept America in the late 1960s. In the brief communication, the FDA indicated that it was considering scheduling ketamine as well, but did not do so until 20 years later. The delay was probably due to the utility of ketamine in anesthesiology practice and the desire not to make it too hard to obtain. And of course government agencies, notoriously, move at glacial paces.

Medical access to recreational ketamine in the United States ended in 1999, when ketamine did become a controlled substance (Schedule III). These days, every vial of ketamine is locked securely. The amount given is documented in the patient's chart, and any unused portion is placed in a plastic bag, labeled with the patient's information, and sent securely to the pharmacy so that the pharmacist can account for every milligram. Stealing ketamine would be difficult unless a lot of medical personnel were involved in a ketamine diversion conspiracy.

The Party Drug Emerges

So when ketamine became a controlled drug, did recreational use disappear as well? Nothing of the sort. As documented by Jansen (2001), recreational ketamine use morphed into an entertainment for young people at raves, dance clubs, and other social events. Ketamine users went from people seeking a higher truth to kids looking for a good time at a party, who used it along with a plethora of other drugs such as stimulants, opiates, and of course, alcohol. Recreational ketamine use has its own jargon: sobriquets for ketamine from the 1979 FDA report included *green* (from its crystalline form), *supergrass* (when mixed with marijuana), *super acid, purple, mauve, special LA coke*, and *super C*. It is often referred to as *special K* (or some other sobriquet with the letter K in it), and going into a deep state of ketamine intoxication is called the *K-hole*. Ketamine became, and still is, a fixture of the club drug scene around the world.

As Jansen (2001) tells the story, in the early 1990s (before regulation), disc jockeys from London visited the party scene in the tony, upscale Goa region of southwest India, where ketamine could be purchased over the counter. These disc jockeys brought supplies back to London and introduced it to raves (club drugging), where it became a big hit. Apparently, for most of the night, typical clubbers would use stimulants (cocaine, methamphetamine, amphetamine, MDMA) to enhance the dancing and excitement they were seeking and then, when it was time to chill out a bit, would quiet down, inhale some ketamine, and enjoy the dissociative buzz. The uninitiated who used ketamine while still trying to dance would fall down and injure themselves. Ketamine was also used to facilitate sexual experiences, and sometimes to render an unsuspecting user helpless against sexual assault: ketamine is known as a date rape drug. Thus the psychonauts' doorway to transcendence became corrupted for vulgar motives.

Jansen (2001) described how addiction to ketamine evolves. Tolerance builds up, so that ever-higher doses are needed to achieve some type of high, but with diminishing returns, thus making the desperate user seek even higher doses. Access to ketamine was a limiting factor, as it still is today, at least in the United Kingdom where Jansen interviewed users, as well as in the United States (in contrast, the supply in some Asian countries is plentiful). There is no physical withdrawal syndrome as with benzodiazepines, alcohol, barbiturates, or cigarettes, but nevertheless over time, the ketamine addict typically has an ongoing mood of dysphoria and anxiety: they are not happy people.

The Scope of Ketamine Use in Modern Times

The evolution of nonmedical, or recreational, ketamine use can be conceptualized as three waves. As discussed earlier, the first wave started in the late 1960s or early '70s in predominantly Western countries where ketamine was used medically. Isolated users were curious about ketamine's effects and either had legal access or stole from medical supplies. That wave essentially ended with regulation in 1999 and the early 2000s.

The second wave of ketamine use was its spread as a club drug starting in the early 1990s in England and spreading to other Western countries. That type of use still exists but is not terribly widespread since regulation. In the United States, ketamine as a club drug has been relatively sparse in comparison to other recreational drugs and is concentrated in large urban areas. Following are some data sets detailing the Western use of ketamine.

Lankenau and Clatts (2002) interviewed 25 young ketamine users (by either intravenous or intramuscular injection) in New York. They tended to inject ketamine as part of a group, with multiple injections and needle sharing, and thus high risk of transmitting HIV and hepatitis. The interviewees were a rather lost, alienated group, unemployed, coming from broken homes, having poor education, and apparently having little interest in life. In a later report, focusing on the same population's first injection experience with ketamine (Lankenau and Clatts 2004), the same authors reported on 23 people, ages 18–25, who took ketamine as a first injection experience. Mostly they were unemployed, underemployed, or selling drugs, prostituting themselves, or panhandling, and many were homeless.

Monitoring the Future is an annual survey of drug use among American teenagers. Along with the data, it documented more street names for ketamine in modern use, such as *cat valium, donkey, jet K, kit kat*, and *wonky*, as well as the eternal *special K*. The proportion of 8th-, 10th-, and 12th-graders who had ever used ketamine were, in 2000, 1.6%, 2.1%, and 2.5%, respectively. By 2011, use had declined to 0.8%, 1.2%, and 1.7%, and in 2022, the number for 12th-graders was 1.2% (National Institute on Drug Abuse 2023). Thus, ketamine usage has declined over time in the United States. This is undoubtedly due to ketamine being placed on Schedule III, with the attendant law enforcement attention to ketamine trafficking and tracking of medical supplies. In a similar European experience, among a sample of 130 French medical students surveyed by Fond et al. (2018), 1.6% had ever used ketamine (1.0% of women and 2.7% of men).

The third wave of ketamine recreational use is the utter epidemic in Asian regions: mainland China, Hong Kong, and Taiwan, with some use in Singapore and Malaysia. In China, numerous factories make astonishing amounts of ketamine to feed the medical world's demand, and a significant part of it is diverted for recreational use. For all intents and purposes, since about the year 2000, ketamine is available in unlimited supplies and is cheap in Hong Kong, Taipei, and China's major cities. Data sets routinely involve hundreds of patients at treatment centers for ketamine addiction. These remarkable numbers are due only partly to the large populations in those regions—additional factors are the ready availability of large supplies of ketamine, its cheap cost on the street, and the inability of law enforcement to rein in illicit trafficking. The situation has become essentially an experiment in unfettered access to ketamine, and the results aren't pretty: ketamine ruins lives.

In this section, we explore relatively recent literature documenting epidemiological aspects of ketamine use in various parts of the world. In the 1990s, ecstasy (MDMA) was the dance club drug of choice, but again ketamine was introduced as a way to top off a night of ecstasy use when it was time to slow down after dancing for hours on end. (See next section, "Ketamine in the Dance Club and Music Festival Scene.") MDMA, unlike ketamine with its legitimate use as an anesthetic, had a limited supply chain. Ketamine soon became the drug of choice in its own right, owing to its addictive nature and low cost in that market. It was most popular among working-class youth and was used socially for the most part.[1]

Joe Laidler (2005) provided some context for the rising popularity of ketamine in Hong Kong in the early 2000s. Historically, heroin and opium dominated that city-state's drug market. The author undertook ethnographic studies to assess the status of club drugs there in the early 2000s. She detailed the transition from ad hoc all-night raves to permanent dance clubs. Ketamine was first known to appear in the Hong Kong drug market in about 2000. Other drugs included heroin, cannabis, cocaine, methamphetamine (smoked in a form there known as *ice*), and MDMA. Joe-Laidler and Hunt (2008) conducted in-depth interviews with 100 Hong Kong youth about ketamine use. They described ketamine's effects as "floating," which gave them a feeling of being free, something desired among youth everywhere.

By 2002, the percentage of clubbers using ketamine reached 70%. Most users were "weekenders," but a small proportion became seriously addicted, inhaling it multiple times every day. A lot of those users said it dulled their thinking skills. Thus, the deadly combination of widespread availability, low cost, and high addictive potential made ketamine a real problem in Hong Kong (and mainland China and Taiwan). The percentage of Hong Kong clubbing youth who said they had used ketamine at least once during the previous year went from 0.1% in 1997 to 73.2% in 2006 (and, incidentally, the respective percentages for heroin fell from 48.0% to 2.0% during the same time frame) (Joe-Laidler and Hunt 2008).

Jia et al. (2015) wrote about the ketamine trends in China from 2003 to 2010. They noted that in April 2005, Chinese President Hu Jintao proclaimed a "People's War on Drugs."[2] Drug users in China are registered by the authorities and tracked longitudinally. Jia et al. analyzed three cohorts: before the People's War on Drugs (2003–2004, $n = 230,278$); Phase I (2005–

---

[1]Joe-Laidler and Hunt (2008) noted that a Hong Kong band called "MP4" had a song with the lyrics "don't sniff K daddy," an allusion to ketamine.

2007, n=518,651); and Phase II (2008–2010, n=435,195) (these are staggeringly large sample sizes by U.S. and U.K. standards). Over time, users were less likely to use heroin and more likely to use synthetics (a class that includes ketamine, methamphetamines, and MDMA) (Jia et al. 2015).

Chang et al. (2019) interviewed a sample of people in Taiwan, median age 26, from 2007 to 2010 (N=1,115). Each participant was given a questionnaire about positive and negative expectations for different drugs. Exclusive ketamine use was found in 2.4% of the sample, and 9.0% of the sample reported polydrug use including ketamine. The users of ketamine, predictably, had high positive and low negative expectations about ketamine.

Hong et al. (2018) presented a graph of the number of estimated ketamine users in Hong Kong from 1999 to 2016. It was essentially zero before 1999 but shot up to around 3,000 in 2001; from 2002 to 2009, it increased to around 5,000. With increased regulation and law enforcement, it fell to around 1,000 in 2016. Tam et al. (2016) surveyed a large number (11,938) of Hong Kong adolescents and found that 1.16% reported ever having used ketamine, which is commensurate with the prevalence in high schoolers in the United States.

Guo et al. (2018)Guo et al. (2018) surveyed a large number of Chinese 10th- through 12th-graders (16 to 18 years old) about a variety of health issues, and 59,518 questionnaires were returned. Pertinent to this discussion, 0.8% of boys and 0.18% of girls had ever tried ketamine. Childhood sexual abuse was associated with later ketamine use, as was physical abuse in boys and emotional abuse in girls. These findings are not surprising, given the known negative outcomes for abused children.

Ketamine in the Dance Club and Music Festival Scene

In modern times, recreational ketamine is for the most part a young person's drug, a party and social drug. As such, it appears at dance clubs and music festivals. Calle et al. (2019), in a data set from a 2015 dance festival in Belgium, found that 121 people had acute intoxications, 6% of which were found to be positive for ketamine (as well as for other drugs; notably, 54% were positive for MDMA).

Hoegberg et al. (2018), using a methodology that probably could be devised only by Scandinavians, collected pooled urine samples in several bath-

---

[2]This harkens to the analogous 1970 proclamation by President Richard Nixon, the "War on Drugs," albeit without the "People's" reference that communist leaders cannot resist.

rooms at a Røskilde, Denmark, music festival in 2016. The investigators actually connected devices to public urinals that extracted samples at selected intervals during the multiday festival. The 44 samples collected from three urinals included pooled urine from probably hundreds (if not thousands) of people. Seventy-seven different drugs were found. Not surprisingly, cocaine and MDMA were found in all 44 samples; ketamine was found in 17 of the samples—definitely not rare.

A group of researchers surveyed 1,045 New York nightclub or festival attendees in 2016. As a whole, a very large proportion were drug users of any kind, mostly stimulants and marijuana, and 5.4% of the sample were ketamine users (Fernández-Calderón et al. 2018). A substudy (Palamar 2018) focused on MDMA use and whether people knew that *molly* was in fact MDMA. Of the MDMA users, 22.5% had ever taken ketamine, an indication that ketamine is still part of the party drug scene in the United States.

Richeval et al. (2019) analyzed saliva samples in drivers around a 2017 music festival in France. Ketamine was found in 3 of 229 samples. Newer cyclohexanones such as methoxetamine and methoxyketamine were also found, indicating that kitchen chemists are getting creative at synthesizing new compounds.

Betzler et al. (2019) surveyed Berlin's party scene by interviewing 877 attendees (mean age 29) of dance clubs in 2017. The proportion who had used ketamine at least once in their lifetime was a whopping 63.6%, with 12-month prevalence being 51.2% and 30-day prevalence 32.2%; 36% wanted to reduce their consumption. One wonders whether, at least at that time, the trafficking of ketamine into Berlin was particularly robust to satisfy such large demands for recreational ketamine.

Why Do People Take Ketamine Recreationally?

As discussed in Chapter 2, "The Birth of Ketamine," when ketamine was first available for relatively widespread use in the early 1970s, anesthesiologists had patients who bitterly complained after they had been given this new "wonder drug." The dreamlike states, out-of-body experiences, visual hallucinations, and emergence distress essentially prevented ketamine from becoming a routine first-line anesthetic in the modern operating room. Why then would people want to take this drug recreationally?

Put simply, not all people who take (or are given) ketamine hate it. Those who do of course never take it again. Those who rather like it might seek it out and even become addicted to it. In this section, we review some of the reports exploring the positive reinforcing experiences people have had with ketamine, accounting for its widespread recreational use.

Dalgarno and Shewan (1996), working from Scotland in the mid-1990s, provided in-depth interview data from 20 ketamine users, mean age 26. The authors found their interviewees based on their work in the drug abuse community and word-of-mouth; thus, the sample is not representative from an epidemiological standpoint but is quite instructive. Two of the users were completing doctoral degrees—far from immature club drug users. Two were drug dealers. Most were gainfully employed and reasonably well educated. All 20 knew that ketamine was used as an anesthetic agent for people and animals. It was believed by the users to have been obtained by their suppliers as a diversion from licit medical sources. Seventeen used it occasionally; three used it quite frequently (one of them used it ~ 100 times; the other two, 15–20 times). It was used at first out of curiosity after hearing about it from friends. The mean dose was about 8 mg (a tiny dose, if accurate). It was powder or liquid, usually inhaled, but sometimes smoked, injected, or swallowed.

Commonly reported experiences included a sensation of light through the body, novel body consistency (e.g., made out of wood or plastic), distorted body shape or size, floating weightlessly in space, colorful visions, absence of time sense (going either fast or slow), sudden insight into the "riddle of existence," being at one with the universe (also referred to as "oceanic boundlessness"), and visions of spiritual or supernatural entities. A typical inhalational trip would last about an hour. All 20 users in the sample took the drug by themselves or with a monitor (again, not club drug users). Scarcity limited how often they used ketamine. None of them felt they were addicted to ketamine, but the three with the highest usage seem suspect in that regard. Tolerance was reported in the repeat users. All 20 agreed that ketamine would be inappropriate for dance club use (which obviously has been belied by rave attendees). All used other drugs and said that they were not prepared for the utter intensity of their first ketamine trip— far more intense than with other drugs of exploration. Ketamine is a drug apart.

Muetzelfeldt et al. (2008) conducted in-depth interviews of current frequent users (n=30, at least 20 days/month), current infrequent users (n=30), and ex-users (n=30, at least 84 days since last use) of ketamine in England. All the participants inhaled ketamine as a powder. At initiation, they were introduced to ketamine by friends and used it out of curiosity. The average number of years of use was 5, with a mean dose of 3.8 g (seven times as much as a first dose, indicating tolerance). Things they liked about it were dissociation, "melting into the surroundings," visual hallucinations, out-of-body experiences, and giggliness. For the most part, they were social users of ketamine, although one participant said ketamine gave them "new ways of thinking and an understanding of the mind-body question which 3 years of a philosophy degree could not match." A true psychonaut!

Things they did not like about ketamine were nausea and vomiting, loss of control, dissociation (some like it, some hate it), impaired memory (cited by 50%), and decreased sociability (cited by 50%). Reasons for stopping included tolerance and psychological effects such as paranoia, decreased sociability, depression, and blunted affect (Muetzelfeldt et al. 2008). Many believed it cured boredom; 28% were concerned about compulsive use. K-cramps (abdominal pain) and cystitis symptoms were reported by 33% of current users. Most frequent users used it until supplies ran out, only to use it again when they could get their hands on it. Ex-users cited getting themselves away from the ketamine-using environment as necessary to stop the drug.

Dillon et al. (2003) provided a nice review of users' experiences with ketamine. They interviewed 100 ketamine users in Sydney, Australia. Mean age was ~30 years. They were recruited by the first author and in advertisements in media used by drug users. Fourteen had access to ketamine from medical settings, reflecting the unregulated state of ketamine in Australia at that time. The "pure" ketamine user was rare in that sample, as in pretty much all other samples: the vast majority of the 100 used alcohol, cigarettes, and other drugs. Twenty-six were regular ketamine users. Eighty-two used it by snorting, 11 by intravenous injection, and the rest by intramuscular injection or swallowing. Twenty-five said they preferred using ketamine alone (i.e., without other drugs). Mostly, however, it was used as a party drug along with other drugs. The best thing about ketamine, according to 78%, was "altered senses." About half reported "euphoric rush" as something about it they liked. About half also said out-of-body experiences were positive. Some said the social aspect was a positive. Many (78%) said they danced while taking ketamine, indicating the dose must have been too low to cause deep dissociation. Fear of the K-hole and "coming down" were negatives associated with ketamine. Some (20%) said regular use caused lowered work performance, and 22% reported tolerance, or a need for increasing dosage. The most common co-drugs were MDMA, MDA (methylenedioxyamphetamine), and amphetamine. Almost all said they intended to use ketamine again. Wilkins et al. (2011), in an online survey of drug users' out-of-body experiences, found that ketamine alone was associated with this particular state and not any of the other drugs used. Thus, it seems specific to N-methyl-D-aspartate (NMDA) antagonists and not to stimulants, cannabinoids, or other drugs.

Psychiatrist and neuropharmacologist Dr. Karl Jansen wrote extensively about users' personal experiences with ketamine in his 2001 book, *Ketamine: Dreams and Realities*, published by the Multidisciplinary Association for Psychedelic Studies (Jansen 2001). Jansen posted solicitations on the internet and gathered many firsthand accounts from around the world. His book contains direct quotations, many of which provide intense and colorful renditions of what ketamine is like. Consistent experiences revolve around the out-of-body experience: disembodied consciousness or dream-like states, a feeling of transcendence (i.e., being in a realm different from social consensus reality), meetings with archetypal religious or spiritual figures or a feeling of spirituality, and near-death-like experiences. Many of the respondents to Jansen's survey indicated a clear addiction to ketamine, either self-reported or as attested by a third party. Jansen's book is very much a cautionary tale about ketamine—this drug provides psychedelic experiences that are quite intense but hard to control, like a novice driver taking the wheel of a Formula One race car.

Morgan et al. (2004a) administered ketamine (either 0.4 or 0.8 mg/kg) over 80 minutes to 54 non-drug-using volunteers to study the reinforcing aspects of ketamine. During infusions, ketamine was generally seen as pleasant, and dissociative symptoms were observed. Mean blood levels were 128.96 ng/mL in the lower-dose group and 261.90 ng/mL in the higher-dose group, which are commensurate with those seen during ketamine treatment for chronic pain and depression, topics to be considered in more detail in chapters 6 and 7. The volunteers were not unconscious and were able to respond to questionnaires at these blood levels. Much higher doses of ketamine, at faster rates, are needed to induce unconsciousness.

Ketamine and the Near-Death-Like Experience

Near-death experiences have been described for centuries and seem to be ubiquitous in the human race. When people lose consciousness and almost die, their reports of what was seen or felt are remarkably consistent; examples include a light at the end of a tunnel, out-of-body experiences, visitation with iconic or archetypal religious figures, and a conviction of their own death (until, of course, consciousness returns). This topic generated enormous publicity in the 1970s with the publication of Dr. Raymond Moody's 1975 bestselling book, *Life After Life*, in which the author detailed cross-cultural descriptions and explanations of near-death experiences. The scientific study of near-death experiences took off, with intense interest in the neurobiological basis of these fascinating transcendental states.

Greyson (1983) developed a 16-item scale to assess the qualitative features of near-death experiences. There were four domains, each with four items:

1. Cognitive (time speeding up, thoughts speeding up, scenes from the person's past appearing, sudden understanding of the meaning of things);

2. Affective (peace, joy, unity or harmony with the universe, a brilliant light);
3. Paranormal (senses more vivid, extrasensory perception, scenes from the future, out-of-body experiences); and
4. Transcendental (being in another world, seeing mystical beings, seeing deceased spirits or religious figures, being on a border of no return).

It turns out that the descriptions of near-death experiences have much in common with those of deep ketamine trips. Jansen (1989; 1997; 2001) became fascinated by the similarity and wrote about it. There seemed to be two themes: first, that ketamine users' descriptions of ketamine trips were quite similar to patients' descriptions of near-death experiences in that literature; and second, that blockade of NMDA receptors may constitute the neurobiological basis of both ketamine's effects and those of near-death experiences. Jansen pointed out similarities between the two: traveling through a tunnel, a light at the end, conviction that one is dead, communication with an iconic religious figure or deity, out-of-body feeling, mystical experiences, and reviewing the events of one's life. Presumably, when somebody does not actually die, but comes close and thus lives to tell the tale, what is remembered reflects some type of neuronal activity, deep in the brain, even in the absence of higher cortical activity (and thus a flat line on a surface EEG). The classic example is cardiac arrest causing cessation of blood flow to the brain for a period of time, with resuscitative efforts bringing back spontaneous heartbeat. Jansen speculated that conditions leading to prolonged unconsciousness from lack of cerebral blood flow or hypoglycemia cause a flood of glutamate to be released from neurons. Glutamate kills neurons in large supply. Perhaps the brain, in a desperate attempt to preserve neurons in the face of a glutamate flood, downregulates NMDA receptors, or releases molecules endogenously that block these receptors, and maybe the latter actions cause the transcendental, out-of-body experiences that are remembered later if the person lives through the event. Perhaps, Jansen hypothesized, ketamine mimics that activity and, as a potent NMDA receptor blocker, directly causes the same experiences.

Corazza and Schifano (2010) recruited 50 ketamine users in the United Kingdom. The authors put the word out in the drug-using community based on their contacts, and 125 people answered. A score of at least 7 on the Greyson Near-Death Experience Scale was needed to qualify for the study, which 50 did. The mean number of lifetime ketamine usages was 140. Interestingly, five had doctoral degrees. The authors interviewed the participants with a special interest in near-death-like experiences while taking ketamine. The most frequent experiences were altered time perception (90%), detachment from the physical body/out-of-body (88%), and a feeling of peace or joy (76%); these usually occurred within the first few usages of ketamine. It is quite likely that Jansen is correct, and that the neurobiological effects of ketamine mimic whatever happens during the low-brain-oxygenation states that are associated with near-death experiences. Thus, a lot of ketamine users, especially those who use only ketamine and study its unique effects with some modicum of introspection (psychonauts as opposed to dance clubbers), are likely to report experiences in common with those who have been near death.

In a later publication, the same group (Corazza et al. 2013) provided further descriptions of the similarities between ketamine trips and near-death experiences. They emphasized the following features: ineffability of the experience, feelings of joy/peace/love, detachment from the body, traveling along darkness toward light, visualization of life experiences (i.e., life review), visions and communications involving deceased loved ones or "beings of light," a decision to return to life, and altered perception of time. It should be noted that these ketamine-related near-death-like experiences involve dosages of ketamine that are high enough to cause lack of responsiveness with the environment—people experiencing these are not interacting with what or who is around them but rather appear unconscious. In an early paper on the topic, Jansen (1990) estimated the minimal dose of ketamine needed to induce a near-death-like state at ~0.7 mg/kg (which approaches the usual anesthesia induction dose of 1.0–1.5 mg/kg).

Legal and Regulatory Issues

Around the world, ketamine has definitely caught the attention of law enforcement agencies. As use increased over time and the dangers and risks of ketamine became apparent, laws and regulations were enacted to stem the illegal synthesis, trafficking, and use of ketamine. Nowhere can ketamine be legally bought over-the-counter. Presumably, law enforcement agencies are tasked with ensuring that all of the ketamine made is accounted for in licit supply chains.

Liao et al. (2017) reviewed international ketamine-related regulations. They noted usage in China, Hong Kong, Taiwan, Indonesia, Malaysia, and Australia. The first large-scale trafficking occurred in southeast Asia in the early 1990s and dramatically increased around 2000. About 99% of all ketamine seizures worldwide in 2009 took place in China and India. Most use in China is in the urban centers of Guangzhou and Shenzhen, two large cities near Hong Kong. In response to the abrupt rise in ketamine trafficking and use after 2000, multiple countries implemented stricter regulations on its dispersion and use: the United States in 1999; Hong Kong in 2000; Taiwan in 2002; Australia in 2003; Canada and North Korea in 2005; Singapore in 2006; China and Japan in 2007; and India in 2013; the United Kingdom re-scheduled ketamine to a more restrictive class in 2014. By 2009, 48 countries regulated ketamine.

There are no ketamine factories in the United States or United Kingdom as of the writing of this book, a situation unlikely to change anytime soon. The nations where ketamine is synthesized in industrial supply are India, Mexico, and most notably, mainland China, where enormous quantities are made. In a summary of ketamine trafficking knowledge, De Luca et al. (2012) reported that five factories were licensed to make ketamine in China at that time.

At some point, much ketamine is diverted to the more profitable, though risky, business of illicit trafficking. It does not take a lot of imagination to conceive how: more ketamine being made than is documented, perhaps, or regulators who can be bribed or threatened to forge paperwork. Clandestine, illicit synthesis does take place as well. In 2009, Chinese authorities seized two secret laboratories with a total of 8.5 million tons of ketamine precursor material, which seems simply gigantic! Such enterprises must be very labor intensive to skirt the law, but presumably the profit margins make it worthwhile. And once ketamine makes its way over a border, the country of origin can no longer control what happens to it.

Thus large supplies—tons—of ketamine make their way into trafficking. Southeast Asia has been particularly hard hit, as detailed earlier. Ketamine has become one of the top three club drugs in mainland China, Taiwan, and Hong Kong (along with methamphetamine and MDMA) (Liu et al. 2016). This epidemic of ketamine use is reflected in the massive amount of ketamine-related research issuing from these regions in the last 20 years.

Most recreational ketamine in the United States is believed to emanate from Mexico (Sassano-Higgins et al. 2016). Whether it is actually synthesized there or simply trafficked there from elsewhere, such as China, is an open question. The source of ketamine for the United Kingdom is China and India, although the illegal trafficking situation is always in flux considering that law enforcement agencies are constantly trying to bust ketamine rings.

Leung et al. (2018) analyzed ketamine levels in 1,771 hair samples taken from people suspected of ketamine use in Hong Kong, from a variety of places interfacing with law enforcement from 2012 to 2016. Ketamine was the most common drug found, in 77.2% of samples. For comparison purposes, cocaine was second at 21.3% and methamphetamine third with 16.5%. Thus, ketamine was clearly the main drug of abuse in this large sample.

Cheng and Dao (2019) analyzed data from Hong Kong consisting of two sets of samples: analysis of drugs seized by law enforcement and drug testing of offenders undergoing urine drug screens from 2011 to 2015. In 2011, ketamine was found in 40.9% of seizures, versus 25.5% in 2015. In urine drug screens, ketamine was present in 10.0% in 2011 versus 4.8% in 2015. They also compared 146,000 survey responses from Hong Kong students in 2011/2012 versus 2014/2015. Use of ketamine dropped from 33.3% of drug users to 16.3%, respectively, and total percentages of students who were drug takers also went down slightly, from 2.2% to 2.0%. Thus, on the whole, it seems as though interest in ketamine is waning in Hong Kong, the world's epicenter of ketamine use in the early 2000s. One reason may be increased regulation and law enforcement. New psychotropic drugs (e.g., cathinones) were on the rise during that time, so another reason may be the ever-changing whims of young people. New generations emerge and view the drugs of their parents' generation as passé. Perhaps this is happening with ketamine.

Reflecting a particularly sinister usage of ketamine, Lee et al. (2018) analyzed urine for drugs in 126 sexual assault victims and found ketamine in 7.9%. Whether the victims had taken ketamine knowingly or were given it surreptitiously, it is clear that ketamine is used as a date rape drug. Ketamine renders its users less aware of their environment and less able to interact with people. If a ketamine user is in a full dissociative state, they may not even be aware of being sexually assaulted.

The Ketamine Celebrities

The history of ketamine has brought about some canonical users, celebrities if you will, whose experiences with and reports of ketamine use have made their way into the annals of this strange and fascinating drug. Three people—who would in modern social media parlance be called "influencers"—became "ketamine celebrities." The two most prominent are John C. Lilly and Marcia Moore, both from the 1970s. In addition, from the 1990s, a mysterious figure wrote under the pseudonym D.M. Turner.

John C. Lilly, M.D.

We start with John C. Lilly. Unemployed trust fund recipient, playboy, womanizer, eccentric, genius, scientist, pseudoscientist, mad scientist, ketamine addict, cocaine addict, intellectual trailblazer, weirdo, communicator with dolphins, inventor of isolation boxes, bon vivant—all these and probably a lot more descriptors are accurate. By all appearances, Lilly led a long, fruitful, fun, happy life. A pretty good summary statement would be that, living off of the trust fund his wealthy father set up for him, John Lilly spent every moment of his life doing exactly what he felt like doing and not one thing more. He did not concern himself with "employment," but he did keep intellectually and physically busy. Unlike the other two ketamine celebrities described here, ketamine itself was not a huge part of Lilly's 86-year-long life, and it was not a part of his death, either. However, for about a year in 1973–1974, he explored its effects intensely, and the record he left contributes to the ketamine story.

Lilly was born January 6, 1915, in St. Paul, Minnesota, to very wealthy parents. He was quite precocious as a child and adolescent, conducting many types of chemistry, biology, and physics experiments of his own design. His classmates called him "Einstein Jr." He went to college at the California Institute of Technology and then medical school, first at Dartmouth, then transferring to and earning his medical degree from the University of Pennsylvania. For some years thereafter, he was involved with many scientific research endeavors that probably would be considered fairly conventional for the time period (e.g., developing various electronics-based physiological monitoring devices).

In the 1950s, there was much interest in the psychological and physiological effects of sensory deprivation. Lilly developed a water-filled isolation tank that people would enter and float in, in the dark, breathing through a tube, not able to hear anything of the outside world. These tanks enjoyed considerable popularity among people such as behavioral scientists, those interested in non-ordinary states of consciousness, and even celebrities of the day. It is not terribly surprising that Lilly would spend a lot of time in an isolation tank: he was a bit of an eccentric, schizoid loner who did not like to be bothered much by others, and one assumes he relished time alone.

By around 1960, Lilly's career took a decidedly nonconformist turn. Living off his parents' trust fund, he explored pretty much anything he wanted, such as the inner world of dolphins, something for which he became notorious. He wrote several books about dolphins, and the 1973 movie *Day of the Dolphin*, starring actor George C. Scott, was loosely based on his work and fame in this area. He is credited with bringing the sophistication of sea mammals like dolphins, porpoises, and whales to the attention of society in general, leading to more compassionate, respectful ways of treating them.

He ended up living on the west coast of America with his third wife, Toni, and they participated in the stylish motivational cults of the day, such as the Esalen Institute in Big Sur, California, which explored ways that bored, upper-middle-class people could pursue "higher consciousness," a term in common use during that era but curiously undefined. Recreational drugs and promiscuous sex figured prominently in the programs (we are talking about the 1970s, after all).

An astonishingly solipsistic person, Lilly enjoyed writing and talking about himself. He seems to have spent most of his time by himself; one gets the impression, reading his books and those about him, that other people, including his wives, were either to help him in whatever endeavor he was pursuing at the time or stay away and leave him alone. He wrote several books, mostly autobiographical in nature. One was *The Scientist*, published in 1978 and consisting of a quirky rendition of his own life written in the third person (Lilly 1978). Some years later, he cowrote another autobiography, *John Lilly So Far...*, which was much more conventional in style (Jeffrey and Lilly 1990). In addition, Karl Jansen, in his book *Ketamine: Dreams and Realities* (Jansen 2001) discussed earlier, interviewed 83-year-old John Lilly in 1998 about his ketamine use.

Lilly's first ketamine experience occurred in 1973, when he was 58, under the care of a doctor he knew, Dr. Craig Enright, who practiced in the Big Sur area. Lilly suffered regularly recurring severe migraine headaches (apparently every 18 days predictably). During one of Lilly's migraines, Enright administered the newly approved "wonder drug" in three serial intramuscular injections, based on the information at that time about its analgesic effects. The injections completely cured the headache and even prevented future ones. That alone impressed Lilly, quite understandably, but what really caught the eccentric doctor's attention was the psychological, dissociative state caused by the ketamine. He was smitten with the idea of dissociation between mind and body, going into trancelike states where his mind would sail off into outer space and the like; he even contacted non-human, non-Earth-based entities. (Of note, Lilly experienced paranormal phenomena and such before ever trying ketamine. He was a strange yet imaginative man.)

He ended up obtaining large supplies of ketamine through physician friends (in those days when licensed doctors could purchase as much ketamine as they liked), injecting himself regularly, and keeping close tabs on his psychological experiences. He implied that he took ketamine regularly for 13 months (intriguingly, however, Jansen wrote that Lilly kept taking ketamine, at unspecified intervals, right up to the time of his interview in 1998). There was even one period where he injected it each hour, around the clock, for 3 weeks, which would amount to some 500 injections of ketamine, all done without supervision. Not surprisingly, Lilly had some near misses, including once, when he nearly drowned in his swimming pool under the influence of ketamine.

Lilly described in minute detail the ideations he experienced under different dosage levels. Initially, at low doses, there was a break from external reality (social consensus reality) to what he called "internal reality," wherein he was oblivious to external stimuli and only preoccupied with internal consciousness. At further dosage increases, he progressed to what he called "extraterrestrial reality," a deeper state of dissociation and complete lack of awareness of having a body at all, along with communication with nonhuman entities. Deeper still, with yet higher dosages, was essentially a comatose state with no mental activity at all.

Eventually, as his wife and his ketamine suppliers got quite concerned with his heavy ketamine use and lack of engagement with other people, he ran out of ketamine. He described using a related compound, undoubtedly phencyclidine (he probably refused to name it given that it was illegal by that time; probably it had been stolen from a veterinary office). Under probably-PCP's influence, he had a bad bicycle accident that caused prolonged painful injuries, and he stopped using such drugs, at least for a while. During a visit from Marcia Moore (see next section), he cautioned her against daily use. She indicated to him her intention of engaging in daily, prolonged use, to which he replied (according to Moore in *Journeys Into the Bright World*, p. 169): "You'd better be damn strong if you're going to play that game."

Lilly lived to age 86, dying of natural causes in 2001. When Jansen caught up with him in 1998 at Lilly's home in Hawaii, Lilly said that in his opinion, he never was addicted to ketamine. He also indicated his distaste for the emerging trend of ketamine as a club drug. Lilly's books are still cited by modern authors in the ketamine literature. His account probably represents the single most-documented individual case report on ketamine recreational use.

Marcia Moore

Marcia Moore is a most intriguing figure, a woman whose life personified the harm that ketamine can do to a person and whose fate is shrouded in mystery. Moore herself, along with her then-husband Howard Alltounian, wrote *Journeys Into the Bright World* (Moody 1975); we also know parts of her story from Jansen's book, *Ketamine: Dreams and Realities* (Jansen 2001). Finally, her cause of death is debated in one chapter of a book by true-crime writer Ann Rule, *A Rage to Kill and Other True Cases* (Rule, 1999).

Marcia (pronounced mar-SEE-uh) Moore was born in Cambridge, Massachusetts, in 1928, into a wealthy family—her father started the Sheraton Hotel chain. Her mother was an enthusiast in paranormal phenomena, and Moore became a believer in astrology and reincarnation. The Buddhist theory of *reincarnation* is that a person's soul is reborn into a succession or iteration of physical bodies over time, and with each new identity, the soul achieves ever-higher levels of spiritual enlightenment, with the ultimate goal of reaching *nirvana*, the highest state. After graduating from Harvard

University, Moore spent essentially her whole adult life traveling around presenting her beliefs to groups of similar-minded people and conducting what she called "regression sessions," whereby she would explore a participant's past lives and horoscope.

Quite successful and popular on this circuit, Moore wrote and cowrote a number of books. She lived fairly simply for an heiress. She married and divorced three times and was single in 1976, when one of her friends introduced her to ketamine. The drug had been procured by a young man called Rama who, in addition to being a 1970s "seeker of higher consciousness," took trips to Mexico to obtain ketamine and bring it back to the States. (In other words, Rama was a drug runner.) At any rate, Moore described her ketamine trip in 1976 in very positive, glowing terms. She felt that she had achieved some kind of special awareness of alternative realities and such. For the time being, she did not pursue any further ketamine trips.

She continued her desultory existence speaking and writing about astrology and reincarnation. In the summer of 1977, she met a man named Howard Alltounian, who was living in Seattle, Washington, and working as a hospital anesthesiologist. These two seemed to be made for each other, in a certain treacly Romeo-and-Juliet sense of tragic love. Alltounian, recently divorced and lonely for female companionship, had a monster crush on Moore. He first saw her picture on the back cover of one of her books in an astrology bookstore, as he was a bit of a believer in that type of stuff himself. He immediately decided he needed to meet this woman of his dreams, made inquiries, and ultimately attended one of her talks in Seattle.

In one way, at least, Alltounian was just what Moore needed: a source of ketamine. In those days, ketamine was not controlled, and any licensed physician could simply buy it directly from the drug company. Thus Alltounian could obtain as much ketamine as he wanted, and legally; plus with his anesthesiology knowledge, he could administer it to Moore and monitor its use. After their meeting at the Seattle astrology talk, Alltounian ravenously pursued her romantically through letters and phone calls (as she traveled during the latter part of the summer of 1977), and she agreed to meet up with him in September. They ended up spending a week together, became engaged, and then married. Anybody observing, with any common sense, would have said the marriage was doomed.

Her own version of these events is her book *Journeys Into the Bright World*. The front cover is purple with two six-sided rings, symbolic of the two rings (phenyl and cyclohexyl) in the ketamine molecule. The subtitle is *Pioneering a New Path to Higher Consciousness—A Personal Account by the Extraordinary Couple Who Risked Everything to Learn Its Secrets* (Moody 1975). (The part about "risked everything" was tragically true.) This was a book she essentially wrote herself, but out of politeness she listed her then-husband as co-author. It is an account of their time together focusing on her increasingly obsessional use of ketamine, procured and administered by her husband. From the very title page all the way to the last paragraph, the book displays an excited and optimistic view of what ketamine could do, not only for an individual but for the world at large.

The opening lines pretty much tell the story: "The theme of this book is the sacramental use of medical technology in raising the consciousness of man." It is "...an intensely personal account of the stages by which we came to believe that [ketamine]...could be safely, easily, and advantageously applied toward the psychospiritual regeneration of planet Earth." High hopes for ketamine indeed!

On the back cover is a picture of Moore in Alltounian's arms, the two sitting side by side, gazing forward. On superficial examination, it is a typical husband-and-wife picture, but upon closer inspection, Moore is looking slightly askance, as if the two are somehow out of sync with one another. It is an odd effect, especially for anybody who knows the denouement of the tragedy.

Moore described her career as astrologer and "regression therapist" who engaged in *hypersentience*, the process by which she explored the past lives of her clients. In her travels, she was a bit lonely (although she does not mention her three previous marriages and divorces). Along came Sunny Alltounian, pursuing her affections in the summer of 1977. She was 49 years old at the time and he was 40. Her conceptualization of their connection was phrased in the language of past lives the two supposedly shared. Incidentally noted was her first experience of ketamine as noted above, which, unlike other psychedelic experiences with LSD and morning glory seeds, was very profound to Marcia. One can only speculate how excited she must have been when she found out her suitor happened to be an anesthesiologist who could procure as much ketamine as she wanted. After their marriage, they (or perhaps more accurately, she) embarked on regular ketamine sessions, which she termed *samadhi therapy* (*samadhi* was a term Moore borrowed from Hindu yoga, meaning intense concentration). Typically, Moore was administered ketamine by Alltounian, who acted as a monitor for safety. He took occasional doses himself but does not appear to have been as smitten with it.

Moore described her ketamine experiences in the language of reincarnation, astrology, psychic phenomena, mysticism, spiritualism, cosmology—the stuff of her life. Her writing abilities were quite impressive. Her ability to use metaphors and similes could easily have been adapted for more conventional books or novels (indeed, one of her brothers was the best-selling novelist Robin Moore). On the other hand, the book was dripping with paranormal beliefs and really beggars the imagination of the non-believing reader. (In fact, as a psychiatrist, I cannot help but speculate that she may have been delusional!) But on the other hand, she was part of a community who shared these beliefs and with whose members she enjoyed some celebrity status. In any case, like John Lilly described earlier, she was a strange person, but brilliant.

In fact, Lilly and Moore had several traits in common: both lived on family trust funds, both had very high intelligence, both had very eccentric ideas and lifestyles, and of course, both became habitual consumers of ketamine. They both had a fondness for exploring what everybody else calls "paranormal" phenomena. Neither was content living in day-to-day reality, meaning the 9-to-5 job with all its tedium and domesticated home life. They wanted something more, and ketamine seemed to fill the bill, along with their other adventures in life. Such people may be particularly likely to find great significance and meaning in psychedelic trips (as opposed to just being entertained). The following quotation captures Moore's attitude toward ketamine (Moody 1975):

> It seemed to us that if captains of industry, leaders of nations, and molders of public opinion could partake of this love medicine the whole planet might be converted into the garden of Eden it is potentially capable of becoming. (p. 118)

Moore presented her ketamine experiences "diary style" by providing the dates, dosage used, and her experience with that session. She was so taken with ketamine that she ended up believing, like so many other psychedelic users of that era, that her drug of choice could make the world a better place. She and Alltounian began offering ketamine to other people, and she described some of their reactions.

In the book, Moore wrote as if her husband was fully on board with her now-daily ketamine use and as if none of her friends were concerned about it. (Although in an oblique reference to possible conflict with Alltounian, she called herself the "Fire Lady" at times in the book and indicated that "boys"—presumably Alltounian—who get involved with Fire Ladies "get burned." What did she mean by this? Was she referring to conflicts and arguments over her ketamine addiction?)

One interesting question broached by Moore is whether a ketamine trip is truly "mind revealing" as the term *psychedelic* implies—in other words, does the trip open up important aspects of that individual's psyche, or is it simply a random scrambling of perception for a period of time? Moore gave her view that ketamine is a type of "truth serum" that does indeed uncover ordinarily hidden or unconscious conflicts of the user (Moody 1975):

> If a person would rather not view the cancerous tissues of his own person-
> ality then he is best advised to stay away from ketamine. (p. 138)

The book ended on a happy note: Moore and Alltounian (who has now quit his conventional job) were going to devote themselves to Samadhi therapy research, the details of which are not specified but which presumably consist of enlisting volunteers to get ketamine and explore the meaning of their trips. Moore and Alltounian even solicited such volunteers from the book's readers by providing an address for inquiries (which, decades later, seems rather quaint). They petitioned the Food and Drug Administration for approval, finding roadblocks along the way and not having final approval as the book went to print in October 1978. Plans were underway for Moore to continue her ketamine explorations, Samadhi therapy, and writings, in her next book to be titled *The Alchemy of the Soul*. Samadhi therapy was going to make the world a better place. She even met with John Lilly to discuss ketamine, and he gave her the warning quoted earlier ("You'd better be damn strong if you're going to play that game"). She could not have been happier or more optimistic, it seems. The future, she indicated, would be a bright one in the "bright world."

But just 3 months later, she was dead.

The mystery of Moore's end may have nothing to do with ketamine, but it deserves to be told here. Her work on ketamine, if misguided, was nothing if not sincere. She had no hidden agendas, she was not trying to make money, and she did not appear to be seeking fame or any kind of narcissistic gratification. She seemed to be motivated by a genuine belief that ketamine was going to make the world a better place. The fact that this simple aryl-cyclohexylamine molecule would make an otherwise highly intelligent person believe such a thing is part of the ketamine story, and ketamine surely played some type of role in the causal chain leading to her disappearance.

To stick with known facts, in the wee hours of the morning of January 15, 1979, Alltounian called the local police department and reported her missing. Two years later, on the first day of spring, 1981, a landowner clearing his land in some woods about 15 miles from the Alltounian/Moore townhouse found a skull that was proven to be Marcia Moore's, based on dental records.

So what happened to her? Our information in this regard, so many decades later, comes from two sources. One is a book by Ann Rule, who has been called the "queen of true crime writing" from her dozens of books detailing the victims and perpetrators of high-profile crimes—most famously, serial killer Ted Bundy. She devoted a chapter of her book *A Rage to Kill and Other True Cases* to the Marcia Moore disappearance (Rule 1999). Rule reviewed police records and interviewed detectives assigned to the disappearance and some of Moore's friends. The other source is the book by Dr. Karl

Jansen, *Ketamine: Dreams and Realities.* Jansen interviewed Alltounian in the late 1990s.

Jansen presented a theory of Moore's disappearance based on what Alltounian told him, which was that she was addicted to ketamine, he objected to this, and that this issue became a source of conflict between the two. Alltounian also accused her of forging his medical license number and signature to purchase ketamine from the drug company, clandestinely (and of course illegally). If true, that would of course indicate addiction. Jansen believed from this account that Moore went outside the night of Sunday, January 14, 1979, deep into the woods by herself, took a large amount of ketamine, and died of exposure—perhaps not an overt act of suicide but reckless nonetheless. Jansen presented no evidence for his hypothesis.

For her part, Rule theorized that Alltounian murdered Moore and hid the body. She wrote that the skull was found in isolation and there was evidence of damage to the frontal portions of it. Alltounian told the police that he attended a movie by himself that evening; when he returned to the townhouse about 1:00 a.m., she was not there; and he spent the next few hours searching for her in vain before finally calling law enforcement. Rule implied that the police believed Alltounian's story and did not pursue him as a suspect—never checked his story or examined his car for evidence.

Marcia Moore's disappearance and death is unsolved. Nobody can state with certainty what happened, and Harold Alltounian died in 2006.

Over time, the stories of John Lilly and Marcia Moore have been instructive, as these two people took a lot of ketamine over a long period of time, and their experiences with it are intelligently and elegantly memorialized in their books. These two cases represent an account of what happens if a person is not burdened by jobs or responsibilities in daily life, has access to unlimited supplies of ketamine, and is able to articulate their experience.

The Mysterious "D.M. Turner"

Last to present is the sad story of "D.M. Turner." His is more mundane and probably more similar to that of most ketamine addicts than the lofty, rarefied ketamine trips of Moore and Lilly, both of whom were at baseline highly eccentric people with odd beliefs. D.M. Turner (a pseudonym) published two books relevant to psychedelia. One was about *Salvia divinorum*, a psychedelic plant found in Mexico and South America, and is not discussed further here. The other, *The Essential Psychedelic Guide* (Turner 1994), described, chapter by chapter, different classes of compounds and how to use them safely (if illegally).

Turner described ketamine as offering intense feelings of dissociation at deep levels, to the point where there is no longer a memory of identity or personality, a feeling of being at one with the universe, with time being fluid. He warned of the addictive effect of ketamine, admitting to his own addiction. He probably represents most users of recreational ketamine (and other psychedelic drugs): the goal is entertainment and release from tedium and boredom, not as part of some quest for spirituality or higher meaning in life.

The concepts of *set and setting* are crucial to an understanding of how psychedelic drug phenomena are interpreted and experienced by the user. What one takes away from a drug trip is deeply influenced by the set of expectations the user has and the setting in which the drugs are used. As an example of the importance of *set* (short for *cognitive set*), one can imagine what would happen if a psychedelic drug were administered to a person surreptitiously, without their awareness. The resulting perceptual changes would be frightening and later on would be recalled as traumatic. Conversely, if the same drug were taken by the same person as part of a culturally sanctioned ritual, its effects would likely be experienced as positive by the user. Thus, a ketamine user's set of expectations strongly influences the ultimate experience. All psychedelics should be taken with an attendant or monitor present, to make sure no accidents happen.

Regarding *setting*, a user's immediate environment can drastically affect the result. On the one hand, taking a drug as part of a party where everybody is high and behaving irresponsibly may influence the experience in negative ways, whereas the presence of a supportive community is likely to skew the user's reactions toward the positive. Regarding ketamine, just as set is important, in that a person needs to be prepared in advance for the types of dissociative phenomena induced, setting is critical for safety because ketamine users are typically near unconsciousness. In such a state, the ketamine user is at risk for accidents or being taken advantage of (date rape, for example).

Apart from anonymous and unreferenced suppositions on the internet, including Wikipedia and the web site Erowid, the identity of D.M. Turner is unknown. He is described as a psychedelic "researcher," although "experimenter" or "enthusiast" may be more appropriate. Tales of Turner have been passed on via oral transmission in the insular and private world of psychedelia. He was described as male, having worked in an office wearing a suit during the week, being interested in lots of hobbies like woodworking, being private and reclusive but quite friendly, and being a relentless psychedelic drug user. His death is said to have occurred on New Year's Eve, December 31, 1996, but his body was not found until several weeks later. Ketamine paraphernalia were said to be found in the bathroom where his body was discovered, face down in a full bathtub, a drowning victim.

Epilogue

Moore, Lilly, and Turner described numinous experiences with ketamine. Further study might elaborate the neurobiological basis of religiosity and spirituality. One of the big controversies in this regard in the field of psychedelic studies is whether there is in fact a "hard-wired" spirituality substrate in the brain or whether the consciousness-altering effects of these drugs are only interpreted by some people with pre-existing religious beliefs or spiritual inclinations as such, something akin to a neuropharmacological Rorschach test: a stimulus devoid of any intrinsic meaning, subject to different interpretations by people based on set and setting. One thing is for certain: unlike any other drug, ketamine inspires people to undergo a fundamental change in world view.

Known Complications and Dangers of Nonmedical Ketamine Use

Clearly, the joys of the K-hole have a price. In this section, we consider the very important question of sequelae of recreational ketamine use. A report from Nutt et al. (2007) provides guidelines with which to consider how harmful a drug is. Three overall classes of harm were considered: physical harm, dependence, and societal harm. The first of these, physical harm, was subclassified into acute, chronic, and intravenous use harm. The second, dependence, was subclassified into pleasure, psychological dependence, and physical dependence. Social harm was subclassified into intoxication harms, social harm, and costs.

A panel of drug addiction experts rated a variety of drugs on a 4-point scale on each of these 12 items: 0 (none) to 3 (severe harm). Thus, a total score could be achieved by adding the 12 item scores (maximum of 36, minimum of 0); or it could be reported as mean individual item score (with a minimum of 0 and maximum of 3). Of the 20 drugs of abuse considered by the panel of experts, heroin scored the highest, with a mean item score of 2.75. Ketamine scored 1.75, lower than cocaine, barbiturates, street methadone, and alcohol. Thus, this panel of experts considered ketamine moderately harmful overall. Its highest item score was 2.1 for harms of acute intoxication and 2.1 for harms associated with intravenous use (Nutt et al. 2007). Of note, as discussed later, the literature on the devastating effects of chronic ketamine use on the urinary bladder were not known at the time: the score for ketamine's chronic use harms would undoubtedly be higher today. Interestingly, the panel gave ketamine a score of only 1.7 for "psychological dependence"; one wonders whether the panel (who were U.K.

clinicians and experts in addiction) were aware of the devastations of unfettered ketamine access going on in Asia.

Cognitive Effects of Recreational Ketamine Use

A common concern about any drug of abuse is disrupted thinking and memory, or cognitive dysfunction. Alcohol used over a long period of time is known to cause dementia, for example, and benzodiazepines have well-documented effects on memory consolidation. Jansen (2001) noted that ketamine users subjectively reported memory problems. In the early 2000s, a fairly large set of research began to document this. There are two predominant sources of data on the cognitive effects of ketamine recreational use: one is from Asia (Taiwan, mainland China, and Hong Kong), and the other is from London, where a group from University College of London (UCL) undertook a series of studies in the early and mid-2000s. In general, the studies from Asia involve large sample sizes with very heavy ketamine use (e.g., 6–8 years of daily or near-daily use of several grams per day), whereas the UCL studies involve smaller sample sizes and lighter ketamine use (e.g., a few times a month).

First, a quick primer on memory. *Semantic memory* refers to information (e.g., recalling facts about history, geopolitical events, or prompts provided as part of a memory test to be recalled later). *Episodic memory* refers to autobiographical events (e.g., recalling a personal experience such as a social occasion). *Procedural memory* refers to remembering how to do things (e.g., driving a car). *Working memory* refers to recalling elements of an ongoing task (e.g., scanning a list of words and saying out loud which have a particular characteristic, such as a certain number of letters). Finally, the *perceptual representation system* refers to memory of the sound or appearance of things without connecting the meaning of them. Most studies of ketamine focus on semantic memory, episodic memory, and working memory.

Ke et al. (2018) studied the cognitive function of 63 chronic ketamine users (mean age ~25, duration of ketamine use ~6 years, using 6.5 days per week, 3.5 g inhaled per day of use) compared with 65 non-drug-using controls. The ketamine users performed worse on several tests, including immediate and delayed visual and verbal memory, working memory, and selective attention. There was no difference between the two groups on measures of *executive function* (a catch-all term referring to the complex cognitive activities that require not only attention and memory but also the use of logic).

Chan et al. (2013) studied people recruited from bars, including 25 ketamine users, 30 non-drug-using controls, and 10 nonketamine polydrug users. Of note, the ketamine users, to meet criteria for the study, had to use ketamine at least twice a month for 2 years, which is not much ketamine in comparison to other studies. Mean age was ~19, so it was a young sample. There was little difference between the various groups on testing of cognition, which is not surprising considering the relatively light usage of ketamine.

Tang et al. (2013), working in Hong Kong, studied 51 current ketamine users, 49 ex-users (>6 months of abstinence from ketamine), and 100 non-drug-using controls by use of a cognitive battery and a depression rating scale. Current users performed worse than the other groups on almost all of the tests, which assessed various aspects of working memory, semantic memory, visual memory, mental speed, attention, and verbal fluency (there were 15 tests in all). These results provide evidence that chronic ketamine use does impair cognition but that abstinence can restore functioning.

Wang et al. (2018a) compared the cognitive testing profiles of 58 ketamine users (mostly in their early 30s; mean of an enormous 6.8 g/day inhaled ketamine; mean duration of use 8.6 years) to 49 methamphetamine users and 58 non-drug-using controls. Almost all the ketamine users had self-reported histories of ketamine-induced psychosis at one point, although a precise definition was not given (a brief period of psychosis around the time of a heavy ketamine binge is not unexpected). The drug users were tested after about a week of abstinence. The test battery included verbal memory, working memory, motor speed, verbal fluency, attention, processing speed, and executive function. For most of the tests except executive function, the ketamine users scored about two standard deviations below the mean for the population at large (which was where the non-drug-using controls scored), indicating substantially lower cognitive function, albeit not necessarily in the formal impaired range. The nonketamine drug users scored in between the ketamine users and the non-drug-using controls. On tests of executive function, the ketamine users scored in the average range, indicating that general thinking or intelligence was more or less unimpaired. Tests requiring intense focus and recall were impaired.

Cheng et al. (2018) compared 51 ketamine users without psychosis, 23 ketamine users with persisting psychosis (beyond 24 hours after last use), and 75 people with schizophrenia. Cognitive tests for delayed recall and visuospatial learning revealed that the ketamine users with persistent psychosis did particularly poorly, and worse than those with schizophrenia, indicating that long-term heavy ketamine use is associated with cognitive disruptions.

Zhang et al. (2018) assessed cognitive function in three groups: ketamine plus low use of other drugs; ketamine plus heavy use of other drugs; and non-drug-using controls. Non-drug-using controls tended to score better on tests of memory but not other cognitive domains. There was no difference in cognition between ketamine users with or without concomitant heavy drug use. The authors concluded that ketamine's effect on cognition is independent of other drug use. This is important, as finding "pure" ketamine users is quite difficult—pretty much everybody who uses ketamine regularly uses other substances such as alcohol, marijuana, stimulants, and opiates.

In sum, these well-conducted Asian studies indicate a cognitive signal of long-term ketamine use, manifesting in young, otherwise healthy people.

We next turn our attention to the studies conducted in London. In the early to mid-2000s, a group of psychologists at UCL, headed up by Drs. Celia Morgan and Valerie Curran, undertook a series of studies of ketamine users recruited from dance clubs to determine the cognitive function of chronic users. These studies constitute one of the most important sets of data on the cognitive and psychopathological effects of long-term ketamine use. The group used the "snowball technique" to recruit participants: they started with known ketamine users and asked them to contact other users who might be interested in joining. They also visited dance clubs on nights of intense parties, asked around, and recruited participants in that way.

Essentially, all ketamine users also used other drugs, most notably stimulants such as cocaine, methamphetamine, and MDMA, in addition to alcohol and marijuana. To control for the effects of the other drugs, the researchers divided their participants into those who used ketamine plus other drugs and those who only used other drugs. This solution was not ideal—if one wants to know the effects of ketamine, one should study those who use only ketamine—but again, a user who partook of ketamine alone was quite rare. Also, they divided ketamine users into those who used infrequently (e.g., weekends only at the dance clubs), frequently (e.g., half the days each month or more), or formerly (ex-users). Control groups consisted of nonketamine polydrug users (i.e., those who used the same drugs as ketamine users except without ketamine) and non-drug-using controls. Not all of the five groups were included in all of the studies.

Curran and Morgan (2000) studied 20 ketamine users and 19 nonketamine drug users several days after ketamine usage. Schizotypal and dissociative symptoms persisted into day 3 of abstinence in this cohort of ketamine users, as did semantic memory problems on the cognitive task. Morgan et al. (2004b), in 20 ketamine users versus 20 nonketamine drug users, assessed *source memory*, the ability to recall the source of learned information, in this case, the gender of the voice that earlier communicated with each participant. Source memory was impaired in the ketamine users, both on the night of use and after 3 days of abstinence.

Curran and Monaghan (2001) compared 18 frequent ketamine users to 19 infrequent users regarding episodic and semantic memory and found that on the night of ketamine use (they studied people who were at a club where there were a lot of drug users), both groups had impairments related to acute ketamine use, but 3 days later, after abstinence, only the chronic frequent users had continued evidence of impairment. This implies that chronic use of ketamine can have cognitive effects outlasting the immediate presence of ketamine or its metabolites in the system. The authors also assessed dissociative and schizotypal signs at the same time points. They were high in the frequent users (using about half the days of the month) on the night of use but not 3 days later, indicating that the effects on these traits are not necessarily long-lasting.

Morgan et al. (2004c) followed up on an earlier-studied cohort 3 years later for cognition. Eighteen ketamine users and 10 nonketamine polydrug users were tested for working memory, episodic memory, and semantic memory. Ketamine use had declined by a mean of 88.8%, so for the most part, the former users were abstinent from ketamine. The amount of reduction in ketamine use correlated with improvements in semantic memory. Episodic and working memory improved in the ketamine users but was still worse than for the polydrug users. Baseline cognitive functioning (before ketamine use started) was not measured, however.

Morgan et al. (2006a) abstracted data from 11 ketamine studies undertaken at Yale University involving 295 normal volunteers. A wide variety of cognitive tests were administered at baseline and after ketamine infusions. The bottom line is that males had greater decrements than females in memory test scores after ketamine infusions. Interestingly, the males had higher ketamine blood concentrations (mean of 161.67 versus 139.82 ng/mL for females), which may have influenced the outcomes.

In non-drug-using volunteers given ketamine and in chronic users, Morgan et al. (2006b) studied *semantic priming* (more quickly responding to a word when it is preceded by a related word; e.g., people react more quickly to the word "butter" when it is preceded by "bread" than if it is preceded by something unrelated such as "book"). The investigators used an extremely complicated four-way variable scheme to test a variety of constructs. The primary purpose of the study was to test whether ketamine users have cognitive profiles that mimic schizophrenia, which is characterized by a certain deficit on semantic priming tasks. The chronic ketamine users had impaired performance on a semantic priming task relative to nonketamine polydrug users.

Whether ketamine use somehow impairs the user's daily cognitive function is difficult to gauge from the UCL studies, as their paradigms do not involve standardized neuropsychological tests with norms for the population at large or any research correlating the results with daily functionality. From their studies taken as a whole, however, it is clear time and again that chronic ketamine users perform less well on a variety of tasks than nonketamine polydrug users or non-drug-using controls. Morgan et al. (2006b) provided a nice review of their studies of ketamine's effects on memory.

In another report from the UCL group, Uhlhaas et al. (2007) administered a visual perceptual organizational task to ketamine users ($n=16$) and nonketamine drug users ($n=16$) on the night of use (testing took place at a club where participants were recruited for the study), and then again after 3 days of abstinence. On the night of use, ketamine users had more perceptual errors than nonketamine users, but by 3 days later, there was no difference. This was taken as evidence that the perceptual disorganization caused by ketamine was an acute but not chronic phenomenon.

Morgan et al. (2008) evaluated attentional bias in groups of infrequent ketamine users, frequent ketamine users, former ketamine users, nonketamine polydrug users, and non-drug-using controls (five groups total). *Attentional bias* refers to the tendency to pay attention to some things while ignoring others: in this case, drug users tend to notice stimuli in their environment that are drug-related. This is often an automatic process and not conscious. The investigators concocted a computer-based scheme whereby each participant had a session at the computer attending to different types of stimuli and responding in certain ways by pressing certain keys on the keyboard. Latency of responding in the appropriate manner was a dependent variable. The frequent ketamine users (some of whom inhaled almost 9 g/day) had the most intense responses to drug-related stimuli (i.e., shortest latencies to pressing keys), indicating attentional bias toward drug-related stimuli. How this translates into day-to-day functioning is not clear, as the test they used was not standardized with published norms. However, the authors believed that, according to the results, frequent ketamine users might be unable in daily life to resist responding to any stimuli that are drug-related, thus making it hard for them to fight addiction.

Morgan et al. (2010) studied 30 each of five similar groups for a variety of cognitive functions. The current frequent ketamine users overall performed the worst, including on tests of spatial working memory, spatial planning, pattern recognition, and source memory. There was no difference among the groups in prose recall or verbal fluency. Of note, the cognitive function of the ex-users was no worse than that of any of the other groups. Thus, abstinence from ketamine may result in cognitive improvement.

Morgan et al. (2010) conducted a 1-year follow-up of five similar groups. For those with continued use of ketamine, cognitive performance correlated with amount of continued use. There were impairments in spatial working memory and pattern recognition memory, as well as increased delusional and dissociative thinking. The abstinent group showed no deficits in the baseline study or at 1-year follow-up, suggesting that the cognitive effects of ketamine may not be permanent. A good summary of their work can be found in their reviews (Morgan and Curran 2006 and Morgan et al. 2011).

In one of their reviews of their extensive studies, Morgan and Curran (2006) pointed out that acute administration of ketamine impairs episodic, semantic, and working memory as well as attention but not executive function (in normal volunteers). With abstinence, problems with semantic memory improve, but there are persisting problems with episodic memory and attention. Of course, it is not possible for this kind of study to be randomized, prompting questions as to whether the ketamine users were different at baseline, whether other drug use (stimulants, cannabis, opiates, alcohol) caused cognitive problems, or whether ketamine-induced psychopathology caused cognitive problems. There seems to be a consistent finding that long-term ketamine users function cognitively at a lower level than never-users or users of other drugs, which certainly provides a cautionary tale about the dangers of ketamine use. It does seem that occasional ketamine users (e.g., weekends only) perform much better cognitively than the really frequent, heavy users. And long-term abstinence does seem to be associated with improvements in cognition.

Addictive Potential of Recreational Ketamine Use

As addicts develop tolerance, use of the drug trumps other activities of daily life such as school, job, or social relationships. Functionality falters, physical and psychological health deteriorates, and life revolves around the drug. Does this happen with ketamine?

The short answer is yes—not for everybody who takes it, but a minority of ketamine users, if they have access to it, will take it compulsively at least until they run out. Where access is unlimited, they will take it until the body breaks down. This is acutely instantiated in the first-person accounts provided by Jansen (2001) discussed earlier.

It is not uncommon for typical ketamine users to start in their late teens or so and use ketamine daily or almost daily for many years. The amount used per day is often 3 g or more (inhaled in powder form, usually, in Asia; such use does not occur in the United States or Great Britain because of the lack of availability). That behavior is compulsive use any way you look at it.

Sassano-Higgins et al. (2016) reviewed some of the proposed neurobiological mechanisms whereby ketamine is addictive, including NMDA receptor blockade (which causes the dissociative effects), dopamine signaling enhancement (which is common to many drugs of addiction), and opioid receptor agonism. Other literature on this topic is worth reviewing.

Tung et al. (2014) studied data from a sample of 80 people (median age 27) seeking treatment for ketamine dependence on the Chinese Severity of Dependence Scale, which contains five questions:

- Did you think your ketamine use was out of control?
- Did the prospect of missing a dose make you anxious or worried?
- Did you worry about your use of ketamine?
- Did you wish you could stop?
- How difficult would you find it to stop or go without ketamine?

The first four questions are answered with *never* (0), *sometimes* (1), *often* (2), or *always/nearly always* (3) and the fifth with *not difficult* (0), *quite difficult* (1), *very difficult* (2), or *impossible* (3). The score range is 0–15. All 80 patients were intranasal (inhalational) ketamine users, most using ketamine more than three times per week. Median score on the scale was 9, so there were plenty of patients who considered ketamine an addictive problem in their lives.

In what seems to be the only follow-up report after a ketamine treatment program, Wang et al. (2018b) compared relapse rates between those with ketamine use and those with stimulant use. Among the 92 ketamine users, the relapse rate was 34.8% over the 7 years of follow-up, much lower than the 60.5% relapse rate among the 43 stimulant users. Relapse was defined by a subsequent positive drug test during mandatory monitoring. The participants were young people (mean age 16 at time of treatment) sent to treatment by courts after being arrested on drug charges.

Fatality With Recreational Ketamine Use

One of the properties of ketamine attractive to anesthesiologists is low respiratory suppression. Ketamine is thus a direct cause of death only in extremely high doses, and such cases are rare. (The 2023 death of actor Matthew Perry was attributed to very high levels of ketamine, which alone might or might not have been fatal, but in his case, led to drowning in a hot tub.) A ketamine-related death is more likely to be caused indirectly via accident (e.g., car crash, falling) or being a victim of a crime while intoxicated.

Schifano et al. (2008) searched various mortality databases in the United Kingdom during 1993–2006 and found four deaths in which ketamine was the only drug detected in the body. Further details about each death were not provided, so it is not known if ketamine did in fact cause the deaths or just happened to be there. What it does confirm is the rarity of ketamine-caused death.

Li et al. (2020) noted that in China in 2016, ketamine accounted for 2.5% of drug use, well behind methamphetamine and heroin. During the years of their study (2004–2017 in Shanghai and 2005–2017 in Wuhan), in which they analyzed police reports, there were two deaths attributed due solely to ketamine: one suicide and one undetermined cause. There were seven ketamine-plus-methamphetamine deaths: four falls and three undetermined drug poisonings (either suicide or accident).

Accidents Arising From Recreational Ketamine Use

Various drugs can dull the senses and render the user liable to accidents such as motor vehicle crashes and falls, and also to victimization from crimes such as sexual assault. Alcohol is particularly notorious for these things. Ketamine, being a sedative and causing dissociation of consciousness from the immediate environment, can be associated with all of these things as well. Cheng and Dao (2017), for example, analyzed toxicological data from fatal driving accidents and those driving under the influence of drugs from 2006 to 2015 in Hong Kong. Ketamine was the most frequently detected drug (after alcohol) in dead drivers. Nine of 223 fatally injured drivers had ketamine in their systems. Of those driving under the influence of drugs from 2010 to 2015, 138 had ketamine detected. Chronic pain and depression clinics treating with ketamine have the patient reclining in a chair, and any recreational ketamine user would be well advised to do the same and also have a trusted adult in attendance to ensure nothing bad happens. Automobile (or other potentially dangerous machinery usage) restrictions should be prescribed for recurrent ketamine treatment in depression or chronic pain clinics after each administration.

Psychopathological Effects of Recreational Ketamine Use

As a group, drugs are often associated with mental health issues such as depression, mania, anxiety, or psychosis. With the epidemic of ketamine use in Asia and to a lesser extent in England, several groups have assessed the presence and severity of these conditions in ketamine users. There is a distinction between studying ketamine to see how it affects users' mental health (which is the subject of this section) versus in the laboratory under standardized conditions as a test of the ketamine/NMDA model of schizophrenia; the latter is covered in Chapter 5, "The Ketamine Model of Schizophrenia."

During the PCP abuse era of roughly the 1970s, when horror stories of violent behavior abounded in American media, there were two predominant fears among the public: precipitation of psychosis and late-onset psychotic elements (flashbacks). These fears permeated the earlier LSD era as well, so the American public was primed to be afraid of ketamine. Three early reports purporting to confirm these fears have been widely cited over the decades. Johnson (1971) described a 29-year-old woman given ketamine for a surgical procedure who complained of hallucinations—consisting of bright lights and "thousands of faces"—off and on for a year. Fine and Finestone (1973) said that three patients reported delayed psychotic phenomena after the procedure (out of 1,400 ketamine administrations in their anesthesiology practice). Perel and Davidson (1976) described an 11-year-old boy given serial ketamine infusions during surgery who had recurrent visual hallucinations for up to 5 minutes at a time over the next 5 days. (This oft-cited report hardly constitutes frightening evidence of persisting psychosis: the amounts of ketamine were rather large, and the effects lasted a fairly short time.) These three reports have been cited repeatedly in the literature in subsequent decades as "evidence" that ketamine causes persisting or delayed-onset psychosis. More modern research has provided higher-quality data sets.

Both Curran and Morgan (2000) and Curran and Monaghan (2001) found schizotypal signs and dissociative symptoms in recreational users on the night of ketamine use; 3 days later, the symptoms were much less in the 2000 study and about the same in the 2001 study. In another data set from this group, Morgan et al. (2004d) found high dissociation and schizotypy on the night of ketamine use but not after 3 days of abstinence. Thus, the weight of evidence from this group is that dissociative and schizotypal effects of ketamine are acute and generally not persistent after just 3 days.

Morgan et al. (2004c), in the follow-up study described earlier, found that after 3 years of near-abstinence, ketamine users still were more likely to have schizotypal and perceptual disorganization symptoms than nonketamine polydrug users, but the degree (severity) of dissociative symptoms was not different. Of note, one of the original 19 ketamine users in this cohort had been diagnosed with schizophrenia in the 3-year interim and was not a participant in the follow-up study, again prompting the question of whether a predisposition to these symptoms may exist.

In the Uhlhaas et al. (2007) study cited earlier, symptoms of dissociation and delusional thinking were assessed on the night of ketamine use and after 3 days of abstinence. Ketamine users showed very high levels of dissociative thinking (derealization, depersonalization, and amnesia) on the night of use but not 3 days later. Delusional thinking scores were higher than for non-users not only on the night of use but also 3 days later, indicating that this particular effect of ketamine is persistent.

Blagrove et al. (2009) administered infusions of ketamine or placebo to volunteers and found over the next 3 nights that the ketamine group had a higher incidence of unpleasant dreams. Thus, this side effect of ketamine noted early in the anesthesia literature turns out to be persistent if patients are evaluated carefully. One interesting possibility is that the effect was really related to loss of positive dreaming in the ketamine group, as opposed to an increase in negative dreaming.

Freeman et al. (2009) studied a phenomenon called *superstitious conditioning*, whereby under laboratory stimulus conditions, development of false ideations (superstitions) may underlie delusion formation. Ketamine users did have more superstitious conditioning in these laboratory conditions than nonketamine polydrug users, but the participants still did not have psychosis.

The five groups studied by Morgan et al. (2009) (30 each of frequent ketamine users, infrequent ketamine users, former ketamine users, nonketamine drug users, and non-drug-using controls), whose cognitive data were presented earlier, underwent psychopathological testing to assess schizophrenia-like experiences, delusional thinking, and dissociative experiences. On all of these, the frequent current users scored the highest, but the former users scored higher than the non-ketamine-using groups as well, indicating some persisting psychopathology even after abstinence. The question again is whether ketamine or a predisposition is responsible.

Tang et al. (2013), also cited earlier with the cognitive data, assessed depression rating scale scores among current ketamine users, ex-users, and non-drug-using controls and found higher scores (i.e., worse depressive symptoms) in the current users compared with the other two groups, lending support to the idea that chronic ketamine use does not help depression, but rather worsens it, and that abstinence leads to lower depression ratings.

Stone et al. (2014), studying British patients, used a comprehensive psychopathological questionnaire for 15 chronic ketamine users and 13 nonketamine polydrug users. Six of the ketamine users had abnormal profiles on the questionnaire, but this was pretty nonspecific. None of the ketamine users were described as having overt psychosis or schizophrenia.

Zhang et al. (2014b) studied users of ketamine only, stimulants only, and both ketamine and stimulants admitted to a psychiatric unit and found lower overall psychopathology scores, lower hostility scores, lower thought disorder scores, and higher depression-anxiety scores in the ketamine-only group than the others. The psychopathology scores of chronic ketamine users matched those of a previous cohort of prodromal schizophrenia patients, adding support to the notion that chronic ketamine use causes signs and symptoms similar to those of schizophrenia.

Stone et al. (2015), in a neuroimaging study, compared psychopathological screening scales between 15 chronic ketamine users and 13 nonketamine polydrug users. They found greater "abnormal thought content" in the ketamine users but, importantly, no overt psychosis. More details on this study are given in the next section.

Liang et al. (2015) studied 129 people at three centers in Hong Kong. On average, age at first use was 17.7 years, and duration of use was 8.7 years. All patients were diagnosed as having ketamine dependence. The authors retrospectively retrieved information about psychopathology from records: 27.7% of the sample had depression, and 31.8% had psychosis, but the definition of psychosis was unclear—was it visual phenomena? auditory phenomena? delusions? Were the psychotic symptoms identical to those of schizophrenia? Or were they essentially toxic phenomena from heavy ketamine use that abated with abstinence? What is remarkable about this and other similar Asian data sets is the large number of ketamine addicts studied, the young age at onset of use, and the long duration of usage. Such large samples with long, intense ketamine usage are unlikely to exist in the United States or United Kingdom.

Tang et al. (2015) screened ketamine users (mean age 22) attending counseling services for psychopathology. Of the 200 screened, 170 scored positive for a mood, anxiety, or psychotic disorder. On full diagnostic interview, 51 had a psychiatric diagnosis, four of whom had psychosis, for a total rate of psychosis of 2%. Forty-two patients had a mood disorder (21% of the total sample).

Xu et al. (2015) conducted psychopathological ratings in four groups: 135 normal volunteers given an infusion of ketamine; 187 habitual ketamine users; 154 patients with "early" schizophrenia; and 522 patients with chronic schizophrenia. The psychosis rating scores were higher in those with schizophrenia than both ketamine groups, who nonetheless had symptom clusters similar to those with schizophrenia. There was better homology between the chronic ketamine users and those with schizophrenia than between the volunteers given ketamine and those with schizophrenia.

Fan et al. (2016) recruited ketamine users from two hospitals in mainland China with programs to treat such patients. The data set contained 187 patients who were dependent on ketamine, mean age of 26.2, mean time since first use of 6.3 years, and mean time of dependence of 3.1 years. The mean daily dose was 3.7 g inhaled, and 75.4% used ketamine daily. These were heavy, chronic, frequent ketamine users, underscoring the unusually easy availability of this drug in Asian countries. Patients were administered psychosis rating scales; all subscales were either less than mildly ill (92%)

or mildly ill (8%). Thus, there was little evidence of psychosis in this group. On a depression rating scale, 44.9% scored moderate and 32.6% scored severe, and 46% scored moderate to severe on an anxiety scale. The latter two scales correlated positively with severity of ketamine dependence. Of note, these were voluntary patients at a ketamine treatment facility who were capable of participating in 2 hours of questioning. If ketamine does cause an ongoing psychotic syndrome that persists beyond a few days since last use (which is probably rare), those patients would probably not be in such a program or capable of participating: they would be on a psychiatric unit. In addition, all patients in this study had been detoxified from ketamine— there was no recent use.

Zhang et al. (2018) studied 67 chronic ketamine users and 40 non-drug-using controls in China with psychopathological rating scales for psychosis, depression, and anxiety. Mean duration of ketamine use was 73.61 months, 6.13 days per week (essentially daily), and 2.8 g inhaled per day.

Cheng et al. (2018), cited above in the section on cognition, also compared psychopathological rating scale scores between nonpsychotic ketamine users, psychotic ketamine users ($n=23$), and patients with schizophrenia ($n=75$) using the Positive and Negative Syndrome Scale (PANSS), a commonly used psychosis scale in the Asian studies (Kay et al. 1987). There were similar elevations between those with schizophrenia and ketamine psychosis; however, the scale is not very specific. We do not really know anything about the qualitative features of their supposed psychosis. The authors estimated that about 3% of chronic ketamine users eventually meet criteria for persisting ketamine psychotic disorder.

Taken together, these psychopathological studies of ketamine users indicate that anxiety and depression are common among chronic users. Elevations are seen on rating scales of psychotic symptoms in some studies, but frustratingly, the specifics of the psychopathology are not given in the studies. Do ketamine users look like they have schizophrenia? Do they get diagnosed with schizophrenia by clinicians who do not know of their ketamine use? Do they require long-term antipsychotic therapy, like those with schizophrenia? The answers seem to be "no," for the most part. Rather, the typical long-term heavy ketamine user may be somewhat odd and eccentric but not blatantly psychotic or disorganized. Additionally, data indicate that abstinence from ketamine over time is associated with improvements in psychopathology, as is the case with cognitive issues. Also, people self-select for ketamine use, so those who are eccentric and prone to odd patterns of thinking may be more likely to use ketamine and enjoy its mind-altering effects.

The NMDA receptor, which is antagonized by ketamine, has been implicated in the etiology of schizophrenia, the so-called *NMDA receptor hy-*

pofunction model. Ketamine has been used as a neuropharmacological probe to test this hypothesis, with the idea that ketamine users may look like they have schizophrenia or that acute administration of ketamine may make a normal person look schizophrenic for a while. This highly investigated topic is covered in more detail in Chapter 5.

Neurologic Effects of Ketamine Use

One of the biggest questions regarding ketamine basic science research is whether it causes "brain damage." This topic is so important that it is covered in some detail in Chapter 9, "Is Ketamine a Neuroprotectant or a Neurotoxin?" Exciting developments in biological psychiatry over the past half century have involved new neuroimaging techniques that allow visualization of brain structure and function. First there was CT scanning (computed tomography), then structural MRI (magnetic resonance imaging), then PET (positron emission tomography) and SPECT (single-photon emission computed tomography), and in more recent decades, fMRI (functional MRI) and MRS (magnetic resonance spectroscopy).

A discussion of each of these is beyond the scope of this book (and indeed, this author!), but the main point is that many investigators have put the ketamine challenge paradigm to good use, recruiting volunteers for one or more of these scans. Here, we discuss the research dedicated to performing brain scans on people who use ketamine chronically from a recreational standpoint to see if there is evidence of brain damage.

Chan et al. (2012) performed fMRI on three chronic ketamine users and found evidence of impaired cerebellar function, a finding that is difficult to interpret. Wang et al. (2013) studied 21 ketamine addicts (duration of use 0.5–12 years). They performed head MRI and found, after 2–4 years of use, a variety of degenerative lesions in various cortical and subcortical regions. Early lesions seemed to be minute patches that progressed to large sites of abnormality and atrophy by 4 years of regular use. Stone et al. (2014) performed MRS (similar to MRI, but results are not as definitive in terms of what constitutes an abnormality) on 15 chronic ketamine users and 13 non-ketamine polydrug-using controls. Of the 15 separate points of comparison between the two groups on the scan, only one differed: the *N*-acetyl aspartate/creatinine ratio in the thalamus was lower in the ketamine group, which supposedly makes them similar to people with schizophrenia. The meaning of this is obscure, however, especially in terms of any implications for day-to-day function.

Liao et al. (2011) analyzed MRI scan data from 41 people dependent on ketamine and 44 non-drug-using controls. The left superior frontal gyrus and right middle frontal gyrus were both smaller in the ketamine group, the differences correlating with duration of use and estimated lifetime ketamine consumption. Those in the ketamine group were in their mid-20s with about 3.5 years of ketamine use, but also a lot of other drug use as well, confounding the data. Again, it is difficult to find a ketamine-only group of drug users.

Liao et al. (2012) also compared fMRI scans between the two groups. Right anterior cingulate cortex and left precentral gyrus differences in activity were found, the meaning of which is, again, obscure. Of note, the authors did not mention time since last ketamine use, so the results may be acute or chronic effects of ketamine. The same groups were also studied with diffusion tensor imaging (DTI), a type of MRI scan (Liao et al. 2010). The authors found bilateral white matter abnormalities in the left frontal lobes and left temporoparietal lobes of the ketamine users, the severity of which directly correlated with degree of ketamine use. The subjects were in their mid-20s with a mean of 41 months of ketamine use. As with other studies of a newer imaging technology that is not available for clinical use, DTI results do not translate into confident statements about whether actual neurological damage was caused by ketamine, or whether the changes are permanent.

Narendran et al. (2005) conducted PET scans in 14 recreational ketamine users. Dopamine receptor binding was upregulated, in a weekly dose–dependent manner, in the dorsolateral prefrontal cortex of the ketamine users in comparison to non-drug-using controls, indicating that chronic use of ketamine may deplete dopamine stores prefrontally. This in turn may be the neurobiological basis of the inhibiting effect of chronic ketamine use on working memory and executive function. Interestingly, however, dopamine binding did not correlate with performance on a working memory task, nor did performance on that task separate the ketamine users from the non-users, thus rendering the meaning of the PET scan data somewhat doubtful.

Roberts et al. (2014) performed both MRI and DTI in 16 chronic ketamine users and 16 nonketamine polydrug users and found abnormal white matter microstructural changes in the right hemisphere of the ketamine users. As with the other modern neuroimaging technologies, the functional meaning of this is not known. The degree of dissociative symptoms did correlate with differences in connectivity between the right caudate and prefrontal cortex, perhaps giving some neurophysiologic credence to ketamine's being called a "dissociative" drug.

Taken as a whole, it is difficult to reach specific conclusions about the effect of chronic ketamine use on brain morphology or function as assessed via these scanning techniques. Almost all the studies found something out of the ordinary in chronic ketamine users, so the results certainly do seem cautionary.

Lower Urinary Tract Effects of Recreational Ketamine Use

With most drugs of abuse, organ damage is feared with chronic use. Well-known examples are cirrhosis of the liver with alcohol and cancer of the lung with cigarettes. Completely unexpected has been the destruction of the lower urinary tract, specifically the urinary bladder, with long-term ketamine use. This effect was not predicted by anybody before the first reports appeared in 2007. Since then, however, the stark reality of this dreadful complication of ketamine use has become clear.

The condition caused by chronic ketamine use is termed *ulcerative cystitis*: inflammation of the inner lining of the urinary bladder. It appears that ketamine and its metabolites, as they collect in the bladder along with urine, cause direct toxic inflammation of the bladder lining, which in early stages presents with painful urination (*dysuria*), frequent urination, and blood in the urine (*hematuria*). If the ketamine use ceases, this is reversible. With continued use, however, the inflammation turns into scarring, and the bladder loses its ability to stretch; affected people need to urinate almost constantly. In addition, urination involves severe pain. Sadly, the scarring is irreversible. Some cases progress to frank renal failure. In the Asian countries where this complication has been seen the most, surgeries have been developed in which prosthetic bladders are fashioned from colonic tissue. There are now numerous case series from a variety of countries documenting the occurrence of ketamine-induced ulcerative cystitis. A few are reviewed here.

The first reports were those of Shahani et al. (2007) from Toronto, Canada, who described nine young people, all chronic ketamine users, who presented to a urological service with complaints of urinary urgency, frequency, dysuria, and hematuria. Computed tomography scans showed small, thickened bladders with evidence of inflammation. Cystoscopy (inserting a video tube directly into the bladder to visualize the lining or epithelium) showed inflamed, denuded urinary epithelium (urothelium). Biopsy confirmed the inflammation. Abstinence and application of pentosan polysulfate to help the lining of the bladder heal provided some improvement in the symptoms.

Chu et al. (2007) in China described 10 chronic ketamine users with lower urinary tract symptoms. They presented with urgency, frequency, dysuria, and hematuria and had, on urological workup, small, contracted non-expansile bladders. Seven had hydronephrosis, markedly abnormal and rare in a young population (mean age mid-20s).

Yee et al. (2015) followed a large cohort of 463 patients with ketamine cystitis from a urology clinic in Hong Kong between 2011 and 2014, 319 of whom returned for follow-up at a later time. The patients were generally in their mid-20s with a mean duration of ketamine use of 80 months. Clearly, abstinence from ketamine was the number one predictor of improvement in symptoms. A few patients had intravesical (inside the bladder) hyaluronic acid or augmentation enterocystoplasty, which was third-line treatment. First-line treatment consisted of non-opiate drugs such as non-steroidal anti-inflammatory agents, anticholinergics to reduce spasm, acetaminophen, or phenazopyridine, and second-line treatment consisted of opiates for pain.

Wu et al. (2016) studied 81 patients with ketamine cystitis from 2008 to 2014. They divided this syndrome into three stages: Stage I consisted of initial inflammation of the bladder lining; Stage II consisted of initial bladder fibrosis (scarring); and Stage III consisted of end-stage bladder fibrosis with bladder contracture. Generally, Stage I was treated with analgesic medications and imploring the patients to stop using ketamine. Stage II patients were given hydrodistension, which involves attempts to install a catheter in the bladder and inject water to try and expand it. Stage III patients were treated with reconstructive surgery. Ureteral wall thickening and dilatation occurred in Stage III, as did hydronephrosis and hydroureter. Renal and liver function tests in the blood were also abnormal at this stage, indicating (along with the other stigmata of Stage III) what a severe and disabling condition it is. Mean duration of ketamine abuse in this sample of 81 patients was 2.9, 3.4, and 4.8 years, respectively, in stages I, II, and III. Mean ages were in the mid-20s, which is rather tragic. Numerous other, similar case series exist of ketamine-associated ulcerative cystitis. This syndrome is so distinct that if a person is diagnosed with ulcerative cystitis, the cause can almost definitely be ascribed to ketamine.

These case series involved recreational ketamine users; it is still an open question whether medically prescribed ketamine regimens, especially those administered over time, might also be associated with ketamine-induced ulcerative cystitis. The two conditions for which ketamine is given that meet these criteria are chronic pain syndromes (discussed in Chapter 6) and psychiatric depression (discussed in Chapter 7). As of this writing, there are no reports in the psychiatric literature reporting ketamine cystitis in depressed patients given ketamine, but it is early days. The ketamine for chronic pain literature contains a few reports of ketamine cystitis (Grégoire et al. 2008; Shahzad et al. 2012; Storr and Quibell 2009).

The importance of the daily oral route of administration should be mentioned here, because with that mode of ketamine consumption, constant levels of ketamine and its metabolites are certain to collect in the urine, contacting and irritating the bladder lining. Intermittent IV ketamine administration, theoretically, would be less likely to cause this syndrome. Thus, any clinician advocating daily oral ketamine administration for either chronic pain or depression should be aware of this risk.

Gastrointestinal Tract Complications of Recreational Ketamine Use

Some time ago, Jansen (1990) described so-called K-cramps, consisting of acute abdominal pain in ketamine users. However, more specific information on gastrointestinal effects of ketamine did not emerge until later. In sum, chronic ketamine use seems to be associated with elevated liver enzymes, bile duct dilatation, and gastritis in some case series (e.g., Liu et al. 2017; Lo et al. 2011; Wong et al. 2014; Yu et al. 2014).

When a drug is inhaled into the nose, nasopharyngeal blood vessels absorb it, but the capacity is not unlimited. With heavy ketamine inhalation, much of the drug bypasses the nasopharyngeal blood vessels, courses down the posterior oropharynx, and is swallowed into the gut. Thus, the swallowed ketamine can directly irritate the stomach lining and cause painful inflammation (gastritis). It is not known if IV or intramuscular ketamine use causes K-cramps; such routes of administration bypass the stomach.

Conclusions

There is no doubt that ketamine is a dangerous substance when used recreationally, without supervision and without monitoring its addictive potential and negative effects. As we continue to explore this molecule's history and future, we turn next to its composition and pharmacological characteristics.

Chapter 4

Pharmacology of Ketamine

- Ketamine has two molecular forms, or enantiomers: esketamine and arketamine.
- Several metabolites of ketamine may be neuropharmacologically active.
- The most potent CNS action of ketamine is uncompetitive blockade of NMDA receptors.

Thus far, this book has followed a chronology of developments in the literature on ketamine. We started with some chemical history leading to PCP, reviewed how ketamine was discovered in the search for an alternative to that drug and was developed as an anesthetic, and then proceeded to the recreational use of ketamine starting in roughly 1970. Before we investigate the use of ketamine as a neuropharmacological probe to study the psychotic process, the use of ketamine for chronic pain syndromes, and the use of ketamine to treat depression and other psychiatric conditions, we review its pharmacology.

Clinical pharmacology is the study of drugs and their effects in humans; animal data are often collected to aid in that process. Pharmacology is generally divided into two parts: pharmacokinetics and pharmacodynamics. Put simply, *pharmacokinetics* refers to what the body does with the drug, and *pharmacodynamics* refers to what the drug does to the body. Regarding the former, we want to know how the body goes about metabolizing and eliminating the drug; regarding the latter, we want to know what makes a drug therapeutic—the mechanism of action—so that we can better understand the illness in question and continue the search for ever-better treatments. First we review the chemistry of ketamine.

Chemistry

Synthesis

Unlike many other psychedelic drugs, nature does not make ketamine for us—nor anything that even closely resembles ketamine (at least discovered so far). As the reader may recall, chemist Calvin Stevens, working as a consultant for Parke-Davis, first synthesized ketamine in 1962 (Stevens 1964). That process is illustrated in Figure 4–1.

To start with, two main reagents are needed: 2-chlorobenzyl-nitrile and cyclopentyl magnesium bromide. Cyclopentyl magnesium bromide can also be referred to as cyclopentyl Grignard: organic moieties attached to metallic halides (in this case, magnesium bromide attached to a cyclopentyl group) constitute a Grignard reagent. The resulting molecule is then brominated (i.e., steeped in liquid bromine). Next, methylamine is added to result in an imine.

It is customary for chemists to refer to an imine modified from a ketone as a *ketimine* (note the spelling). This ketimine is heated carefully and morphs into the molecule of interest here, *ketamine*. Along the way, chemical reactions need to take place in various organic solvents and in certain conditions of temperature and pH; the skilled chemist extracts the chemical of interest from byproducts along the way. All this makes ketamine synthesis very difficult and unlikely to be achieved by kitchen chemists as are other drugs of abuse (such as methamphetamine and PCP). This drug is almost always synthesized industrially in specially equipped factories.

Chemistry Nomenclature

Ketamine, like a lot of other organic chemicals, is not a unitary molecule. It comes in two forms with identical sets of atoms and the same chemical formula, but not in the same configuration. Herein we introduce the concept of *chirality* (pronounced "ky-RAL-i-tee"). Imagine a set of hands, a right hand and a left hand. They are mirror images of one another but are not superimposable. Organic chemicals, often pictured as two-dimensional stick drawings, as in the figures here, are really three-dimensional. Sometimes, especially with regard to carbon atoms in ring formations, two moieties bonded to that carbon can be going in two directions (say, south and north). Then in another form, imagine the same two moieties have switched places: the formerly northward-going one now goes south, and the formerly southward-going one now goes north. Visualizing this, we realize that these two forms of the molecule are mirror images

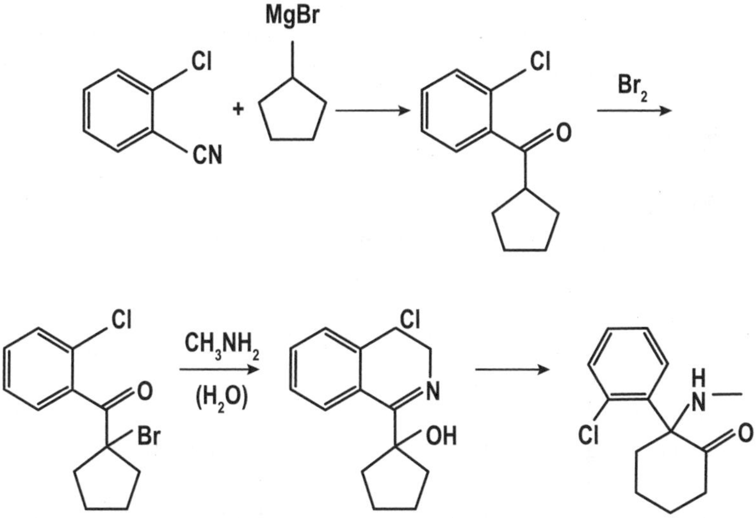

FIGURE 4–1. The process to synthesize ketamine

of one another. The phenomenon of a carbon atom having two attached moieties, each capable of going in either of two directions, is called *chirality*, and the carbon atom in question is referred to as a *chiral center*.

In ketamine, the carbon atom bonded to the methylamino and chlorophenyl groups is a chiral center: in one form, the methylamino points up (figuratively speaking, out of the paper or screen toward the reader), while the chlorophenyl group points down (away from the reader). In the other form of ketamine, this arrangement is reversed. When ketamine is synthesized in the usual way as described above, the resulting molecules are half in one configuration, half in the other (*racemic*, pronounced "ray-SEE-mik").

This matters because the two molecular forms, called *enantiomers*, do not affect the human body identically. They do not bind to neuroreceptors with the same binding affinities. If the receptors were gloves—right- or left-handed—the two enantiomers of ketamine would be right and left hands. A left-handed ketamine molecule fits best into a left-handed receptor and not very well into a right-handed receptor, and vice versa. Now let's suppose that all types of a given receptor in the brain are left-handed: thus only left-handed ketamine binds well and has the resultant neurophysiologic actions. Such is the case with *N*-methyl-D-aspartate (NMDA) receptors (discussed in more detail later): one enantiomer of ketamine binds very tightly to this receptor, but the other binds only weakly.

This analogy of the two enantiomers as right or left extends to their nomenclature. Several structures in chemistry involve Latin words for left and right, and confusingly, there are multiple pairs of terms used. In Latin, the directional terms for left and right are *sinister* and *dexter*. (Given the historical superstition about left-handedness being evil, the words took on more value-oriented connotations over time.) Latin has two more terms roughly meaning left and right: *laevus* ("awkward" or "wrong") and *rectus* ("straight" or "correct").

When an organic compound such as ketamine has a chiral carbon atom, one of the two enantiomers is referred to as rectus (or R) and the other as sinistral (or S). Thus, we have (R)-ketamine and (S)-ketamine. For ease of communication, these two enantiomers are commonly spelled *arketamine* and *esketamine*. (In this book, when *ketamine* is used without specification of enantiomer, the reader can assume it is racemic ketamine.)

When ketamine is administered to a patient, the usual form of it is called racemic, meaning that half the ketamine molecules are the (R)-ketamine and the other half are (S)-ketamine enantiomers. However, because chemists are a clever lot, it is possible to take a batch of racemic ketamine and split it into batches of pure (R) and pure (S) forms, or even to synthesize batches of pure enantiomers de novo. (Indeed, esketamine has been commercially available in some European countries for decades and is even approved now in intranasal form for the treatment of major depression in the United States and the European Union. More on that in Chapter 7.)

Another chemical custom the reader may run into in the ketamine literature is *optical rotation*, specified by the + (plus) or – (minus) sign placed in front of the word. This refers to which direction that light is rotated if it shines straight through the molecule. If a light source is converted into a two-dimensional sliver (essentially a plane of light) and shone on a sample of a molecule, a special device can detect that as it passes through the molecule, the perpendicular plane of light is rotated somewhat. If the rotation, from the observer's standpoint, is to the right (clockwise), then the sample of molecule is called *dextrorotatory* (from Latin *dexter*) or +. If the rotation is to the left (counterclockwise), then it is said to be *levorotatory* (from Latin *laevus*) or –. This property (two forms of a molecule rotating plane polarized light in opposite directions) is called *optical isomerism*, and the two forms are called *optical isomers* of one another.

In the case of the ketamine enantiomers, (S)-ketamine is dextrorotatory and (R)-ketamine is levorotatory. Thus, occasionally, they are spelled S(+)-ketamine and R(–)-ketamine in the literature, but this will not be used further in this book.

There is one more chemical nomenclature issue. This refers to specifying the *molecular configuration* of amino acids. Aspartic acid, or aspartate, is relevant to the NMDA receptor. Amino acids can come in two configurations prefixed with either D (from *dexter*) or L (from *laevus*), in small capitals. The NMDA receptor binds strongly to *N*-methyl-D-aspartate and not *N*-methyl-L-aspartate.

Pharmacokinetics

The processing and elimination of drugs by the body is called pharmacokinetics (*pharmaco* meaning drug, *kinetics* meaning movement). This is divided into four phases: absorption, distribution, metabolism, and excretion. The fundamental procedure for understanding the pharmacokinetics of a particular drug is to administer doses and then measure concentrations of the drug and its metabolites in the bloodstream, urine, and stool, as well as organs such as liver and kidneys. It is much more difficult to measure how much of an administered dose makes its way to the brain, as there is no easy way to sample brain tissue in a living person. Animal studies are crucial to help understand organ distribution of administered drugs.

Absorption

Absorption refers to the transfer of the drug from outside the body into the vascular space (systemic circulation). For intravenous (IV) administration, absorption is taken to be immediate. For other routes of administration, absorption varies. Typical routes in addition to intravenous include oral, sublingual (drug placed under the tongue and absorbed through vasculature located there), intranasal (i.e., snorting, in which case the drug is absorbed through the posterior nasopharyngeal blood vessels), intramuscular (IM), subcutaneous, and other rare and somewhat exotic routes that do not pertain to ketamine. Of all these, the oral route is typically associated with the slowest absorption into the vascular space.

An important aspect of drug absorption is the concept of bioavailability. This refers to the percentage of an administered dose that makes its way to the general circulation. The bioavailability of the intravenous route for any drug is taken to be 100%—that is, all of a dose injected into a vein is in the circulation. For the oral route, some of a dose that is swallowed does not get absorbed and simply passes unchanged through the gastrointestinal tract. Additionally, that portion of an orally administered dose that is absorbed into the small intestines goes first to the liver, where *first-pass metabolism* takes place, limiting the amount of the administered drug that makes its way to the general circulation. First-pass metabolism may not reduce the drug's effectiveness if the metabolite of that drug is also pharmacologically active. For the nasal route, not all of a dose may be absorbed through the nasopharyngeal vasculature and may be either sneezed out or swallowed.

One study showed for ketamine that the IM route was associated with 93% bioavailability, and the oral route, a paltry 17% (Clements et al. 1982). Another study showed that both subcutaneous and IM routes were associated with 66% bioavailability (Abuhelwa et al. 2022). The nasal route for ketamine, which has become quite important of late with the advancement of an intranasal preparation of esketamine for major depression (Spravato), is associated with ~50%–55% bioavailability (Perez-Ruixo et al. 2021). Thus, for ketamine, if the majority of an administered dose is to make its way to systemic circulation, the IV route is best. Further, the bioavailability of the IV route will always be 100%, assuming proper placement of the IV catheter. However, with the other routes, one can expect interindividual variability in bioavailability depending on body composition. For example, a person with small muscle mass may not yield the same blood levels by the same IM route as a person with larger muscle mass. Similarly, a person's body fat percentage influences gluteal IM dosing. One can also assume that variation in inhalational technique influences absorption and that subcutaneous absorption varies from person to person. For all these reasons, the IV route is preferred to guarantee predictable, reliable absorption of the entirety of a ketamine dose.

Distribution

After absorption of a drug into systemic circulation, the next pharmacokinetic step is *distribution* from the vascular space to the various organs of the body. This is difficult to assess in living humans; usually, scientists must extrapolate from animal studies. Research has shown that once a drug gets into the vascular space, it rapidly transfers to highly perfused organs (those intimately involved in circulation) such as the brain, heart, and lungs. Such is true for ketamine and other drugs that are highly lipid soluble, as water-soluble compounds do not pass through the blood–brain barrier. Once the drug settles into these highly perfused organs, it starts to distribute back out into the vasculature again, and over time, it more slowly makes its way into less vascularized bodily spaces such as muscle, bone, and fat. One can conceptualize for each organ a back-and-forth action of the drug: some drug makes its way eventually into that organ but then goes back into the vasculature (called *redistribution*), where it courses through the body and may make its way back into the organ for a time. As drug and drug metabolites leave the body, eventually the drug leaves all these organs as well. Drugs like ketamine are said to follow *two-compartment kinetics*. Compartment 1 is the blood vessels plus the highly vascularized organs that rapidly get high levels of the drug, and Compartment 2 is the less-perfused organs such as bone, muscle, and fat that get levels of the drug slowly.

Zanos et al. (2018) found that peak blood levels of IM-administered ketamine occur 5–30 minutes after the shot. With oral administration, the peak ketamine levels occur in 20–120 minutes.

One factor influencing the distribution of a drug in the body is the degree of protein binding in the blood. Blood proteins can bind to some drugs to different degrees—the greater the protein binding of a given drug in the blood, the less the tissue distribution, as the drug gets spent in the bloodstream. Hijazi and Boulieu (2002) studied the protein binding of ketamine, norketamine, and another metabolite called dehydronorketamine (DHNK) and found protein binding percentages of 60%, 50%, and 69%, respectively, which is moderate protein binding of ketamine and metabolites, thus explaining at least in part the wide tissue distribution of this drug. Ketamine also makes its way to hair. Leung et al. (2016), working in Hong Kong looking for methods of detecting surreptitious ketamine use, analyzed hair samples from drug users at treatment centers. Among 1,371 samples, 977 were positive for ketamine and norketamine. The minimal limit of detection for both compounds was 20 pg/mg of hair.

Metabolism

Many drugs, ketamine being one of them, are highly soluble by fats (lipids) and not easily excreted by the body. The liver contains collections of enzyme complexes called *microsomes* that chemically alter drugs to be more water soluble and thus more easily excreted into the urine and bile. In particular, the *cytochrome P450* (CYP450) enzymes metabolize many commonly used drugs such as ketamine. Portmann et al. (2010) found that *N*-demethylation of ketamine to norketamine involved multiple cytochromes: 3A4, 2C19, 2B6, 2A6, 2D6, 2C9, 3A4, and 2B6 being the major ones. Hydroxylation of norketamine to the OH-NKs was achieved with CYPs 2B6 and 2A6.

These altered versions of the drug are called *metabolites*. Another hepatic mechanism of rendering drug products water soluble enough for excretion is called *conjugation*, whereby either the parent drug or one of its metabolites is connected to a chemical known as glucuronide, with the resulting complex easily excreted in the urine.

Ketamine has several metabolites, and some of them undergo glucuronide conjugation. The first metabolic pathway of ketamine is demethylation to *norketamine* (see Figure 4–2). It is essentially ketamine without the methyl group (*demethylation* is a common metabolic step of many drugs). Norketamine in turn undergoes *hydroxylation*, which is the addition of a hydroxyl group (–OH) to a carbon atom, which further increases the water solubility of a compound and thus its excretability. The hydroxyl group can be added to the 4-, 5-, or 6-carbon atom of the cyclohexanone ring of the norketamine molecule. These

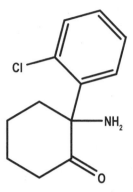

FIGURE 4–2. The molecular structure of norketamine

hydroxynorketamines in turn undergo glucuronide conjugation and are excreted in the urine mostly. Studies have shown that ~91% of a dose of ketamine ultimately is excreted in the urine, with most of that being in the form of hydroxynorketamines. Norketamine can also undergo metabolism to *dehydronorketamine*, or DHNK. Finally, a small amount of ketamine itself is hydroxylated to *hydroxyketamine*, which is further demethylated to hydroxynorketamines. A small percentage of a dose of ketamine is recovered in the urine as ketamine itself or norketamine, but the vast majority is hydroxynorketamines and DHNK. See Figures 4–3, 4–4, 4–5, and 4–6 for molecular structures of the hydroxynorketamines and dehydronorketamine.

Prepared for the situation to get more complicated? Recall the concept of *chirality*, whereby two moieties bonded to a carbon atom can occur in two different orientations. When a cyclohexanone carbon atom (number 4, 5, or 6) is hydroxylated, it is rendered chiral, with resultant (S) and (R) enantiomers possible. Thus, 4-hydroxynorketamine (or 5- or 6-) can be either (S) or (R) at the 4 position (in addition to the two possibilities at the number 2 position, as discussed previously). For hydroxynorketamines, then, there are 2 × 2 × 2 × 2 (for 4, 5, and 6 as well as 2 carbon atoms) = 16 possible combinations. The customary nomenclature for reporting the enantiomers where two carbon atoms have chirality is to report the number of the carbon atom first, then R or S, and then the next chiral carbon atom number and its associated R or S isoform. Thus, a hydroxynorketamine metabolite that is in the R isoform at the number 2 carbon atom and the S isoform at the number 6 carbon atom would be described as (2R,6S)-hydroxynorketamine. (Imagine all the various combinations possible.)

This issue is important, as one of the hot theories is that (2R,6R)-hydroxynorketamine may be the metabolite responsible for ketamine's antidepressant action (which is elaborated in Chapter 7). The existence of

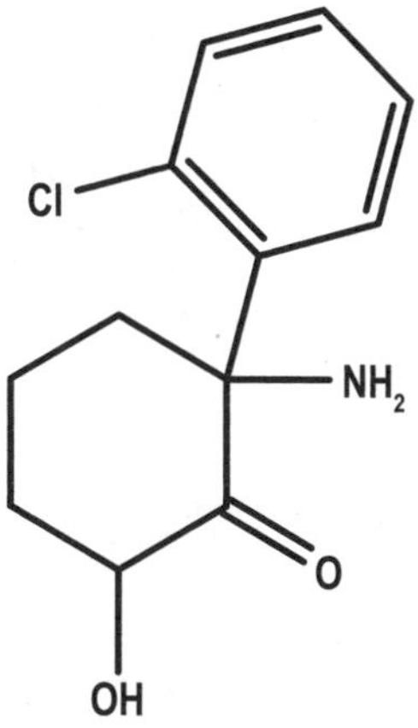

FIGURE 4–3. The molecular structure of 6-hydroxynorketamine

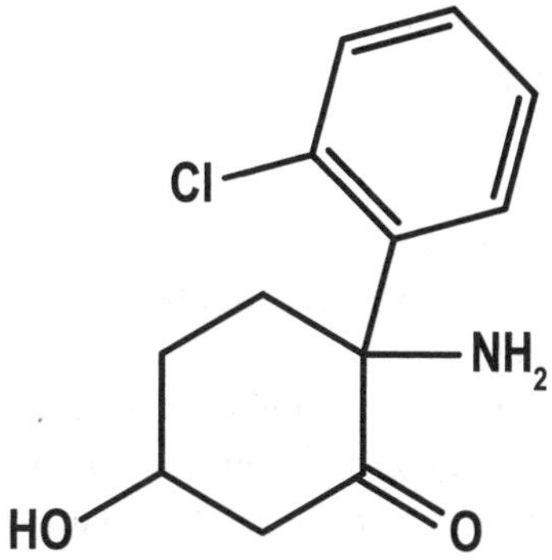

FIGURE 4–4. The molecular structure of 5-hydroxynorketamine

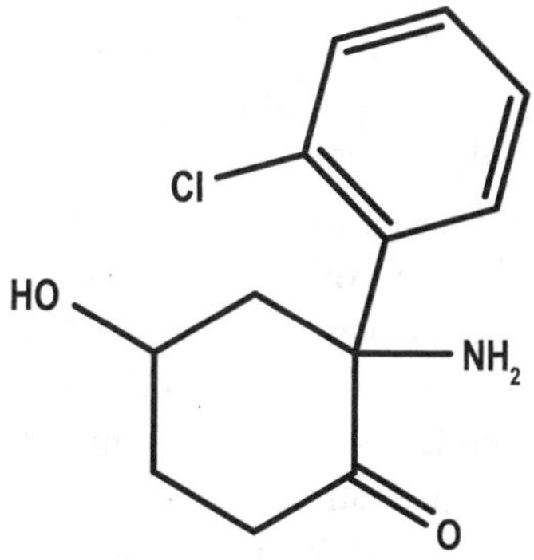

FIGURE 4–5. The molecular structure of 4-hydroxynorketamine

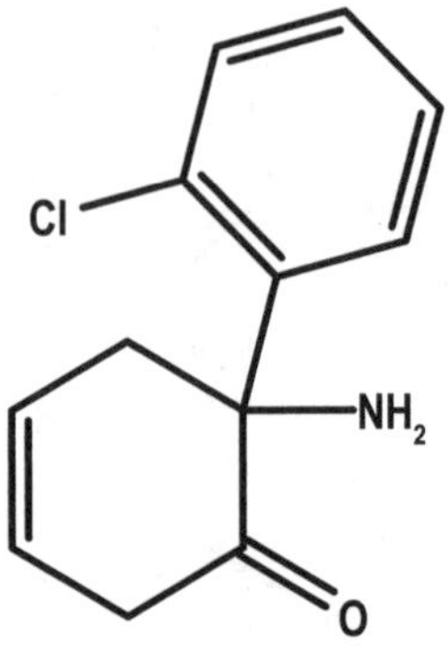

FIGURE 4–6.   The molecular structure of dehydronorketamine

these metabolites in humans exposed to ketamine was confirmed by Turfus et al. (2009), who exposed ketamine to pooled human liver microsomes (enzymes that metabolize drugs) and identified metabolites via liquid chromatography/tandem mass spectrometry. The hydroxyl group can be attached to the 4-, 5-, or 6-carbon atom on the cyclohexanone ring or, in much lesser concentrations, to the phenyl ring (in which case the resultant compound is referred to as a phenol). That study, the most comprehensive analysis of ketamine metabolites to date, was the first to identify hydroxylated phenolic ketamine metabolites, which were found not only in the microsomal preparations but in the urine of volunteers given ketamine.

Zarate et al. (2012b) measured serial ketamine, norketamine, hydroxyketamine, hydroxynorketamine, and dehydronorketamine levels for ~4 hours after an infusion of 0.5 mg/kg administered over 40 minutes as part of a treatment trial for major depressive disorder and bipolar depression. The major metabolite, 230 minutes post-infusion, was norketamine in 46 of 66 patients, dehydronorketamine in 9 patients, and 6-hydroxynorketamine in 11. Other hydroxynorketamines (namely, 4- and 5-) were found in very small quantities, indicating that 6-hydroxynorketamine is the major hydroxylated metabolite. Of note, 6-hydroxyketamine was detected in tiny amounts. It appears that as soon as ketamine is hydroxylated, it is quickly N-demethylated to hydroxynorketamine.

Mion and Villevieille (2013) provided a nice description of the pharmacokinetics of norketamine: it appears in blood ~2–3 minutes after an IV injection of ketamine, blood levels peak at ~30 minutes, and it is less potent as an analgesic and anesthetic than ketamine. Like ketamine, it comes in (R) and (S) enantiomers. Hydroxynorketamines are largely conjugated to glucuronic acid, which renders them even more water soluble and easy to excrete in the urine. Zanos et al. (2018) confirmed that hydroxyketamine is barely detectable in human serum following ketamine administration. It appears that almost as soon as it is formed, by direct hydroxylation of ketamine, it undergoes *N*-demethylation to hydroxynorketamine.

In the modern ketamine literature, there is little enthusiasm for hydroxyketamines as important contributors to neuropharmacological effects owing to its transient existence and rapid transformation. The metabolic pathway for transformation of ketamine to hydroxyketamine is minor. The majority of ketamine is metabolized to norketamine, and from there to either DHNK or hydroxynorketamines. DHNK is formed mostly from metabolism of norketamine by an organic chemistry reaction called *dehydrogenation*. Zanos et al. (2018), reviewing their studies, indicated that DHNK does not penetrate the blood–brain barrier (thus does not enter the brain). For that reason, it is not currently a molecule of interest in the neuropharmacological actions of ketamine. Several studies have shown, however, that it is the longest-lasting metabolite in the urine, being detected up to several days after ketamine administration, long after other metabolites are gone. Parkin et al. (2008) used ultra-high-pressure liquid chromatography/tandem mass spectrometry (the best technology available for drug detection) to study serial urine samples of six volunteers given a single 50-mg oral ketamine dose. Ketamine could be detected in the urine for 5 days, norketamine for 6 days, and DHNK for 10 days, indicating the utility of DHNK for detecting ketamine use from urine. Thus, in settings where detection of surreptitious ketamine use is needed, such as law enforcement, DHNK is of high interest. Also note that, given that DHNK stays in the urine for so long, it might contribute to ketamine-associated ulcerative cystitis.

A final note on metabolism critical for understanding the differential pharmacodynamics of ketamine enantiomers and their metabolites is that for a molecule of esketamine, meaning that the chiral configuration at the number 2 carbon atom on the cyclohexanone ring is in the (S) form, the metabolites are also in the (S) form at the number 2 carbon atom. (Similarly, metabolites of arketamine will all be in the (R) form at the number 2 carbon atom.) Thus, when discussing (2R,6R)-hydroxynorketamine as a possible antidepressant compound, one must understand that it emanates only from arketamine as the parent compound. If one administers a person esketamine, there will be no metabolites that are in the 2R configuration.

Elimination (Excretion)

Most of an administered dose of ketamine is accounted for by renal (kidney) excretion, with a small percentage excreted in the stool. The latter occurs via collection of some metabolites in small ducts in the liver that ultimately collect in a large duct that leads to the gall bladder, which over time expands (much like the urinary bladder does with urine) and finally emits its contents into another duct leading to the intestines, and then to the stool.

Data indicate that ~80% of an administered ketamine dose is ultimately accounted for by conjugated hydroxy metabolites (mostly hydroxynorketamines) in the urine. About 2% each of unchanged ketamine and norketamine are also found in the urine. The rest, ~16%, is DHNK in the urine. A very tiny fraction of ketamine dosing is ultimately found in the stool.

The *half-life* of a drug refers to the amount of time for half of it to dissipate; in general, a phase takes about four to five half-lives to complete. In pharmacodynamics of a substance such as ketamine, there are three half-lives: distribution, redistribution, and elimination. After IV administration, in the distribution phase, ketamine disburses through the vascular bed and highly vascularized organs quite quickly. The half-life of this phase is less than a minute (Mion and Villevieille 2013). During the redistribution phase, ketamine's half-life is 10–15 minutes, and the redistribution phase lasts about 45 minutes (U.S. Food and Drug Administration 2024), at the end of which an anesthetized patient will begin to awaken as the drug redistributes out of the brain. During the last phase, ketamine is metabolized into its metabolites, which are then excreted mostly into the urine and a bit into the gastrointestinal tract. The half-life of the elimination phase is 2–3 hours (Mion and Villevieille 2013); thus, for ketamine, complete elimination takes place in about 8–15 hours. Please note that these half-lives refer to the parent compound, ketamine, and not to the metabolites, which take longer to be excreted.

Ketamine Blood Levels

Zanos et al. (2018) reported that blood levels of ketamine needed to induce anesthesia (by way of comparison to other clinical effects) are 1,200–2,400 ng/mL. In that group's studies of ketamine for depression, 0.5 mg/kg was administered over 40 minutes. At peak blood levels, just after completion of the infusion, levels of ketamine were ~185 ng/mL. Mion and Villevieille (2013) noted that ketamine levels upon awakening from anesthesia are in the range of 600–1,100 ng/mL.

Pharmacodynamics

Whereas the pharmacokinetics of ketamine are usually fairly easy to study and straightforward to interpret, ketamine pharmacodynamics are quite complicated.

As indicated earlier, pharmacodynamics refers to what the drug does to the body. What is typically of interest here is the mechanism of action of a drug. Because ketamine has so many noted clinically detectable effects, this task is even more difficult. What is the mechanism of ketamine's anesthetic effect? Analgesic effect? Antidepressant effect? Anti–status epilepticus effect? Psychotomimetic effect? Anti-addictive effect? And how on earth must one deduce the neuromechanistic basis of ketamine's ability to make some people believe they go to outer space and meet with God?

Furthermore, most drugs have biological effects beyond those involved in therapeutic effects. This is especially true of neuroactive agents. Just because a laboratory study reveals that ketamine does something to a rodent brain, for example, does not mean that the same effect happens in humans—or if it does, that it pertains to any outcome measure of interest. It may be an extraneous finding. The brain is inordinately complex, with levels of analysis starting at the genetic and molecular levels, proceeding up to the cellular level, further to the circuitry level, and then on to outward manifestations of the nervous system such as motor function, sensory function, autonomic function, and mental functions such as thought, behavior, and affect. This way of looking at neuroscience studies phenomena at the levels of molecules → cells → circuits → behavior. Studying the pharmacodynamics of neuroactive agents is also difficult because the technology for studying the intact human brain—in real time, safely, and at all these levels—is not currently possible. The field of neuropharmacology relies quite heavily on the study of animal brains. With ketamine, the study of its neuropharmacological actions at the molecular and cellular levels relies on thousands of studies in mice and rats. In this section, I highlight a few important studies of the pharmacological actions of interest in ketamine, rather than attempt an exhaustive review.

Consider neuropharmacological study of drugs at the four levels mentioned: molecular, cellular, circuit, and behavioral (for convenience, *behavioral* describes all clinical manifestations including thought, behavior, affect, consciousness, perception, and cognition). When a drug enters the brain, it first binds to some type of binding site—a receptor, transporter, or other molecular complex. Next, a cascade of molecular and intracellular events take place, ultimately leading to changes in the structure or function of the cell (termed *neuroplasticity*). This in turn leads to functional changes in the circuitry of the brain, as all cell groupings communicate with other cell groupings; finally, this manifests outwardly as changes in thought, behavior, and affect. The key word here is *cascade*. An initial receptor occupancy of a drug in the brain is the beginning, not the end, of its mechanism of action. To say "ketamine is an NMDA receptor inhibitor" may be accurate, but that is only the first step in a complex cascade. Probably there are no drugs in all of neuropharmacology for which the entire cascade of steps from binding to behavior is known—certainly not ketamine's.

NMDA Receptor–Based Pharmacodynamic Effects of Ketamine

Recall that the first thing that ketamine does across the blood–brain barrier at the brain or spinal cord is to bind to something. By far the most important binding site is the NMDA (*N*-methyl-D-aspartate) receptor. This site is also called the PCP receptor, because that was the first ligand noted to bind there. Hashimoto (2017) conducted a thorough review of what NMDA receptors look like and how they function. Suffice to say that NMDA receptors are located throughout the brain and are involved in many processes such as consciousness, perception, learning, memory, and emotion. It is no surprise that a ligand that alters their function has profound effects on all these things.

NMDA receptors are located postsynaptically on neuronal membranes. Glutamate released by the presynaptic neuron is the ligand for NMDA receptors. These receptors are *tetrameric*, meaning they have four components. They are also *transmembranous*, meaning they have parts located extracellularly, intramembranously, and intracellularly. There is a central channel in each NMDA receptor through which ions such as calcium, sodium, and potassium flow. Thus, these receptors are termed *ligand-gated ion channels*: a ligand (glutamate, as well as co-agonists glycine or D-serine) binds to them and causes them to allow calcium and sodium ions to flow into the cell and potassium ions to flow out of the cell, thus depolarizing the membrane, as glutamate is an excitatory neurotransmitter. In the NMDA receptor, magnesium ions sit on the ion channel leading into the cell, blocking the flow of the calcium, sodium, and potassium as described above. When the cell membrane is electrically depolarized by one of a variety of factors, magnesium pops off the channel, leaving it open and making it easier for the ions to flow when glutamate and a co-agonist sit on their respective binding sites. Ketamine and PCP bind to a site inside the ion channel and can get there only when the magnesium ion has been extricated by membrane depolarization. Further, ketamine and PCP block the ion channel only when glutamate and one of the two co-agonists are occupying their (extracellular) receptor sites on the NMDA receptor. Thus, ketamine and PCP are voltage- and use-dependent NMDA receptor blockers: they only block the receptors at certain membrane voltages and when the receptors are being used by glutamate and a co-agonist.

In addition, ketamine and PCP are said to be noncompetitive (or uncompetitive) blockers of the NMDA receptors: they do not compete with glutamate at its binding site (in other words, when ketamine binds, it does not prevent glutamate from binding). Ketamine, when bound to its site on the NMDA receptor inside the ion channel, prevents the flow of ions into (calcium and sodium) or out of (potassium) the neuron—it antagonizes the function of the NMDA receptor and is thus referred to as an *antagonist*. David Lodge and colleagues in the early 1980s first reported that ketamine had this effect (Anis et al. 1983). This was a monumental finding and has driven neuropharmacological research on ketamine's mechanism of action ever since. The blockade by ketamine of NMDA receptors has been theorized to be the basis for several of ketamine's clinical characteristics, such as anesthesia, analgesia, psychedelic effects, and antidepressant effects. These issues are discussed more thoroughly in the relevant chapters.

Of all the known binding sites for ketamine, that of NMDA—with consequent antagonism of the receptor's actions—is by far the most potent, well studied, and well replicated. Ketamine in research papers is so commonly referred to as an *NMDA receptor antagonist*, in fact, that one might forget it does bind to other sites, albeit not nearly as strongly. Esketamine binds much more strongly to the NMDA receptor than arketamine—in fact, about four times more strongly. Neither the hydroxynorketamines nor DHNK block NMDA receptors.

NMDA receptor blockade is probably the initial basis for ketamine's dissociative and anesthetic effects. The reason ketamine has been so successful is probably that it has just the right potency and selectivity of blockade at the PCP site of this receptor. PCP itself, as well as another compound often studied in the lab, MK-801 (also called dizocilpine, which is even more potent at that site than PCP), are too potent and cause toxic *psychotomimetic* effects (e.g., dissociation, perceptual changes, emotional changes). Other NMDA receptor compounds studied, such as lamotrigine, memantine, and riluzole, have all failed as antidepressants, probably because they have too little NMDA receptor blockade to affect the outcome of interest, and none of them is an anesthetic or dissociative agent at typical doses.

A further issue with NMDA receptors is that the subunit composition appears to play a role in their function. As mentioned earlier, NMDA receptors are tetrameric, consisting of four subunits. NMDA receptor subunits (abbreviated *GluN*) come in three types: GluN1, GluN2, and GluN3 (and each of these has further subunits). All NMDA receptors have two GluN1 subunits to which the co-agonists glycine or D-serine bind. Glutamate binds to GluN2 subunits. Ketamine blocks NMDA receptors regardless of subunit composition, but recent research suggests that different subunits of GluN2 (GluN2A, GluN2B, GluN2C, and GluN2D) may confer different functions, and that selective pharmacological action at these subunits may result in desired behavioral effects (Khlestova et al. 2016).

Another concept worth noting is that postsynaptic NMDA receptor location is important. A collection of such receptors is located where the glutamate that is released presynaptically binds most densely: this is referred to as the *postsynaptic density*. Other NMDA receptors are located on the outer fringes of this area, are not usually occupied by glutamate under normal conditions, and are termed extrasynaptic receptors. It appears that, depending on a variety of conditions, NMDA receptors that are normally part of the postsynaptic density may move to the extrasynaptic area and vice versa. The postsynaptic density and extrasynaptic receptors at baseline may contain different GluN2 subtypes. Lateral movement along the neuronal membrane of NMDA receptors (with potential different subunit compositions) leads to dynamic changes in glutamatergic signaling depending on states such as hypoxia or status epilepticus. Much research is currently focused on elaborating NMDA receptor subunit physiology.

Ligand-gated ion channels for glutamate also come in three types. In addition to NMDA receptors (based on laboratory ligands that bind them) are *AMPA* (α-amino-3-hydroxy-5-methyl-4-isoxazolepropionic acid) and *kainic acid*. Kainic acid receptors have received little attention, but AMPA receptors appear to coexist along with NMDA receptors on dendritic surfaces. When agonized by glutamate, they cause depolarization of the NMDA receptor and removal of the magnesium ion from the ion channel, effectively unplugging it so that ions can flow (and blockers such as ketamine can get into the channel and block the PCP site). According to the GABA-ergic disinhibition hypothesis of ketamine's action, when NMDA receptors on GABA-ergic interneurons (which are normally inhibitory neurons) are blocked by ketamine, the GABA-ergic interneurons do not fire; thus their normal inhibition of downstream glutamatergic neurons is lost, so the latter have increased firing, and their input into the prefrontal cortex causes increased glutamate levels. It is thought that these increased glutamate levels in the prefrontal cortex agonize AMPA receptors and thus increase AMPA throughput. This is theorized to be a mechanism of ketamine's antidepressant action.

Neuromolecular Cascades With Ketamine

What happens after either NMDA receptor blockade or AMPA receptor activation with ketamine? Presumably, intracellular neuromolecular cascades are initiated, series of chemical reactions that ultimately lead to altered gene products and changes in cellular function (i.e., neuroplasticity). Neuroplastic changes are thought to include formation of new synapses (*synaptogenesis*) and dendritic sprouting. The exciting thing about ketamine, based on animal data and the antidepressant response in humans, is that these neuroplastic changes outlast the presence of ketamine in the brain, thus obviating the need for daily, ongoing ketamine dosing.

Rodent research has elucidated some of the possible neuromolecular intracellular targets of ketamine's receptor blockade. The most commonly mentioned is a complex known as *mTOR* (mechanistic [formerly "mammalian"] target of rapamycin). Activation of this interesting molecular complex appears to be critical for many neuroplastic changes in neurons, and rodent data using depression models with ketamine implicate mTOR activation as part of ket-amine's cascade of effects leading to relief from depression. Other neuromolec-ular targets of ketamine that have been implicated in animal models include *brain-derived neurotrophic factor* (BDNF) and its cell surface receptor *tropomyosin kinase B* (TrK-B), activation of which by ketamine is correlated with improved depression symptoms in rodent models. Another commonly mentioned neu-romolecule is *eukaryotic elongation factor 2* (eEF$_2$), downregulation of which with ketamine is correlated with antidepressant effects in rodent models.

The study of these neuromolecular cascades has really only just begun. Undoubtedly, with further refinements in neurodiagnostic technology al-lowing the study of neuromolecules in the living human brain, the story will become much more complicated.

It is worth noting that the psychomimetic effects of ketamine occur im-mediately after ketamine administration and disappear when ketamine lev-els go down. Acute administrations of ketamine, as will be seen in Chapter 5 ("The Ketamine Model of Schizophrenia"), causes these effects as long as the infusions continue. When infusions are stopped, the psychotomi-metic effects abate quickly. In contrast, equal dosing regimens of ketamine (e.g., 0.5 mg/kg IV over 40 minutes) for depression often lead to antide-pressant effects, the subject of Chapter 7, but these effects typically take a few hours to occur and last much longer than the presence of ketamine in the brain. Thus, neuropharmacologists must explain the time course differ-ences of these two types of effect (i.e., the effects that depend on ketamine's presence in the brain and those that outlast such presence).

The immediate psychotomimetic effects in all likelihood emanate from, and are dependent on, the potent NMDA receptor blockade of ketamine; the delayed antidepressant effects might be due to non-NMDA receptor blockade, or at least actions that are downstream of such blockade (Zorumski et al. 2016). A further pharmacodynamic aspect of ketamine's antidepressant ef-fect is postulated reliance on (2R,6R)-hydroxynorketamine, mentioned earlier. However, the potent antidepressant effects of esketamine, which is not metabolized to that hydroxy metabolite, weigh against this theory.

Non–NMDA Receptor Actions of Ketamine

Opioid receptors, which are divided into μ, κ, and δ subtypes, deserve at-tention in the ketamine conversation. Ketamine is sometimes thought of as an opioid agonist, although evidence for this is surprisingly scarce after all these years. *Opioid agonism* (which means that ketamine promotes, rather than antagonizes, the function of the receptors) is often invoked as the mechanism behind ketamine's analgesic effects.

Sigma receptors (σ-receptors) are another widely dispersed receptor type in the brain involved in several cognitive processes. Interestingly, esketamine has an approximately 15-fold lesser binding affinity for these receptors than does arketamine. These receptors have attracted attention in the neurobiology of depression, but then again, so have many other receptors, signaling processes, and transporters. Sigma receptors are studied because they are known to exist and the technology for studying them exists, which is true for most other systems as well.

Monoaminergic neurotransmitters (dopamine, serotonin, and norepinephrine) have received enormous attention in psychiatry for many decades. In fact, the monoaminergic hypotheses of mood and psychotic disorder etiology dominated biological psychiatry for almost half a century. Thus, whether ketamine affects the monoaminergic systems has received research attention. Surprisingly, as was the case with opioid receptors and ketamine, the literature is not unanimous on this issue. Even in studies that purported to show some effect on one of these receptors, the effect was weak at best. Again, any effect of ketamine on monoamine systems is probably indirect, starting elsewhere, rather than direct.

Another long-popular proposed target for ketamine is the *cholinergic receptor* system, consisting of muscarinic and nicotinic receptors. Speculation about these receptors goes back to the 1970s. At best, there is weak binding of ketamine to either of these receptor systems. However, the 6-hydroxy-norketamines do potently block the α7 nicotinic receptor, a mechanism possibly involved in its antidepressant effects.

Some other recently described possible receptor binding affinities for ketamine include such esoteric and exotic systems as hyperpolarization-activated cyclic nucleotide-gated channels, voltage-gated sodium channels, and L-type voltage-dependent calcium channels. Only scarce data exist for each of these regarding whether ketamine or any of its metabolites bind to these channels, which all are widely dispersed in the brain and involved in many different metabolic pathways.

Recall the four components of neuropharmacology: molecular, cellular, circuitry, and behavioral. We have covered a few theories of ketamine's first molecular step, namely, where it binds in the central nervous system. The most robust finding in this regard is NMDA receptor antagonism. The next step is to deduce how initial binding translates into intracellular process changes ultimately leading to neuroplasticity (long-lasting cellular changes induced by a drug). After that, neuroplastic changes in some cell groupings translate into neurocircuitry changes, which we study via fMRI. Finally, these changes are manifested in thought, behavior, affect, cognition, perception, and consciousness. Numerous functional neuroimaging studies of ketamine in humans have not yet cohered into a unified set of conclusions.

Chapter 5

The Ketamine Model of Schizophrenia

KEY POINTS IN THIS CHAPTER:

- Ketamine causes a temporary return of psychotic symptoms in schizophrenic patients.

- In those without mental disorders, ketamine causes symptoms that partially mimic those of schizophrenia.

- Ketamine challenge studies have been used to study the pathophysiology of and potential new treatments for schizophrenia.

In this chapter, we consider a unique usage of ketamine. In all the other chapters, ketamine is used to gain some desired effect: anesthesia, pain control, relief from depression or other psychiatric disorders, augmentation of psychotherapy, or a recreational drug high. In contrast, here we discuss the use of ketamine as a neuropharmacological probe to study brain processes. The dependent variable in such studies is not a therapeutic effect, but rather the study of molecular, cellular, or neural circuitry correlates of behavior and cognition. Ketamine has been used in this context for several decades since its discovery as a potent and selective antagonist of the NMDA receptor. Ketamine is easily available, well tolerated by animals and humans, and cheap, and it has short-lived effects. All these characteristics make it useful for the laboratory neuropharmacologist wishing to study mechanisms of brain and behavior.

In humans, ketamine has been used in this context primarily to study neurobiological mechanisms of schizophrenia. In fact, there is a robust literature on this topic. The general idea here is that if the mechanisms of ketamine in the brain share similarities with biologic mechanisms in schizophrenia, then perhaps studying the molecular, cellular, circuitry, and behavioral effects of this drug might teach lessons about schizophrenia.

A couple of prefatory notes are in order. First, we will focus solely on human use of ketamine in this regard, not the animal literature, which is simply too large to cover here. Second, as has been the case so often, the road to the use of ketamine as a neuropharmacological probe began with PCP. We start with a quick review of schizophrenia to bring into focus the importance of this topic and the nature of this disorder.

Introduction to Schizophrenia

Formerly known as *dementia praecox* in the days of the German psychiatrist Emil Kraepelin (late 19th and early 20th centuries), the modern concept of schizophrenia (from Greek words *skhizein* "to split" and *phren* "mind") began to take shape in the 1940s and '50s. In 1980, it was formally distinguished from its main differential diagnostic companion, bipolar disorder, in DSM-III (American Psychiatric Association 1980). The diagnostic features have undergone relatively few changes in the various editions of DSM since that time. The three main features include the following: *positive symptoms*, the presence of psychopathological phenomena that are not supposed to be present; *negative symptoms*, the absence of features that normally are present; and *cognitive impairment*. The diagnostic criteria from DSM-5 do not include cognitive features, but research over the last 50 or so years has documented cognitive impairments in schizophrenia patients that often are the most disabling feature of the illness.

Common positive symptoms include hallucinations (classically auditory, consisting of one or more voices addressing the patient or talking about the patient in the third person), bizarre delusions (conspiracies of persecution, others' controlling one's thoughts, putting thoughts into one's head, or controlling one's actions), grossly disorganized behavior, disorganized thoughts, and catatonia (posturing, rigidity, mutism, and stupor as catatonic signs, reminiscent of the cataleptoid state described in animals given PCP). Common negative symptoms include lack of motivation, lack of emotional expression, poverty of thinking, and blunted emotionality. Cognitive abnormalities in schizophrenia are less well characterized, and less specific to the disorder, than positive and negative features but tend to involve impairments in complex episodic, semantic, and working memory as well as executive dysfunction. Negative features and cognitive impairments tend to be resistant to commonly used antipsychotic medications, while positive symptoms tend to respond robustly if the patients take the medications.

Schizophrenia usually manifests overtly in late adolescence or young adulthood and takes a chronic, lifelong course. Prodromal features in earlier adolescence or childhood consisting of awkward social competence, behavioral oddities, and physical incoordination are common, especially if a parent looks back on a now-diagnosed obviously psychotic young adult's earlier life. Schizophrenia often leads to profound disability, necessitating that its sufferers obtain publicly funded disability payments. Patients often live in subsidized, structured housing such as group homes and foster homes or with their parents; the more severely ill live chronically in government-funded long-term institutions. They often need guardians to handle their financial and living arrangements. Noncompliance with medications is common, leading to hospitalization recidivism.

Commonly used rating scales for schizophrenia signs and symptoms include the Brief Psychiatric Rating Scale (BPRS) (Overall and Gorham 1962), the Positive and Negative Syndrome Scale (PANSS) (Kay et al. 1987), and the Scale for the Assessment of Positive Symptoms (SAPS) and Scale for the Assessment of Negative Symptoms (SANS) (Andreasen 1982; Andreasen et al. 1995). With these rating scales, quantifications of positive and negative symptoms of psychosis can be conducted at serial intervals. They all have proven reliability and validity.

Treatment consists of antipsychotic medications and psychosocial rehabilitation, which tend to be time- and money-intensive. Schizophrenia devastates lives and costs a lot of money. Psychiatric science is (and has been) desperate to cure or prevent this awful illness. With global population prevalence rates of ~0.5%–1.0%, and onset early in adulthood, schizophrenia has an enormous public health significance. Patients with this condition are often impaired in their thinking and judgment skills, and they are considered especially vulnerable when it comes to scientific study. Thus, a neuropharmacological probe, such as ketamine, to model schizophrenia when given to normal volunteers, obviously would be very valuable.

The Concept of "Model Psychosis"

A first attempt to investigate the neurobiology of schizophrenia came from what was called the *model psychosis*. This meant administering various drugs and carefully recording the clinical effects. If the effects mimicked the clinical presentation of schizophrenia, then the drug's biological effects may also mimic the pathophysiology of schizophrenia—thus, the drug's effects would constitute a model of the disease. Drugs that have been studied to varying degrees for this purpose include LSD and other classic psychedelics (e.g., mescaline, psilocybin, *N,N*-dimethyltryptamine or DMT), amphetamines and other stimulants, and cannabinoids such as tetrahydrocannabinol (THC).

The psychosis symptoms caused by amphetamines were noted to be similar to the positive symptoms of schizophrenia, and the amphetamine model of psychosis has had impressive staying power in biological psychiatry. It was eventually discovered that amphetamines caused dopamine release in the brain and that drugs that blocked dopamine receptors (specifically D2 receptors) would be highly efficacious in treating delusions, hallucinations, disorganized thinking, and disorganized behavior and rendering the patient more socially appropriate. Such drugs would become, and continue to be, the mainstay of pharmacological management of schizophrenia. Much research in the 1960s all the way to the present has focused on dopamine mechanisms in the brain as they relate to the pathophysiology of schizophrenia.

As popular and inspiring as the dopamine hypothesis of schizophrenia was during those early years, it was not complete, because the well-known negative and cognitive features of schizophrenia could not be explained by it and were not helped, or were even worsened, by the dopamine-blocking antipsychotic drugs. Beyond stimulating pharmaceutical companies to keep synthesizing new dopamine blockers over a multidecade period, the dopamine hypothesis just did not solve the riddle of schizophrenia. Biological psychiatry was hungry for something else—which brings us to PCP and ketamine.

The PCP Model of Schizophrenia

After the scientists at Parke-Davis synthesized ketamine, word got around. In some of the academic centers in Michigan, psychiatrists took a keen interest in this most unusual drug. Specifically, pharmacologist Dr. Edward Domino, whom we met earlier conducting pharmacological work on humans with PCP as a consultant for Parke-Davis, collaborated with psychiatrist Dr. Elliot Luby and colleagues at the Lafayette Clinic, a mental health facility affiliated with Detroit's Wayne State University, on whether PCP could mimic the signs and symptoms of schizophrenia. Back in those days, it was pretty easy (too easy) to conduct human experiments, and this group (Luby et al. 1959) administered PCP to 18 people: nine volunteers and nine patients (four with chronic schizophrenia, one with acute catatonic schizophrenia, two with pseudoneurotic schizophrenia, and two with "character disorders"). The dose was 0.1 mg/kg IV over 12 minutes, a subanesthetic dose. The participants were interviewed during the hour after infusion.

The first noted effect was alteration in body image, consisting of lack of awareness of body or feelings of the body being foreign, a dissociated feeling. This was followed by a feeling of detachment from the surroundings, a further manifestation of dissociation. Next was thought disorganization, negativism, hostility, apathy, drowsiness, dream-like states (*hypnogogy*), inebriation, and repetitive motor behaviors such as rocking or head-rolling. All four of the patients with chronic schizophrenia experienced exacerbations of behavioral and emotional dysregulation persisting for at least a month, a complication that alarmed the investigators. Interestingly, the formerly mute, stuporous catatonic patient did not react acutely to PCP but came out of the catatonic state (which he had been in for several months) 4 days later, an improvement that lasted for at least 6 weeks. The authors concluded that PCP caused signs mimicking schizophrenia and that PCP caused a better model psychosis than LSD, which caused a purely visual hallucinatory state. This paper has been much cited for more than 60 years and inaugurated the PCP model (and later variously the ketamine model or NMDA receptor hypofunction model) of schizophrenia. It has spawned legions of publications and a theory of schizophrenia that is currently the dominant one. It is genuinely a landmark article in the history of modern psychiatry.

Another early report from this group (Rodin et al. 1959) examined EEG data from 14 nonpsychotic psychiatric patients and 6 volunteers who were given one of three dosages of PCP (referred to as Sernyl): 0.03, 0.1, or 0.2 mg/kg over 12 minutes. The participants given the two larger doses showed prominent slowing of EEG frequencies; most of the low-dosage participants did not display this effect. Eighteen of the participants displayed prominent psychotomimetic effects including, as in the other reports, body image disturbance, depersonalization (dissociation), mood lability, and disorganized thinking. Two of the low-dose participants did not display such effects. Interestingly, the psychotomimetic effects occurred 1–2 minutes before onset of the EEG effects; the latter abated within an hour, whereas the former lasted up to several hours. This report provides more support for not using PCP as a pharmacological challenge agent—it is simply too toxic.

Nonetheless, the group was not finished with the PCP model of schizophrenia. Rosenbaum et al. (1959), which included Luby, studied 10 volunteers with the same dose of PCP, namely, 0.1 mg/kg; 10 other subjects had a drug session with LSD, and 5 subjects, with the anesthetic barbiturate sodium amytal. In this report, the authors focused on tests of attention, motor coordination, and proprioceptive function while subjects were under the influence of one of the three drugs, all of which were compared to similar tests in 10 chronic schizophrenia patients (who did not receive PCP—these authors knew by then not to give PCP to schizophrenics). The effects of PCP on the testing mimicked the functioning of schizophrenia better than the effects of LSD or sodium amytal.

In the next phase of this group's comparison of the effects of PCP with those of LSD and sodium amytal, Cohen et al. (1962) used the same groups as in the previous study, and the outcome measures included proverb interpretation and the ability to count backward from 100 by 7's (called *serial sevens* in mental health work). For both these tests, the authors believed that the PCP-treated volunteers performed similarly to schizophrenia patients. One wonders whether their previously existing belief in the accuracy of the PCP model of schizophrenia may have influenced their conclusion about the subjects' responses to something as subjective as proverb interpretation.

Reflecting the popularity of sensory deprivation experiments in that era, the group gave PCP to five normal volunteers and placed them in an isolation room (Cohen et al. 1960). There was a dampening of the usual PCP effects. The volunteers were questioned after the drug effects wore off and said the experience was like "nothingness" or even death, interestingly, perhaps presaging the observation that Karl Jansen would write about decades later regarding the similarity of ketamine effects to near-death experiences. The subjects in the Cohen et al. (1960) study felt a pleasant calmness with PCP in the isolation tank, not fear or dysphoria. Of note, the authors pointed out that these were the same volunteers given PCP in their earlier study, so the subjects could compare their PCP experiences outside and inside the isolation room, and the latter apparently was distinctly more pleasant. The authors also noted that schizophrenia patients tended to like the isolation tank. This led the authors to postulate that sensory input is required for PCP to have its effects and that disintegration of this process was involved in PCP and schizophrenia. Modern researchers continue to study sensory integration processes in schizophrenia.

Other groups during that time period were smitten with the PCP model of schizophrenia. Bakker and Amini (1961), at the University of Michigan at Ann Arbor (the same institution where Edward Domino was working), described seven volunteers given PCP. Alterations in body image and dissociation were noted. In a separate limb of the study, 25 prison inmates were given PCP and a variety of tests. The authors concluded that the effects of PCP did not really mimic the signs of schizophrenia but were interesting enough to study nonetheless. This opinion reflects that of a number of investigators over the subsequent decades, that PCP and later ketamine, although quite fascinating in their effects, do not really mimic schizophrenia that closely. This has been a point of contention in that literature.

Parke-Davis had a European branch that supplied PCP and encouraged research on the drug. In one such project, Davies and Beech (1960), working from the Bethlem Royal and Maudsley hospitals in London, gave PCP in subanesthetic doses to 12 volunteers. They started with 0.1 mg/kg; because a few patients got severe nausea and vomiting at this dose, they lowered it to 0.075 mg/kg in subsequent subjects. Effects of PCP were carefully noted. Changes in perception of limbs were common, while analgesia, detachment, body image distortion, and mild dissociation were other effects. One subject became catatonic, being mute with a fixed stare for 23 minutes. Feelings of detachment from others, which is reflective of mild dissociation, lasted for some hours. Nystagmus, ataxia, and feelings of inebriation were commonly reported. The authors were not convinced that the effects of PCP mimicked the signs of schizophrenia. In a subsequent study from this group (Beech et al. 1961), 21 volunteers were studied: 10 were given sodium amytal and 12 were given PCP 7.5 mg, all by mouth instead of intravenously as in all the other studies. The outcome measure was a rather idiosyncratic method of testing "thought disorder" using the methods from an unpublished doctoral dissertation. The authors again did not feel that the effects of PCP matched the signs of schizophrenia.

Ban et al. (1961), a group from Verdun, Quebec, Canada, including academic Canadian psychiatrist Dr. Heinz Lehmann, gave PCP to 43 schizophrenia patients and found a marked return of psychotic symptoms. This constitutes the largest published sample of PCP given to schizophrenia patients and clearly shows that they do poorly with this drug. Levy et al. (1960) gave PCP to four schizophrenia patients and provided further evidence that it aggravates their symptoms.

In what appears to be the final purposeful administration of PCP to schizophrenia patients, Itil et al. (1967) gave the drug to 29 subjects: 10 who had been lobotomized and 19 who had not, a rather interesting twist. All patients had been unmedicated for at least 8 weeks before PCP administrations. There were increases in the core signs of schizophrenia, much more pronounced in the nonlobotomized patients. The lobotomized ones did not react that much to PCP. The authors related this to the sensory integration model of schizophrenia, prevalent at that time, and hypothesized that the cutting of thalamocortical connections by lobotomy prevented the PCP from having its disintegrating effect. Whether there is accuracy to this view or not, this study appears to have put the final, merciful end to the practice of administering PCP to those with schizophrenia.

Eventually, in the 1970s, people who took PCP recreationally often got so psychotic and agitated that they presented (or more accurately, were hauled in by law enforcement) for psychiatric care indistinguishably from those with schizophrenia. That added even more fuel to the notion that the study of this drug could lead to insights into the pathophysiology or treatment of schizophrenia. But if it cannot be deliberately given to people for

such study, how could it be used? This leads to the second 1970s development in the history of PCP, namely, its laboratory use on animals with studies of neurotransmitters and receptors. Even today, an occasional study is
published that used the PCP model in animals.

Luby was a rather young psychiatrist during the years of his PCP studies
at the Lafayette Clinic in Detroit, and he lived long enough to provide some
interesting retrospective thoughts in later decades. For example, in 1980,
he noted the continuing controversy as to whether PCP really provided a
good model of schizophrenia (Luby 1980). Regarding the toxic reactions of
humans to PCP, he said "It is unlikely that research in model psychoses using volunteer subjects for patients will ever be done again." Did that ever
turn out to be a wrong prediction! As we will see later in this chapter, when
the world discovered ketamine as a model psychosis drug, that field ex-
ploded and there have been more than 100 reports of the use of ketamine
in humans, mostly normal volunteers but a few with schizophrenia, as a test
of the ketamine model of schizophrenia. Some three decades later, Domino
and Luby (2012) reflected back on the influence of the early PCP research
and indicated that its main effect was to stimulate further research on model
psychoses, rather than provide a theory that stood the test of time.

Schizophrenia and the 1980s:
A New Decade, a New Theory,
and a New Drug Model

So by the end of the 1960s, everybody seemed to agree not to do any more
PCP challenges in humans because of the prolonged psychotic reactions. It
would be unethical and downright cruel. Because of the innovations in the
study of molecular neuropharmacology of the 1960s and beyond, it was
now possible to give PCP to animals in the laboratory and study their brains
at the neuroreceptor and neurotransmitter level. Such research did thrive
(reviewed extensively in Domino 1980) but during most of the 1970s really
did not lead anywhere. Thus, going into the 1980s, the PCP model of
schizophrenia had stalled. A commentary from renowned psychiatrist and
neuropharmacologist Dr. Solomon H. Snyder from Johns Hopkins University nicely summarized the problem (Snyder 1980). He mentioned that
according to the PCP challenge studies of the 1950s and '60s, as well as the
results of the recreational abuse epidemic of PCP in the 1970s, it seemed
that PCP represented the best pharmacological model for schizophrenia,
but nobody knew its brain mechanism in spite of intense work in the 1970s.
Two papers published more or less simultaneously in 1979 (Vincent et al.
1979; Zukin and Zukin 1979) did establish that there was in fact a binding

site in the central nervous system for PCP, and that it was not related to monoamine, opioid, sigma, or cholinergic receptors. But what was it? Snyder pointed out that it would be important to identify this binding site to continue pathophysiological research on schizophrenia, and he was right.

Meanwhile, a group from the University of Ulm, in Germany, took the theorizing on the pathophysiology of schizophrenia in a new direction (Kim et al. 1980a, 1980b). The dopamine hypothesis—that either too much dopamine or too many or hypersensitive dopamine receptors caused schizophrenia—was the predominant model but did not explain the negative symptoms of schizophrenia. Kim et al. (1980a, 1980b) reasoned that the parts of the brain implicated in schizophrenia, such as the prefrontal cortex and limbic areas, contained a lot of glutamate receptors and that perhaps biological psychiatry should start looking at the glutamatergic system to discover the pathophysiology of schizophrenia. To get things started in that direction, those investigators measured cerebrospinal fluid (CSF) glutamate levels in schizophrenia patients and normal volunteers and found that the patient samples had much lower levels. That led them to reason that glutamate hypofunction might be at the core of schizophrenia. Later studies did not replicate the findings, however (Gattaz et al. 1985; Korpi et al. 1987; Macciardi et al. 1990). The Kim et al. (1980a, 1980b) methodology for measuring glutamate was probably flawed. Furthermore, it appears that studying CSF glutamate is not a good way to test for glutamatergic functioning in the brain; there are simply too many factors influencing CSF levels other than synaptic glutamatergic function.

Most modern investigators of glutamatergic function in schizophrenia discount the Kim et al. (1980b) paper. However, from the standpoint of history, this was the first group to point in the direction of the glutamate system in the study of schizophrenia, and their rationale for doing so was sound—modern theorists and investigators indeed focus on the brain areas mentioned by Kim and colleagues. The technology of the day allowed nothing more sophisticated than CSF analysis, which subsequently was found to be too crude to study the intricacies of the glutamatergic system in a living person, but the group deserves credit for surmising that the glutamate system was important. Of note, they mentioned nothing of the PCP/glutamate/NMDA model of schizophrenia, because at that point, nobody knew that PCP had anything to do with the glutamate system or NMDA receptors.

In 1983, that situation changed with a groundbreaking publication from a group headed by David Lodge (Anis et al. 1983) from the Royal Veterinary College in London. The group found that ketamine and PCP blocked the NMDA receptor (the authors referred to it as the NMDLA receptor, as at that time the distinction between D and L isomers was not appreciated; however, it was the same receptor as is now named NMDA). It did not take Lodge long to make a connection between PCP/ketamine, NMDA receptors, and the pathophysiology or treatment of schizophrenia (Lodge and Berry 1984). That report was the first to speculate that NMDA receptor hypofunction may be involved in the pathophysiology of schizophrenia. Consider this sentence from that paper: "It therefore seems that any future considerations of the etiology of schizophrenia should include possible disturbances in amino acid-mediated excitatory synaptic transmission" (pp. 512–513). There it was, what would much later be referred to as the *NMDA receptor hypofunction* model of schizophrenia. They even correctly predicted that there would be interest in using NMDA agonists to treat schizophrenia. Here is the last line of the paper: "The exciting possibility remains that a specific NMDLA-like agonist which crosses the blood–brain barrier might ameliorate the symptoms of schizophrenia and of phencyclidine intoxication" (p. 514). Decades later, neuropharmacologists are feverishly looking for just such drugs.

Thus, Lodge and colleagues from the Royal Veterinary College in London in 1984 were the first to propose a link between schizophrenia, NMDA receptors, and NMDA antagonists such as ketamine or PCP. Interestingly, the only place I have seen this 1984 reference is by Lodge himself in a decades-later review of ketamine (Lodge and Mercier 2015). Nobody else cites this paper, probably because it was published in an esoteric journal not captured by internet literature searches (*Neurology and Neurobiology* published in Tallinn, Estonia). Thus, few know that it was Lodge who first developed the model. However, Lodge's paper revolved around several other themes, such as σ-receptors; the NMDA involvement in schizophrenia was not the highlight of that paper and was only tangentially mentioned. The first person to devote a whole paper to the notion of a link between the glutamate receptor NMDA, schizophrenia, and NMDA receptor antagonists was Dr. Daniel C. Javitt, then a fourth-year psychiatry resident at Albert Einstein College of Medicine (Javitt 1987). Interestingly, the paper was also published in an obscure journal (the *Hillside Journal of Clinical Psychiatry*, probably read only by people who worked at Hillside Hospital in New York). It too is almost never cited except in later papers written by Javitt himself. In this fine paper, he explained first the drawbacks of the then-dominant dopaminergic model of schizophrenia, which did not explain negative symptoms or cognitive aspects of schizophrenia. He then reviewed aspects of the glutamate system that are better suited to this purpose and provided some rodent data documenting a link between glutamate function and mesocortical dopamine function, the first-ever such data establishing that modulating the glutamate system also affects dopaminergic tracts to the prefrontal cortex and might account for the all-important negative symptoms of schizophrenia. He then pointed out that NMDA receptors are blocked by PCP, the most schizophrenogenic of the drug models of schizophrenia, and he concluded that this is where research efforts should be focused.

His was an accurate observation, as in subsequent decades, the focus on NMDA receptors has been furious. Another suggestion he made was to focus on the hippocampus as an area richly endowed with glutamate receptors; indeed, the hippocampus has been an area of intense interest in schizophrenia research. A few years later, Javitt, along with his neuropharmacology mentor Dr. Stephen Zukin (who had discovered a PCP binding site some years earlier), published a nice review of the PCP model in the *American Journal of Psychiatry*, which was read by a lot more people and is the one widely cited in later literature (Javitt and Zukin 1991).

At that point in the 1980s, a connection between NMDA receptors, their antagonists (such as PCP and ketamine), and the pathophysiology of schizophrenia had been mentioned by a veterinary physiology researcher in London (Lodge) and a psychiatry resident in New York (Javitt). The third person to invoke these connections was Dr. John W. Olney, a psychiatrist and neuropharmacologist at Washington University in St. Louis, Missouri (Olney 1988; 1989). His two publications, one a book chapter probably read by very few people and the other a paper in a mainstream psychiatric journal (*Biological Psychiatry*), are essentially identical. In these publications, Dr. Olney pointed out the dual nature of NMDA receptor functioning. On the one hand, excessive NMDA signaling leads to brain damage, which Olney famously termed *excitotoxicity*. On the other hand, too little NMDA signaling, he theorized, may lead to signs of schizophrenia. He pointed out the necessary balance in normal functioning. Excitotoxic-related conditions were hypothesized to be ischemic/anoxic injuries (e.g., stroke, cardiac arrest), severe and prolonged hypoglycemia, status epilepticus, and some neurodegenerative disorders (e.g., Huntington's disease). An NMDA antagonist such as ketamine theoretically could treat such conditions (and this topic will be discussed in Chapter 9, "Is Ketamine a Neuroprotectant or a Neurotoxin?"). Correspondingly, diminished functioning of the NMDA receptor was hypothesized to be part of the pathophysiology of schizophrenia, which NMDA antagonists like ketamine or PCP would worsen. Olney called for more research on the NMDA hypofunction hypothesis to explore schizophrenia further.

Later, in the 1990s, Olney and colleagues would expound on this NMDA hypofunction model of schizophrenia, including discussions of possible counteracting treatments and downstream effects, such as disinhibition of GABA-ergic cortex inputs leading to excessive glutamate signaling in the cortex, in several publications (Olney and Farber 1994; 1995a, 1995b;

Olney et al. 1999). Olney et al. (1989) discovered vacuoles in certain brain areas after NMDA antagonists were given to rodents. These were later dubbed *Olney lesions* and are believed to represent brain damage. In papers during the 1990s on the NMDA hypofunction model of schizophrenia, Olney and colleagues speculated that these lesions may occur in humans as well. There is no way to prove or disprove that, because no technology exists for histological studies in living humans. Nonetheless, they further theorized that the vacuoles are responsible for schizophrenic neuropathology, and concluded that if medications given concomitantly with NMDA blockers (such as ketamine or PCP) in rodents prevented the lesions, then perhaps those medications would do the same in humans and might therefore be useful for schizophrenia.

Importantly, these investigators proposed a methodology of giving putative antischizophrenic drugs along with PCP or ketamine as a test of the efficacy of such drugs—a methodology that has been often used in the ketamine model of schizophrenia studies.

As the 1990s started, the use of PCP had been relegated to animals only, and research did occur with rodents to pursue a new focus on glutamatergic mechanisms. However, a human model was desperately needed using a drug much better tolerated than PCP. Of course, we know what that drug would be—ketamine.

Psychiatry Discovers the Ketamine Challenge Model

Starting in the early 1990s, a large number of studies administered ketamine to see whether the results in any way mimicked schizophrenia (in volunteers) or made the core symptoms of that disorder worse (in patients). What is there to be learned by giving people ketamine? Four general outcome measures are used in the ketamine challenge studies: psychopathological, cognitive, neurophysiological, and neuroimaging. It is reasoned that if any one of these outcomes seems to mimic schizophrenia, then the ketamine model is valid and further studies with it might yield clues to the neurobiological basis of schizophrenia and targets for future drug development. Back in the 1950s and 1960s, the outcome measures were crude by modern standards. By the 1990s and into this millennium, newer technologies emerged for studying neurophysiology and neuroimaging.

A group at Yale University led by psychiatrist Dr. John Krystal were the first investigators to use ketamine explicitly as a test of relevance to schizophrenia. This group began what has now become a standard procedure: giving subanesthetic doses of ketamine to research volunteers to study its effects as they might relate to schizophrenia. In the first-ever use of ketamine to normal volunteers to test this hypothesis (Krystal et al. 1994), 19 volunteers were studied on three separate days with one treatment each of saline infusion (placebo), ketamine 0.1 mg/kg IV over 40 minutes, and ketamine 0.5 mg/kg IV over 40 minutes. Outcome measures included assessments of positive psychotic symptoms (delusions, perceptual distortions, hallucinations, thought disorganization), negative symptoms (apathy, lack of motivation, lack of emotional expression), dissociation (disembodied consciousness, abnormal body sensation), and cognition (memory, attention, vigilance, executive function).

The highest dose of ketamine (0.5 mg/kg) was associated with prominent positive symptoms (mostly disorganized thoughts, visual perceptual distortions, and suspiciousness), negative symptoms (mostly amotivation and lack of emotional expression), dissociative symptoms, and small but detectable effects on cognitive vigilance and perseverence on tasks in the absence of gross disturbance of level of consciousness. Importantly, all ketamine-induced symptoms abated completely within 15 minutes or so of intravenous cessation. The authors noted that the effects of ketamine were somewhat similar to the symptoms of schizophrenia but were not identical, in that ketamine did not cause auditory hallucinations (which are classic in schizophrenia) or bizarre delusions. Furthermore, the prominent dissociation caused by ketamine was not considered typical of schizophrenia. The most important findings were that ketamine was well tolerated, and the effects were quite transient, meaning that ketamine challenge studies, at least in normal volunteers, appeared acceptably safe.

A few years later, this group essentially replicated the original study (Krystal et al. 1998), only this time a slightly higher ketamine dose was used, and pretreatment with lorazepam was attempted to see if it mitigated the psychotogenic effects of ketamine. Earlier, in Chapter 2, we discussed the use of benzodiazepines in anesthesia to lessen the emergence panic caused by ketamine. One of the theories of the schizophrenogenic effect of ketamine is that by blocking NMDA action on GABA-ergic interneurons that project to the cortex, disinhibition of the cortical neurons occurs, leading to their unmitigated excitement and the symptoms of schizophrenia (Olney and Farber 1995a, 1995b). If that theory is true, then adding a GABA-ergic agonist such as a benzodiazepine might mitigate the psychotogenic effects of ketamine. Krystal et al. (1998) found that lorazepam did not do that, but it did lessen the emotional reaction to ketamine by causing sedation. At any rate, Krystal and colleagues in the 1990s made groundbreaking progress in the study of schizophrenia by introducing the ketamine challenge paradigm, which has been used in decades of constant research.

Ketamine Challenge Studies in Schizophrenia Patients

Several groups in the 1990s became interested in studying the psychotomimetic effects of ketamine challenges in schizophrenia. For example, a group headed by Drs. Carol Tamminga and Adrienne Lahti at the Maryland Psychiatric Research Center, affiliated with the University of Maryland School of Medicine, began what would be a several-year fruitful study of ketamine challenge paradigms in both volunteers and schizophrenia patients. In their first study (Lahti et al. 1995a), nine schizophrenia patients taking haloperidol 0.3 mg/kg daily for at least 4 weeks were given (in randomized order) 60-second infusions of placebo saline, 0.1 mg/kg ketamine, 0.3 mg/kg ketamine, and 0.5 mg/kg ketamine. (The high dose was not used first for any participant.) Outcome measures included assessments of psychotic symptoms, which rose sharply for about an hour and then abated, although several patients had psychotomimetic effects of ketamine lasting 8–24 hours, which is of some concern. Negative symptoms such as amotivation and lack of emotionality were not noted to rise with ketamine, as distinct from the Krystal et al. (1994) study. Similar to the findings of Luby et al. (1959), who gave PCP to schizophrenia patients, in the Lahti et al. (1995a) study, the psychotic symptoms in several patients bore a striking similarity to their previous psychotic symptoms (e.g., similar delusional systems or the same type of auditory hallucinations). The authors concluded that the ketamine challenge in schizophrenia patients was a good model with which to study this condition. Because haloperidol did not blunt the ketamine-induced psychotomimetic effect, it was hypothesized that those effects are mediated neurobiologically upstream from dopamine receptors.

In the group's next study (Lahti et al. 1995b), another nine schizophrenia patients medicated with haloperidol were given the four same infusions as before with the same effects: namely, transient rise in psychosis ratings with qualitative features similar to the patients' usual psychotic symptoms. Another five patients were given this ketamine/placebo regimen (three different doses of ketamine and one placebo) with before-and-after PET scans to assess cerebral blood flow. It was found that ketamine induced greater blood flow in the anterior cingulate cortex (a part of the limbic system) and decreased flow in the hippocampus and visual cortex. These results seemed to represent support for an altered glutamatergic system in schizophrenia. The same group (LaPorte et al. 1996) reported on the cognitive testing done as part of the previous studies (Lahti et al. 1995a, 1995b) and found that information provided before the infusion of ketamine was recalled at a later time (30–45 minutes after the infusion) as well as when saline placebo had been given. The long interval after a subanesthetic injection of ketamine probably accounted for the lack of effect on memory for what was a fairly simple recall task. At any rate, the investigators hypothesized that if the schizophrenia patients already had a compromised glutamatergic system, then effects on cognition of further NMDA blockade may not be substantial.

A final publication from this group on the use of ketamine challenges in schizophrenia consisted of a brief abstract (Lahti et al. 1999). Five normal volunteers and an unspecified number of schizophrenia patients were pretreated with placebo or the antipsychotic agent olanzapine and given ketamine challenges (0.3 mg/kg). Olanzapine did not reduce ketamine-induced psychosis ratings. Thus, it seemed that olanzapine's antipsychotic effect is mediated through mechanisms other than glutamatergic.

Another group took a keen interest in using the ketamine challenge test in schizophrenia patients. Dr. Anil Malhotra and colleagues at the National Institute of Mental Health (NIMH, Bethesda, Maryland) started by giving 13 neuroleptic-free schizophrenia patients an infusion of 0.77 mg/kg ketamine administered over 1 hour; each patient also had a session with a saline (placebo) infusion for comparison purposes (Malhotra et al. 1997a). Outcome measures included psychopathology and some measures of cognition including attention and memory (the latter consisted of recall and recognition of word lists provided before the infusions started). Results showed that ketamine infusions, versus saline, caused decrements in free recall of words as well as recognition. The same thing occurred in a comparison group of 16 volunteers undergoing the same protocol. Thought disorganization and body image distortions took place in all study participants, but the schizophrenia patients had recrudescence of their particular psychotic symptoms such as auditory hallucinations or delusions, just as in the Lahti et al. (1995a, 1995b) studies. The latter did not occur with normal volunteers given ketamine; they experienced only essentially dissociative symptoms (body image distortions) and some relatively minor thought disorganization.

The group's next study involved 10 schizophrenia patients treated with one ketamine and one saline infusion in a blind manner, both while not taking neuroleptic medication and then later while taking stable doses of clozapine, an antipsychotic agent (Malhotra et al. 1997b). Alterations in thought disorganization caused by ketamine were blunted with clozapine in 8 of the 10 patients, and there was more increase in thought disorganization with ketamine while taking clozapine than in the other two patients. The authors concluded that the mechanism of action of clozapine for schizophrenia may include effects on the glutamatergic system.

The final ketamine challenge study in schizophrenia from this group involved an attempt to correlate the ketamine-induced psychotic changes with the apolipoprotein E ε4 (ApoE-ε4) allele (Malhotra et al. 1998). Everybody has two such alleles of one of three types (2, 3, or 4). Those with allele 4 were considered to have a lesser chance of ketamine-induced psychotic changes, and indeed, in 18 schizophrenia patients, the 7 who had at least one type 4 allele had blunted increases in psychosis with ketamine than the 11 who did not have the type 4 allele. The meaning of these findings is so far obscure.

One report not involving the ketamine challenge but rather anesthesia for schizophrenia patients was published by Ishihara et al. (1997). In this case series, 14 schizophrenia patients requiring surgery for various conditions were anesthetized with ketamine for induction and maintenance of anesthesia. Two of the patients died after surgery from complications of their severe illnesses (burns). In the other 12 patients, no psychotic exacerbations were noted in the recovery room or during 1 month of follow-up, indicating that schizophrenia patients can be anesthetized safely with ketamine if that is otherwise deemed the anesthetic agent of choice.

Of course, some people were not exactly thrilled by the idea of giving schizophrenia patients drugs to make them presumably more schizophrenic for a while. In the late 1990s, just when the ketamine challenge studies for schizophrenia took hold in the psychiatric research community, some of those outside the community became outraged that patients would be given a medication specifically designed to make their symptoms worse. The opponents consisted of two groups mostly: those who consider themselves advocates on behalf of the mentally ill (e.g., parents of children with schizophrenia, bioethicists) and journalists. (Journalists are always looking for good controversies to write about, and psychiatric topics seem to fill that bill.) Tishler and Gordon (1999) published a review of what they considered ethical lapses in the research on ketamine challenge studies, but the paper is rather sophomoric and unconvincing. Much more influential was a series of articles in late 1998 and early 1999 published in the *Boston Globe* to the effect that plenty of "mental health advocates" were outraged by ketamine challenges and other similar types of psychiatric studies (Kong 1998a, 1998b, 1998c, 1998d; 1999a, 1999b; Whitaker and Kong 1998). The accusation was that people with schizophrenia are in no position to understand the true risk of undertaking a ketamine challenge, and that such tests should be done only in volunteers who are clear-headed enough to know what they are getting into. Plenty of horror stories were presented, with quotes from various parties. Kong's articles proved effective. By the end of the *Boston Globe* series, as reported by Kong in February 1999, some 29 of 108 studies at NIMH had been suspended on account of the bad publicity. NIMH, the main source of research grant money in American psychiatry, essentially stopped funding ketamine challenge studies in schizophrenia.

There is nothing like intense public embarrassment to stop scientists from doing their thing, and psychiatry relented. This was probably the right thing to do, as any attempt to resist public pressure and continue ketamine challenges in schizophrenia would have been a Sisyphean task. Psychiatric research has always been on shaky grounds in the public eye anyway. There was some attempt on the part of psychiatry to defend itself. For example, the Yale group, which had performed the first-ever ketamine challenge study (in normal volunteers) specifically referencing its relevance to schizophrenia (Krystal et al. 1994), wrote a long paper on the concept of symptom provocation studies in medicine and psychiatry, pointing out the uses of such studies to elaborate the pathophysiology of disease and to test new treatments (D'Souza et al. 1999). In that paper, the authors noted that for much of its existence, cardiac stress testing, which can provoke electrocardiographic or symptomatic evidence of myocardial ischemia and even rare deaths, was not associated with any clinical relevance. They argued that even though psychiatric symptom provocation studies had no clinical relevance, that situation could change with continued research.

Dr. William T. Carpenter, then director of the Maryland Psychiatric Research Center where many of the ketamine challenges in schizophrenia patients had been conducted, wrote a thoughtful paper on this debate (Carpenter 1999). He reviewed the experiences of all known sites where ketamine challenge studies had been undertaken: Maryland Psychiatric Research Center (26 patients), NIMH (18 patients), and Yale University (12 patients, but the data were not published). At Yale, where the ketamine had been infused at a dose of 0.5 mg/kg over 40 minutes, two of the 12 patients had their infusions stopped prematurely because of severe psychotic and emotional distress symptoms. This probably reflected the more severe state of patients enrolled at that institution. Overall, among the three locations, no long-term problems occurred as the result of the ketamine challenges. The ketamine-induced symptoms lasted only 30–60 minutes. The author did lament the rather weak response from psychiatry to the media hysteria. He believed that the use of ketamine challenges in schizophrenia was on solid ethical and scientific ground.

Lahti et al. (2001a) provided long-term follow-up (mean of 8 months) on schizophrenia patients given ketamine challenges at Maryland Psychiatric Research Center in the 1990s. The sample size was 30, with follow-up available on 25. These patients were compared to follow-up data on 25 other schizophrenia patients in their research studies who did not receive ketamine, and there was no signal indicating the ketamine challenges caused any worsening of the patients' longitudinal course. No serious adverse events occurred acutely with any of the sample of 30 patients given ketamine. Thus, it looked like ketamine challenges in schizophrenia patients were safe.

However, the public relations damage had been done—thenceforth, ketamine challenges would be used only in normal volunteers, not schizophrenia patients, with three exceptions as reported in Holcomb et al. 2005; Lahti et al. 2001b; and Medoff et al. 2001. The Maryland group published these studies, probably based on data collected before the *Boston Globe* series. The first (Lahti et al. 2001b) compared the effects of ketamine challenges in schizophrena ($n = 17$) to those in volunteers ($n = 18$). The schizophrenia patients had increases in positive symptoms (thought disorganization, psychosis) but not negative ones (poverty of thought, blunted emotionality), unlike the volunteers, who had increases in both types of symptoms. As with previous data sets, the schizophrenia patients experienced recrudescence of their own auditory hallucinations or delusional thoughts. The authors concluded that the use of volunteers in place of schizophrenia patients was acceptable as a means of studying psychotic processes in schizophrenia.

The second post-1999 publication (Medoff et al. 2001) compared PET scans in 13 volunteers versus 10 haloperidol-medicated schizophrenia patients, focusing on the hippocampus. They found that blood flow in the middle hippocampi of schizophrenia patients was significantly decreased 16 minutes after ketamine infusion of 0.3 mg/kg versus no change in that region for the volunteers. Also, neither group had significant hippocampal blood flow changes after ketamine in the anterior or posterior hippocampi. The meaning of these results is somewhat obscure but does point to possible pathology in the hippocampi of schizophrenia patients, something that the investigators in this group have emphasized repeatedly in their research in schizophrenia over the decades.

Next, in what would be the final study (at least in the English language, as far as I can tell) of ketamine challenges in schizophrenia patients, Holcomb et al. (2005) conducted PET scans in 10 patients and 13 volunteers after ketamine infusions of 0.3 mg/kg. One suspects this was the same group whose hippocampi were reported in 2001 (Medoff et al. 2001). In both groups, there was increased blood flow in the frontal lobes and anterior cingulate region, which the authors interpreted to mean that GABA-ergic inhibitory neurons in the anterior thalamus were not being stimulated by NMDA receptors with the ketamine on board, thus leading to disinhibition of cortical glutamatergic neurons and subsequent thought disorganization and cognitive symptoms. They theorized that the GABA-ergic neurons are compromised in schizophrenia and that ketamine administration, by blocking NMDA receptors, exacerbates that situation.

Ketamine Challenge Studies in Volunteers Without Schizophrenia

Covering the studies of ketamine challenge in schizophrenia patients is straightforward, given how few of them there have been. The literature on the ketamine challenge paradigm in normal volunteers contains at least 137 separate publications in which a group of nonschizophrenic research participants were given ketamine with some kind of outcome measure. It would be extremely tedious (for both reader and author!) to review all of them. Thus, this section captures the gist and gives the range of methods and conclusions in tables.

The basic idea for this type of study is to administer a subanesthetic dose of ketamine—that is, a dose sufficiently small that the subject does not lose consciousness and can therefore complete rating scales and other outcome assessments. Because the psychological effects of ketamine may mimic at least partially the signs of schizophrenia, there may be neurobiological similarity in ketamine's effects to the neurobiology of schizophrenia. If this assumption holds true, then investigators might be able to assume that any neurobiological effect of ketamine may shed light on the neurobiology of schizophrenia and reveal neurobiological targets for potential therapies. If in turn ketamine's effects in control subjects are blocked by a new pharmaceutical therapy, it might be worth testing with further trials in clinical samples.

As mentioned earlier, four broad types of outcome measures are used: psychopathological, cognitive, neuroimaging, and neurophysiological. The most common is psychopathological. Typically, investigators will assess the effects of ketamine on mood, dissociation, thought organization, delusional thinking, hallucinations, and negative symptoms such as amotivation, lack of emotional expression, and emotional withdrawal. Several standardized rating scales yield quantifiable measures of psychopathological effects of ketamine, as mentioned earlier in this chapter (BPRS, PANSS, SAPS, and SANS). Cognitive effects of ketamine include memory, attention, and executive function. Third, highly sophisticated neuroimaging modalities have assessed the effects of ketamine and seek similarities to neuroimaging studies in schizophrenia, and whether any of the cognitive or psychopathological changes correlate with neuroimaging findings. Such studies may yield insights into the neurobiology of not only ketamine's effects but schizophrenia's as well. Fourth, some interesting neurophysiological tests have shown similar findings in schizophrenia patients and volunteers administered ketamine.

A few points about the research methodology. The most common study design involved administering to each participant, on separate occasions, a dose of ketamine and a dose of saline (a biologically inert placebo). At each session, outcome measures were taken at baseline and after ketamine or saline administration. Thus, each participant's ketamine administration outcome data were compared to their own saline administration outcome data (a crossover trial, in which patients serve as their own controls). Another design, a bit simpler, compared the outcome measures at baseline and then again after ketamine administration; thus, there was no placebo control. Finally, a few studies involved randomly assigning volunteers to receive either saline or ketamine, but not both, and then at the end the two groups were compared for outcome measures.

The dose of ketamine used in these studies deserves mention. All involved subanesthetic dosing of ketamine, so volunteers were able to interact verbally, answer questions about their experiences, and cooperate with cognitive testing, neuroimaging, or neurophysiological testing. Generally, the blood levels of ketamine were less than 500 ng/mL. Blood levels much higher than this tend to cause diminution of conscious awareness and decreased ability to cooperate with testing paradigms. Doses of ketamine were usually administered as an ongoing infusion over a few minutes (up to 1–2 hours) to allow for all outcome measures to be obtained while there was still ketamine in the system. Of note, most studies involved racemic ketamine, but a few used esketamine.

Psychopathology

A good summary statement of the findings is that at baseline, normal volunteers had essentially no psychopathological features, and after ketamine administration, they had features of psychotic or prepsychotic phenomena such as suspiciousness without full delusion formation, mild thought disorganization, affective blunting, poverty of thinking and speech (*abulia* and *alogia*, respectively), and a variety of emotional reactions including fear in some, irritability in others, and mild euphoria in still others. Dissociative symptoms, as measured by the Clinician-Administered Dissociative States Scale (CADSS, described in Chapter 3), also increased with ketamine. A robust, consistent finding was that as soon as the ketamine infusions were stopped (within, say, 15–30 minutes), these schizophrenia-like, emotional, and dissociative features disappeared, and the volunteers' mental states were back to baseline. Nobody was left with persistent dysphoria or psychosis.

Beck et al. (2020) conducted a meta-analysis of ketamine challenge studies that involved either BPRS or PANSS and used a crossover comparison to placebo (i.e., all subjects received infusions of ketamine and saline at different time points). There were 36 studies included in the analysis that fit the inclusion criteria, involving 725 participants in total. Ketamine resulted in large effect sizes of increased total psychopathological symptom scores on these scales. Positive symptoms increased significantly and robustly with ketamine. Negative symptoms were also significantly increased with ketamine over placebo, but not by as large a margin. Mean score difference between ketamine and placebo in PANSS after infusion was 18.4, which would correspond to marked illness severity increases in a patient with schizophrenia. Thus, ketamine indeed causes substantial, temporary, psychotic-like psychopathology, dependent on its presence in the brain (as opposed to its antidepressant effect, which is delayed several hours after the end of infusion of the same dose and which is longer lasting; more in Chapter 7).

A good question, however, is whether the ketamine-induced psychopathological features truly mimic those of schizophrenia. A consensus among most of the investigators is that they do not. For example, the sine qua non of schizophrenia is auditory hallucinations, in which voices talk about the person or make a running commentary on the person's thoughts. This simply does not happen with ketamine administered to normal volunteers. Additionally, the delusions of schizophrenia tend to be highly persecutory or bizarre, such as the feeling that one's thoughts are taken away (thought withdrawal), inserted into one's mind (thought insertion), or read by others (thought broadcasting). These also do not occur with ketamine. A notion that has been bandied about is that what ketamine may really mimic with regard to schizophrenia is the prodromal features of the illness—that is, the symptoms people have in the months or years leading up to frank psychosis. This notion deserves further study, which is difficult because prodromal schizophrenia is hard to find: at this early stage of the illness, frank psychopathology has usually not been identified, and nobody can tell if a person at this stage is going to become psychotic or not.

Further, the prominent and fascinating dissociative effects of ketamine, well known for many decades and shown as assessed with CADSS, do not occur with schizophrenia. What can be said is that the acute effects of ketamine in normal volunteers have a few things in common with schizophrenia (mild positive and negative symptoms) for an hour or two but do not mimic the condition to the point where normal volunteers are identical with schizophrenia patients. In other words, ketamine does not cause "temporary schizophrenia." An experienced mental health professional asked to assess a person with schizophrenia or a normal volunteer who has just had ketamine will easily be able to make the distinction.

Cognition

Dozens of ketamine challenge studies involved some type of cognitive assessment as an outcome variable. Cognition encompasses a wide array of skills. Attention and memory are the most commonly studied. In Chapter 3, we learned that memory is divided into five domains: *procedural memory, perceptual representation system, working memory, semantic memory*, and *episodic memory*. Procedural memory is memory for how to carry out a learned activity, such as putting on clothes or driving a car. The perceptual representation system refers to the immediate memory of a perception, in any modality, that only lasts a few seconds or so. These two are rarely studied. More commonly studied in the ketamine challenge literature are working memory (the ability to carry out a sustained task requiring memory of what is to be done), semantic memory (memory of general knowledge without any context of the learning), and episodic memory (memory of specific incidents including the context of the incident). *Executive function* refers to complex cognitive activities that require attention, memory, and logic.

Here we review some of the major findings. The studies revealed no adverse effect of ketamine, at the doses used, on basic attention. (Of course, if higher doses had been used, closer to anesthetic effect, attention would have been impaired.) The studies did show that ketamine impairs working memory performance. This is one area of deep similarity between the effects of ketamine and schizophrenia. Another fairly robust finding was that ketamine also impairs episodic memory, another area of similarity with schizophrenia. Only a few of the ketamine challenge studies tested for semantic memory, and generally no impairment by ketamine was found. Executive function was impaired in the ketamine studies as well, also a similarity with schizophrenia.

The ketamine challenge paradigm has been used creatively to investigate whether its effects mimic cognitive aspects of schizophrenia or to pursue the glutamatergic basis for cognitive functions. For example, it has been hypothesized that auditory hallucinations in schizophrenia may emanate from misattributions of one's own thoughts as being external. In experimental studies in which self-generated speech is played back to the participant in a distorted manner, schizophrenia patients are more likely to misattribute the speech as being generated by somebody else. Stone et al. (2011) tested volunteers under saline versus ketamine and found the same tendency with ketamine, suggesting that the basis for auditory hallucinations in schizophrenia may be mediated by NMDA receptors.

Sense of body ownership may be impaired in schizophrenia. In an ingenious research paradigm, the rubber hand test has been used to assess a participant's ability to tell whether a picture of a hand is theirs or not. In this test, the participant is sitting at a desk, and one of their hands resting on the table is hidden from their view, with a screen showing another hand made of rubber located very close to their actual hand. Under certain experimental conditions, it is actually possible for volunteers to misidentify the rubber hand as their own. Morgan et al. (2012), utilizing this test, found that ketamine caused a greater tendency to misattribute the rubber hand as one's own, just as in schizophrenia.

Negative symptoms of schizophrenia such as amotivation can be disabling. Faulty reward anticipation in daily life has been postulated as core to schizophrenic negative symptoms. Francois et al. (2016) developed a laboratory-based reward anticipation test in which participants gazing at a computer screen were to press a button as fast as possible after having been given different types of information about the consequences of pressing fast enough (e.g., they would either be given money or not, presumably thus altering the motivation component for pressing the button fast enough). While ketamine did not alter the reaction times, versus saline, it did alter functional neuroimaging results in a pattern that mimicked that for schizophrenia patients taking the same test. The authors concluded that this provides evidence in favor of the ketamine model for schizophrenic negative symptoms.

Javitt et al. (2018), in an ambitious multisite study of the neuroimaging effects of ketamine versus saline infusions, used a cognitive measure known as the *RISE task*, which stands for relational and item-specific encoding. In this task, participants are shown a sequence of pairs of pictures. For each pair, the participant is asked one of two questions: "Is one of the pictures something that is living?" or "Can one of the items be placed inside the other one?" The first type of question involves item-specific encoding, meaning that the question can be answered by looking at the picture by itself without looking at the other one. The second type of question involves relational encoding, meaning that the relationship of the pictures to one another must be taken into account. It turns out that schizophrenia patients have trouble remembering relationally encoded material versus item-specific encoded material, and that each one correlates with specific neuroimaging findings. Relational encoding difficulties may be involved in delusion formation in schizophrenia, so a neurophysiological understanding of it may lead to treatments. Javitt et al. (2018) wanted to know if ketamine replicates this finding in control subjects—it did not. That is, ketamine in control subjects did not selectively impair memory for relationally encoded material.

Neuroimaging

To propel the field of schizophrenia research forward, what is needed most is a new technology that can detect brain function at the levels of molecules, cells, and circuits, in real time, in the living human brain, safely.

Such a technology is yet to be discovered, but as can be seen in Table 5–1, 55 of the studies involved some type of neuroimaging as part of the

TABLE 5–1. Ketamine neuroimaging studies using radionuclides in volunteers without schizophrenia

Study	Imaging modality	Radionuclide	Ketamine results
Breier et al. 1997	PET	[^{18}F]FDG	Increased prefrontal blood flow correlated with ketamine-induced thought disorganization
Vollenweider et al. 1997a	PET	[^{18}F]FDG	Increased metabolic rate in frontal cortex and anterior cingulate cortex
Vollenweider et al. 1997b	PET	[^{18}F]FDG	Esketamine caused increased cortical metabolic rates; arketamine tended to decrease them
Smith et al. 1998	PET	[^{11}C]raclopride	Radioligand binding to striatal dopamine receptors was decreased
Breier et al. 1998	PET	[^{11}C]raclopride	Radioligand binding to striatal dopamine receptors was decreased and correlated with increases in BPRS
Kegeles et al. 2000	SPECT	[^{123}I]IBZM	Ketamine alone did not displace dopamine-binding radioligand but enhanced amphetamine-induced displacement
Vollenweider et al. 2000	PET	[^{11}C]raclopride	Radioligand binding to striatal dopamine receptors was decreased
Holcomb et al. 2001	PET	H$_2$^{15}O	Increased blood flow in anterior cingulate and prefrontal areas which correlated with increases in BPRS
Aalto et al. 2002	PET	[^{11}C]raclopride	No effect on striatal ligand binding; thus ketamine does not appear to enhance dopamine release

TABLE 5–1. Ketamine neuroimaging studies using radionuclides in volunteers without schizophrenia *(continued)*

Study	Imaging modality	Radionuclide	Ketamine results
Kegeles et al. 2002	PET	[^{11}C]raclopride	No effect on ligand binding in spite of causing robust psychotomimesis
Stone et al. 2005, 2006	SPECT	[^{123}I]CNS-1261	Ketamine displaced this novel NMDA receptor ligand
Matusch et al. 2007	PET	[^{18}F]altanserin	No evidence that ketamine displaced binding of this 5-HT$_{2A}$ binding ligand; thus ketamine does not appear to cause serotonin release
Stone et al. 2008	SPECT	[^{123}I]CNS-1261	Degree of ketamine-induced ligand displacement correlated with ketamine-induced negative symptoms
Rowland et al. 2010	PET	H$_2$^{15}O	Increased blood flow in the anterior cingulate and frontal lobes
Vernaleken et al. 2013	PET	[^{18}F]fallypride	Ketamine did not alter binding of this D2/3 binding ligand; degree of baseline ligand binding correlated with ketamine-induced psychotomimesis

BPRS=Brief Psychiatric Rating Scale; FDG=fluorodeoxyglucose; IBZM=iodobenzamide; NMDA=*N*-methyl-D-aspartate; PET=positron emission tomography; SPECT=single-photon emission computed tomography

outcome assessment during ketamine infusions. Coupling these studies with the now-large literature on neuroimaging in schizophrenia, similarities can be sought, enhancing the utility of the ketamine challenge paradigm as a method to deduce biological mechanisms, explore potential new targets of treatments, and test putative treatments themselves using this easy-to-conduct paradigm.

In Table 5–1, 15 studies used radionuclide scanning with PET or SPECT. In these studies, some type of radioactive compound is injected intravenously into the volunteer, enough time elapses until the compound is dispersed in the brain, and then a scan is done to see where in the brain the radioactive compound went. In the case of radioactive fluorodeoxyglucose (FDG), the radioligand is dispersed according to glucose uptake and thus reflects metabolic activity. The areas of the brain that are lit up during FDG PET show where the most intense metabolic activity takes place. Three FDG studies (Breier et al. 1997; Vollenweider et al. 1997a, 1997b) generally showed increased frontal lobe activity with ketamine, and also anterior cingulate activity.

Five studies used radioactive raclopride, a dopamine receptor ligand, to study ketamine effects. When raclopride binds to dopamine receptors, and then something affects increased presynaptic dopamine release, the increased dopamine in the synapse displaces the raclopride binding, which can be detected on the scans. Raclopride binding was decreased by ketamine in three studies (Breier et al. 1998; Smith et al. 1998; Vollenweider et al. 2000), indicating that ketamine resulted in increased dopamine release, something that has been postulated to be part of its mechanism of action in psychotomimesis. In two other studies, however, this effect was not found (Aalto et al. 2002; Kegeles et al. 2002).

Kegeles et al. (2000) used a novel radioligand to bind to dopamine receptors, radioactive iodobenzamide ($[^{123}I]IBZM$), and found that ketamine alone did not displace the ligand but did enhance amphetamine-induced displacement of the ligand. Yet another ligand to study dopamine binding, radioactive fallypride ($[^{18}F]$fallypride), was used by Vernaleken et al. (2013), who found that ketamine did not displace binding of it. Thus, in sum, it is not clear that subanesthetic dosages of ketamine affect dopamine release in the striatum.

Holcomb et al. (2001) and Rowland et al. (2010) used radioactive water ($H_2{}^{15}O$) to measure cerebral blood flow effects of ketamine and found increased frontal and anterior cingulate flow. Radioactive altanserin ($[^{18}F]$altanserin), a serotonin receptor binding radioligand, was not displaced by ketamine, providing no evidence that ketamine causes increased serotonin release. Finally, radioactive *CNS-1261* ($[^{123}I]$CNS-1261), a novel NMDA receptor–binding ligand, was shown to be displaced by ketamine, not surprisingly (Stone et al. 2005, 2006). In a later study by the same group, Stone et al. (2008), the degree of ligand displacement by ketamine was shown to correlate with increases in negative symptom scores with ketamine.

Table 5–2 lists magnetic resonance-based neuroimaging studies with subanesthetic ketamine in volunteers without schizophrenia, including fMRI and magnetic resonance spectroscopy (MRS) studies. Obviously, fMRI has piqued the curiosity of investigators in brain science, probably because of the relative ease of its scans vis-à-vis PET or SPECT. Also, fMRI allows study of cortical connectivity, an area of intense focus in modern clinical neuroscience. Summarizing the large number of fMRI studies with

TABLE 5-2. Ketamine magnetic resonance-based neuroimaging studies in volunteers without schizophrenia

Study	Imaging modality	Ketamine results
Abel et al. 2003a	fMRI	Facial recognition task: a plethora of difficult-to-explain results
Fu et al. 2005	fMRI	Verbal fluency task: increased metabolic activity in the frontal lobes and anterior cingulate, said to be similar to results in schizophrenia
Honey et al. 2005	fMRI	Episodic memory task: ketamine associated with prefrontal and hippocampal activation
Northoff et al. 2005	fMRI	Episodic memory task: ketamine associated with posterior cingulate activation, correlated with psychotomimesis
Corlett et al. 2006	fMRI	Prediction error task: volunteers with most prefrontal activation had highest psychotomimesis
Deakin et al. 2008	fMRI	Plethora of fMRI signals, some of which were antagonized by lamotrigine
Honey et al. 2008	fMRI	Cognitive tasks: signals correlated with subsequent ketamine-induced psychotomimesis
Daumann et al. 2008	fMRI	Inhibition of return task: variety of frontotemporal areas were activated
Daumann et al. 2010	fMRI	No consistent correlation with ketamine-induced psychotomimesis
Stone et al. 2011	fMRI	Self-generated speech interpretation task: left superior temporal gyrus activation, said to be similar to schizophrenia
Nagels et al. 2011	fMRI	Verbal fluency task: signal patterns said to be similar to schizophrenia
Musso et al. 2011	fMRI	Oddball task: event-related potentials said to be similar to schizophrenia
Nagels et al. 2012	fMRI	Psychotomimetic effects correlated with various fMRI findings, said to be similar to results in schizophrenia

TABLE 5–2. Ketamine magnetic resonance-based neuroimaging studies in volunteers without schizophrenia *(continued)*

Study	Imaging modality	Ketamine results
Driesen et al. 2013a	fMRI	Multiple areas of increased hyperconnectivity on fMRI correlated with ketamine-induced psychopathology
Driesen et al. 2013b	fMRI	Working memory task: change in task performance correlated with connectivity changes
Doyle et al. 2013	fMRI	Lamotrigine and risperidone cotreatment blunted some ketamine-associated fMRI changes
De Simoni et al. 2013	fMRI	Dose-response effect of ketamine on fMRI signals was established
Dandash et al. 2015	fMRI	Various blood flow changes correlated with psychotomimetic effects
Pollak et al. 2015	fMRI	Variety of blood flow changes correlated with various psychotomimetic effects
Grimm et al. 2015	fMRI	Increase in prefrontal-hippocampal connectivity at rest, in contrast to results in schizophrenia
Kleinloog et al. 2015a	fMRI	Ketamine-induced perceptual changes, said to be similar to those in schizophrenia
Shcherbinin et al. 2015	fMRI	Lamotrigine had no effect on, and risperidone increased, ketamine-induced fMRI effects
Joules et al. 2015	fMRI	Same data set as Shcherbinin et al. 2015 with different analyses; effects result from NMDAR blockade and not downstream effects on glutamate release
Anticevic et al. 2015	fMRI	Global functional connectivity increases better model early course than chronic schizophrenia
Höflich et al. 2015	fMRI	Increased corticothalamic connectivity partially mimics findings in schizophrenia
Stone et al. 2015	fMRI	Parietal lobe and anterior cingulate changes correlate with psychopathology

TABLE 5–2. Ketamine magnetic resonance-based neuroimaging studies in volunteers without schizophrenia *(continued)*

Study	Imaging modality	Ketamine results
Steffens et al. 2016	fMRI	Several changes said to be similar to findings with schizophrenia
Francois et al. 2016	fMRI	Reward anticipation task: performance in ventral striatum said to be similar to findings in schizophrenia, postulated to be basis for negative symptoms
Kraguljac et al. 2017	fMRI	Hippocampal and other area connectivity mimics findings in schizophrenia (see also MRS below)
Javitt et al. 2018	fMRI	BOLD fMRI differentiated ketamine from placebo better than MRS (see later in table) or pharmaco-fMRI
Becker et al. 2017	fMRI	Panoply of fMRI changes unrevealing in this study of emotion processing
Mueller et al. 2018	fMRI	Decreased connectivity involving the salience network correlated with ketamine-induced negative symptoms
D'Souza et al. 2018	fMRI	Experimental GLYT1 transporter inhibitor did not attenuate ketamine effects on fMRI or working memory
Nagels et al. 2018	fMRI	Right temporal cortex was activated similarly by natural speech with ketamine and schizophrenia
Steffens et al. 2018	fMRI	Ketamine-induced eye movement changes were dissimilar to those of schizophrenia, with uncompelling fMRI findings
Bryant et al. 2019	fMRI	Whole-brain regional cerebral blood flow and connectivity analyses, some of the numerous fMRI findings similar to those of schizophrenia
Fleming et al. 2019	fMRI	Psychotic symptoms did not correlate with fMRI findings
Yurgelun-Todd et al. 2020	fMRI	Increased BOLD signal in most brain regions, attenuated by phosphodiesterase inhibitor (TAK-063)

TABLE 5–2. Ketamine magnetic resonance-based neuroimaging studies in volunteers without schizophrenia *(continued)*

Study	Imaging modality	Ketamine results
Rowland et al. 2005	MRS	^{1}H-MRS: increased glutamate turnover in anterior cingulate cortex, no correlation with ketamine-induced psychopathology
Kraguljac et al. 2017	MRS	GLX changes mimic those of schizophrenia, focusing on the hippocampus (see fMRI above)
Javitt et al. 2017	MRS	No difference versus saline beyond first 15 minutes of scanning
Bojesen et al. 2018	MRS	Esketamine did not affect glutamate metabolite in anterior cingulate cortex
Abdallah et al. 2018	MRS	^{13}c-MRS: increased GLX cycling with ketamine in the prefrontal cortex, correlated with CADSS score increases

BOLD=blood oxygenation level–dependent; CADSS=Clinician-Administered Dissociative States Scale; fMRI=functional magnetic resonance imaging; GLX=glutamate-glutamine; MRS=magnetic resonance spectroscopy; NMDAR=NMDA receptor

ketamine is difficult because of the variability in methodology. Functional neuroimaging is very much influenced by whatever the volunteer is thinking about during the scan, and as can be seen from a perusal of Table 5–2, a variety of cognitive tasks were used during ketamine administration while the volunteers underwent fMRI scanning. Some of the studies seemed to find similarities between the fMRI findings in subjects taking ketamine and schizophrenia patients, but some did not. Regarding MRS, the findings of the studies were generally uncompelling and do not seem to provide much useful information for the ketamine model of schizophrenia.

Neurophysiological Outcome Measures With Ketamine

Schizophrenia researchers have looked for neurophysiologic markers, or *endophenotypes*, that reliably co-occur with the disorder or in family members of probands with schizophrenia to obtain clues to the disease's pathophysiology. A few of these have been studied in normal volunteers given ketamine to see whether there is any resemblance to the findings in people with schizophrenia. Table 5–3 lists such studies in which volunteers without schizophrenia were administered ketamine and at least one outcome measure constituted a neurophysiological parameter.

Prepulse inhibition (PPI) was examined in five studies. This phenomenon is normal and consists of the tendency of the orbicularis oculi muscle surrounding the eye to contract reflexively when a sudden auditory stimulus is presented in a repeated, unpredictable way (Parwani et al. 2000). If there is a relatively soft-toned stimulus (the prepulse) before the one causing the eye muscle contraction (essentially acting as a predictor stimulus telling the person "there is soon to follow a louder stimulus"), then the resulting eye muscle contraction is less intense. This phenomenon is normal but does not occur to the same degree in those with schizophrenia. As can be seen from four studies in Table 5–3, ketamine actually enhances PPI (that is, has an effect opposite that of schizophrenia). What to make of this, nobody knows.

Event-related potentials (ERPs) consist of EEG responses to stimuli, usually either auditory or visual. Schizophrenia is conceptualized as a disorder of information processing, and ERPs are used by neuroscientists to study preconscious information processing in the brain. The testing paradigm for ERPs is to present a defined stimulus to the participant and measure responses from an EEG lead. Usually, there are several EEG responses over time, with positive or negative deflections. For many different types of stimuli, there are multiple negative and positive ERP deflections at several time points, and some of these have been studied in schizophrenia and after ketamine administration. Table 5–3 lists a number of studies with varied results. In some studies, ketamine seems to have no effect on ERPs; in others, it has effects that mimic those of schizophrenia.

One type of ERP called *mismatch negativity (MMN)* has special relevance to the study of schizophrenia. The MMN testing paradigm consists of a visual or auditory stimulus repeatedly presented to the participant, with each one resulting in a more or less stereotyped ERP on the EEG. After a set pattern of ERPs is determined, if a different stimulus is presented (one that differs in intensity, quality, or duration from the stereotyped one), then a different ERP deflection is noted with a greater electrically negative deflection amplitude. This is called a *mismatch* because the new stimulus does not match the previous one, and *negativity* because the deflection amplitude is greater in the negative direction. MMN is a normal phenomenon that is blunted in schizophrenia, much like PPI. In normal volunteers given ketamine, the MMN effects are quite similar to those of schizophrenia (see Table 5–3). This has caused quite a bit of interest, as it may provide clues to the neurobiology of information-processing deficits in schizophrenia—namely an NMDA receptor basis for it.

TABLE 5–3.   Ketamine neurophysiological outcomes in
volunteers without schizophrenia

Study	Modality	Ketamine results
Radant et al. 1998	Eye movements	Effects on eye tracking similar to schizophrenia
Oranje et al. 2000	MMN; P300 ERPs	Did not replicate MMN findings of schizophrenia; did replicate findings of P300 ERPs and processing negativity
Umbricht et al. 2000	MMN	Blunted mismatch negativity as in schizophrenia
Weiler et al. 2000	Eye movements	Did not replicate eye movement findings in schizophrenia
Kreitschmann-Andermahr et al. 2001	MMN	Reduced mismatch negativity as in schizophrenia
Duncan et al. 2001	PPI	Enhanced prepulse inhibition, opposite of schizophrenia
Oranje et al. 2002	PPI; P50 ERPs	Did not affect PPI or P50 ERPs
Avila et al. 2002	Eye movements	Mimicked saccadic eye movement findings of schizophrenia
Umbricht et al. 2002	MMN	Preketamine MMN amplitude correlated with ketamine rise in BPRS
Abel et al. 2003b	PPI	Ketamine increased prepulse inhibition, opposite of schizophrenia
Passie et al. 2003	Binocular depth inversion	No improvement of binocular depth perception
Ahn et al. 2003	P300 ERPs	Abolished late positive component of P300
Murck et al. 2006	P200 and N100 ERPs; eye movements	Decreased the ERPs (hypericum reversed effect); did not affect eye movement tests
Knott et al. 2006	Multilead EEG	Affected multiple aspects of EEG, did not seem to resemble schizophrenia
Gouzoulis-Mayfrank et al. 2006	IOR	Normal finding was blunted, similar to schizophrenia

TABLE 5–3. Ketamine neurophysiological outcomes in volunteers without schizophrenia *(continued)*

Study	Modality	Ketamine results
Heekeren et al. 2007	PPI	PPI was increased, in contrast with schizophrenia
Boeijinga et al. 2007	Various ERPs; EEG; MEG	Diminished normal inhibition of signal amplitude after auditory stimuli
Daumann et al. 2008	IOR	No effect on IOR
Heekeren et al. 2008	MMN	Diminished MMN
Watson et al. 2009	Visual ERPs; oddball paradigm	Reduced parietal lobe ERP amplitude, uncertain significance
Oranje et al. 2009	P300; processing negativity	Lessened both ERP outcomes; haloperidol reversed effect only for processing negativity
Hong et al. 2010	Auditory ERPs	Increased gamma and decreased low-frequency oscillations, correlated with ketamine-induced negative symptoms
Horacek et al. 2010	EEG	Decreased theta cordance in prefrontal lobes; uncertain significance
Roser et al. 2011	MMN	Slightly diminished MMN latency but not amplitude; rimonabant reversed this effect
Musso et al. 2011	Visual EEG oddball paradigm; skin conductance	P300 much reduced; skin conductance increased; said to be similar to schizophrenia
Knott et al. 2011	P300 ERP	Decreased P300 ERP
Schmidt et al. 2012	MMN	Diminished MMN
Gunduz-Bruce et al. 2012	P300 ERP; auditory MMN	Diminished both, similar to schizophrenia
Schmechtig et al. 2013	Eye movements	Effects of ketamine on eye movements were different from schizophrenia's
Mathalon et al. 2014	P300; MMN	Did not reduce MMN amplitude; did reduce P300 amplitude

TABLE 5–3.   Ketamine neurophysiological outcomes in
volunteers without schizophrenia *(continued)*

Study	Modality	Ketamine results
Kleinloog et al. 2015b	PPI; eye movements	Enhanced PPI, opposite of schizophrenia; impaired various eye movements
Rivolta et al. 2015	MEG	Complex, whole-brain MEG results said to be similar to schizophrenia
de la Salle et al. 2016	EEG	Various frequency changes on EEG correlated with ketamine-induced dissociative symptoms
Steffens et al. 2016	Eye movements	Results on smooth pursuit eye movements said to be similar to schizophrenia
Koychev et al. 2017	P100 and P300 visual ERPs	P100 amplitude greater, and P300 lesser
Kort et al. 2017	N1 ERPs	Complex talk-listen paradigm with auditory ERPs: results said to be similar to schizophrenia
Grent-'t-Jong et al. 2018	MEG ERPs	Highly complex brain connectivity data different from psychotic patients
Hamilton et al. 2018	MMN	Attenuated MMN
Thiebes et al. 2017	Auditory EEG	Altered interhemispheric gamma band connectivity; proposed to be model of auditory hallucinations
Steffens et al. 2018	Eye movements	Did not induce any eye movement patterns as seen in schizophrenia
Rosch et al. 2019	MMN	Dampened MMN
Curic et al. 2019	Auditory EEG responses	Gamma band oscillation effect said to be similar to schizophrenia

BPRS=Brief Psychiatric Rating Scale; EEG=electroencephalography; ERP=event-related potential; IOR=inhibition of return; MEG=magnetoencephalography; MMN=mismatch negativity; PPI=prepulse inhibition
Note.   Capital N or P preceding a number refers to a negative (N) or positive (P) event-related potential occurring a certain number of milliseconds after the onset of a stimulus.

Eye movement analysis is an area of intense interest in schizophrenia research, as those with schizophrenia and their relatives tend to have certain abnormalities of eye movement. The paradigms are numerous and highly complicated. In general, research volunteers visually follow a stimulus moving on a screen, and special equipment connected to their eyes can track the eye movements. Ketamine replicates some aspects of these abnormalities, but not in every study, as noted in Table 5–3. The findings have not been consistent in this regard.

In a small number of other studies, other neurophysiological parameters have been studied with ketamine, such as binocular depth perception, a concept called inhibition of return, skin conductance, and various EEG and magnetoencephalography measures. Findings generally are vague and contribute little to the question of whether ketamine provides a good neurobiological model of schizophrenia.

Pharmacological Modulation of the Effects of Ketamine

One of the most substantial and practical tests of the ketamine model of schizophrenia is whether any putative antipsychotic agent that follows from that model blunts any of the effects of ketamine. In the dopamine hypothesis of schizophrenia (the dominant model for decades), dopamine receptor-blocking agents ameliorated some of the symptoms and signs of schizophrenia, mostly positive ones. For the NMDA receptor hypofunction model of schizophrenia to gain credibility, some agent that promotes NMDA receptor function should be antipsychotic. Many agents have been tested to see whether they alter ketamine's effects. These studies are listed in Table 5–4.

Nicotine has garnered substantial interest in this field because an unusual proportion of people with schizophrenia smoke; it has been hypothesized that they are self-medicating. Six studies in Table 5–4 feature nicotine administered along with ketamine, with varied results. Some of the other agents tried include clozapine, lorazepam, olanzapine, haloperidol, lamotrigine, and risperidone. These agents generally had little effect on ketamine responses. In addition, some experimental agents have been used to test the NMDA hypofunction model of psychosis within the ketamine challenge paradigm but have thus far shown little promise for clinical development.

One of the disadvantages of pharmacological modulation of ketamine challenges in normal volunteers is that usually only a single dose of the putative antipsychotic agent is administered before ketamine. In clinical psychopharmacology, daily administration of medications for days or weeks is

TABLE 5-4. Studies combining another drug with ketamine in volunteers without schizophrenia

Study	Concomitant drug	Results
Lipschitz et al. 1997	Clozapine	Clozapine (one small dose) did not blunt ketamine-induced psychopathology
Krystal et al. 1998	Lorazepam	Lorazepam reduced ketamine-induced emotional distress, did not help psychosis or cognitive effects
Lahti et al. 1999	Olanzapine	Olanzapine did not block ketamine-induced psychosis
Madonick et al. 1999	Naltrexone	Naltrexone had no effect on ketamine effects on cognition or psychopathology
Krystal et al. 1999	Haloperidol	Haloperidol mostly did not blunt ketamine-induced effects, except proverb interpretation and Wisconsin Card Sorting Task
Newcomer et al. 1999	Guanabenz	α-Adrenergic agonism with guanabenz before ketamine administration blocked effects on positive but not negative symptoms
Anand et al. 2000	Lamotrigine	Lamotrigine dampened ketamine-induced rises in positive, negative, and dissociative symptoms and cognition
Kegeles et al. 2000	Amphetamine	Ketamine enhanced amphetamine-induced striatal dopamine release but not when given alone
Krupitsky et al. 2001	Nimodipine	Nimodipine blunted ketamine-induced psychopathology and memory impairment
Oranje et al. 2002	Haloperidol	Haloperidol plus ketamine (not haloperidol alone) diminished PPI and P50 ERPs
Krystal et al. 2005a	Metabotropic glutamate receptor type 2 agonist	LY354740 reduced ketamine-induced effects on working memory but not attention, delayed recall, or psychopathology

TABLE 5–4. Studies combining another drug with ketamine in volunteers without schizophrenia *(continued)*

Study	Concomitant drug	Results
Krystal et al. 2005b	Amphetamine	Immediate memory effects of ketamine attenuated by amphetamine
Krystal et al. 2006	Naltrexone	Naltrexone had no effect on ketamine-induced mood or verbal learning effects, did blunt rise in PANSS
Murck et al. 2006	LI-160 (hypericum extract)	LI-160 reversed ketamine's effect on P200 and N100 ERPs
Knott et al. 2006	Nicotine	Nicotine did not alter ultra-low-dose ketamine effects on EEG
Deakin et al. 2008	Lamotrigine	Lamotrigine blunted some of ketamine's effects on psychopathology and fMRI
Oranje et al. 2009	Haloperidol	Haloperidol blocked ketamine's effect on processing negativity (ERP) but not P300
Rowland et al. 2010	Nicotine	Nicotine attenuated ketamine-induced BPRS rises and increased anterior cingulate blood flow
Roser et al. 2011	Rimonabant	This cannabinoid receptor antagonist altered ketamine's effects on MMN but not psychopathology
Hallak et al. 2011	Cannabidiol	This weak cannabinoid receptor agonist had no significant effect on ketamine-induced psychopathology
Knott et al. 2011	Nicotine	Nicotine partially enhanced ketamine's effect on information processing and P300
Gunduz-Bruce et al. 2012	*N*-acetyl cysteine	*N*-acetyl cysteine did not alter ketamine's effects on psychopathology, MMN, or P300 ERPs
D'Souza et al. 2012a	GlyT1 inhibitor ORG 25935	ORG 25935 reduced ketamine-induced psychopathology but not cognitive effects

TABLE 5–4. Studies combining another drug with ketamine in volunteers without schizophrenia *(continued)*

Study	Concomitant drug	Results
D'Souza et al. 2012b	Nicotine	Nicotine did not diminish ketamine-induced psychopathology or cognitive effects
Schmechtig et al. 2013	Risperidone	Risperidone did not reduce ketamine effects on psychopathology or eye movements
Doyle et al. 2013	Lamotrigine; risperidone	Both drugs attenuated ketamine's effects on fMRI
Mathalon et al. 2014	Nicotine	Nicotine did not blunt any ketamine effect on psychopathology or event-related potentials
Shcherbinin et al. 2015	Lamotrigine; risperidone	Same sample as Doyle et al. 2013; lamotrigine did not affect ketamine's effect on fMRI, but risperidone increased it
Joules et al. 2015	Lamotrigine; risperidone	Further discussion of samples reported in Doyle et al. 2013 and Shcherbinin et al. 2015
Ranganathan et al. 2017	AMPAR potentiator PF-04958242	Reversed ketamine's effects on cognition but not psychopathology
D'Souza et al. 2018	GlyT1 transporter inhibitor PF-03463275	Did not attenuate cognitive or fMRI effects of ketamine
Hamilton et al. 2018	Nicotine	Nicotine did not attenuate the ketamine effect on MMN
Yurgelun-Todd et al. 2020	Phosphodiesterase 10A inhibitor TAK-063	Attenuated ketamine's effects on fMRI

AMPAR=α-amino-3-hydroxy-5-methyl-4-isoxazolepropionic acid receptor; BPRS=Brief Psychiatric Rating Scale; EEG=electroencephalography; ERP=event-related potential; fMRI=functional magnetic resonance imaging; MMN=mismatch negativity; PANSS=Positive and Negative Syndrome Scale; PPI=prepulse inhibition
Note. Capital N or P preceding a number refers to a negative (N) or positive (P) event-related potential occurring a certain number of milliseconds after the onset of a stimulus.

usually necessary to achieve the desired effect. Just because one dose of a medication does not blunt subsequent ketamine-induced psychotic symptoms does not necessarily mean that a more persistent regimen would not accomplish more.

Assessing the Ketamine Challenge Literature

Has the ketamine challenge model been a success? The answer of course depends on the definition of success. At the most practical level, success may be defined by the number of papers published or grants obtained. There have been a lot of these, so according to this definition, the ketamine challenge model has indeed been very successful, and many research neuroscientists and psychiatrists have furthered their careers with it. A more salient definition of success, however, concerns whether the ketamine challenge model has improved the lives of people with schizophrenia; in this regard, the model has been a failure. No treatments have flowed directly from the ketamine-NMDA receptor hypofunction model of psychosis.

Has the model led to any confident knowledge of the pathophysiology of schizophrenia? If it has, better treatments might still be on the horizon. I am skeptical, however, that the ketamine model has led to such knowledge. It seems more prudent to say that it has allowed sophisticated neuroscientists to elaborate and fine-tune their thinking and hypothesizing, and to circle their wagons (so to speak) around certain notions (such as the theory that schizophrenia represents failure of the dentate gyrus of the hippocampus). However, pretty much every technology used to study any aspect of neurological function in schizophrenia has been abnormal, which hardly inspires confidence in our understanding of the pathophysiology of this condition.

Chapter 6

Ketamine for Chronic Pain

KEY POINTS IN THIS CHAPTER:

- Ketamine has been used to treat a variety of chronic pain syndromes.

- Acute reductions in subjectively reported pain occur with ketamine but are often transient.

- Whether ketamine can enhance function in chronic pain patients is unknown.

As we've learned, early investigators of ketamine quickly realized its potent analgesic (pain-reducing) activity. Anesthesiologists put this analgesic quality to good use in the management of acute pain syndromes and thus administered ketamine before, during, and after surgery to combat surgical pain and also before painful procedures such as suturing a wound, changing a burn dressing, and many others. Ketamine for acute pain is almost always given to hospitalized patients for surgery or in the emergency department to assist with painful procedures (see Schwenk et al. 2018a for a concise consensus review).

In contrast to acute pain, chronic pain refers to long-standing pain syndromes, typically lasting months, years, or even decades. Patients with chronic pain are often highly refractory to multiple interventions, and thus, the field of pain medicine has been quite hungry for alternatives over the years. Given ketamine's excellent efficacy in acute pain, it was only a matter

TABLE 6–1.   Chronic pain syndromes

Chronic arthritic pain
Chronic low back pain
Complex regional pain syndrome (Types I and II)
Fibromyalgia
Intractable headache (e.g., migraine, cluster)
Neuropathic pain
Orofacial pain (e.g., temporomandibular joint pain, trigeminal neuralgia, glossopharyngeal neuralgia)
Painful limb ischemia
Phantom limb pain
Postherpetic neuralgia
Post–spinal cord injury pain
Post-stroke thalamic pain
Post-whiplash injury pain

of time before practitioners began wondering whether ketamine could effectively treat chronic pain.

Table 6–1 lists some of the more common chronic pain syndromes, of which there are many. Most of these will be at least somewhat familiar. Mention should be made of *complex regional pain syndrome (CRPS)*, which brings together several types of chronic pain into a single category. The essential feature of CRPS is persistence of pain beyond an initial pain-triggering event, such as an injury, illness, or surgery. CRPS often involves a limb and starts with one of the triggers listed and persists even after the initial wound heals. Associated features include vascular insufficiency manifesting with edema, autonomic nervous system dysfunction such as excessive sweating, and skin trophic changes. The two types of CRPS are Type I (no neuropathic component) and Type II (neuropathic component, meaning some type of nerve damage). Many of the studies on ketamine in chronic pain involve CRPS patients. If the neuropathic pain syndrome source is an ongoing known pathophysiological process (such as diabetes mellitus or amyloidosis), then the diagnosis is neuropathic pain.

Also worth mentioning is *shingles*, a disease of the herpes zoster virus in people who had chickenpox as children. The virus lives and stays dormant in the dorsal root ganglia of the spinal cord; decades later in adult life, for unknown reasons, it can become activated and travel down the peripheral nerves all the way to the skin, causing painful blisters and sometimes persistent pain even when the skin lesions clear up, a condition called *postherpetic neuralgia*. This can be a debilitating condition for some people.

With the wide variety of chronic pain syndromes, the question arises whether ketamine has equal efficacy for all of them or selective efficacy for a subset of them. A further related question is whether the pathophysiology of pain for these syndromes occurs with a unitary final common pathway in the central nervous system or is heterogeneous. The answers to these questions are not known.

Chronic pain manifests with several types of symptoms. Of course, the most common and easily understood is spontaneous, unprovoked pain. This is the pain that people complain of at rest without any stimulus to induce pain. Spontaneous pain is often rated by patients on a visual analog scale (VAS), which is a line drawn on a piece of paper, with the left end corresponding to absence of pain and the right end corresponding to the most severe pain they can imagine. The patient is instructed to mark an X somewhere along the line. The distance from the left end to the X is then taken as the rating. Such measures can then be subjected to statistical analysis when part of a study or to track an individual patient's progress in routine clinical care. Presumably, with effective treatment over time, the patient's X is closer and closer to the left end of the line. Another method of rating spontaneous pain is the numerical pain rating (NPR), which is a rating on a whole-number scale from 0 (absence of pain) to 10 (worst pain imaginable), as with the VAS but in increments of whole numbers. NPR values can also be subjected to statistical analysis in studies of pain intervention efficacy.

Other more subtle manifestations of chronic pain include allodynia, hyperalgesia, and wind-up. *Allodynia* means the experience of pain to a stimulus that normally does not cause pain, such as brushing skin with a cotton swab. *Hyperalgesia* means excessive pain response to a normally painful stimulus such as heat or a needle point. *Wind-up* is an interesting phenomenon whereby a repetitive stimulus, such as tapping a part of the skin, causes increasing pain as the tapping continues. It is a manifestation of exaggerated temporal summation of a stimulus. These various aspects of chronic pain can be tested through quantitative sensory testing (QST) techniques that are a bit beyond the scope of this book. Suffice it to say here that with ketamine, the most substantial improvements in pain in chronic pain patients—the ones most felt by patients and the ones most statistically significant in the studies of ketamine for chronic pain—are spontaneous pain as rated by VAS or NPR and not the specific other types of pain measured by QST.

Chronic pain patients develop secondary complications such as psychiatric disorders (mostly anxiety and depression), cessation of work and disability status, dropping out of school, failure to attending household responsibilities and caring for others such as children or elderly parents, and dropping out of social and recreational activities. These are probably the most devastating consequences of chronic pain and the most resistant to intervention. Thus, any goal of treatment should go beyond mere symptom reduction. In fact, a good question is whether sustained symptom reduction can, in itself, cause a reversal of the secondary complications. If that is to be the case for a patient with years of disability, then the symptom reduction probably has to be long lasting to result in improvements in daily function (not just an hour or two after infusion of a drug). This point is quite relevant to the literature on ketamine for chronic pain.

An additional reason to try ketamine for chronic pain emanated from a series of findings that began in the early 1980s from a group in England headed by the neuroscientist David Lodge and colleagues (see Lodge 2009 for a thorough review of this topic); earlier in Chapter 5, we discussed his discovery that ketamine blocks NMDA receptors. The essence of these laboratory animal studies was that in experimental models of chronic pain, upregulation of NMDA receptors seemed to be involved, a process blocked by administration of ketamine. Thus, a basic science rationale for use of ketamine in humans with chronic pain was born. The totality of this complex set of syndromes surely is not explained solely by NMDA receptors. But some role of NMDA receptors in chronic pain in animal models seems well established, and the study of ketamine for chronic pain constitutes rational pharmacotherapy.

The Main Literature on Ketamine for Chronic Pain

Ketamine for chronic pain has generated enormous interest. Here I review those that represent the basic methodologies and findings. As is the case with most of the other topics related to ketamine in this book, the story here really begins with PCP, in a case report by Kurtzke (1961) of a patient with post-stroke thalamic pain successfully treated with PCP, the analgesic properties of which had become known. However, the use of PCP for chronic pain never gained popularity (for obvious reasons, as we've seen), and that lone case report seems to have been the end of it. Two decades later, Mankowitz et al. (1982) described several patients with a variety of chronic pain syndromes treated with epidural ketamine. That appears to be the first mention of ketamine for chronic pain, albeit with a route of administration that is not clinically practical.

One descriptor is particularly apropos of this large literature: heterogeneous. It is heterogeneous in patient population (more than a dozen different syndromes treated with ketamine), in mode of delivery and dosing (IV versus other routes, small versus high doses, single versus multiple doses), and in study design (randomized versus open-label, outcome measure variance, short-term versus long-term efficacy).

Most of the studies had patients rate severity of pain at baseline via VAS or NPR. Then ketamine was administered (either open-label in the studies without controls or in comparison to placebo or active controls such as lidocaine or alfentanil [a potent opioid] in the controlled, randomized studies), and the pain rating was obtained again. Ketamine almost always was associated with lowering of the pain scores acutely in the open-label studies and in a greater magnitude than with placebo (or at least equal to an active control) in the randomized studies. Again, this pertains to acute response— that is, response right after the administration of ketamine.

The question of how long these responses last has been broached by a few studies. The literature began with the report by Mankowitz et al. (1982) cited earlier, but was stagnant until the mid-1990s, when a great rush occurred. To grasp what has been learned about ketamine in this population, I discuss several dimensions: type of chronic pain syndrome studied, randomization versus open-label design, route of administration, use of intense ketamine dosing, follow-up assessments to see how long ketamine's effects last, and use of serial ketamine dosing to prevent relapse.

Type of Chronic Pain Syndrome

The majority of reports involved CRPS Type I or II or neuropathic pain. Several of the reports had mixed or unspecified pain syndromes. A smattering of other syndromes are represented, such as postherpetic neuralgia, chronic intractable headaches, post–spinal cord injury pain, phantom limb pain, and ischemic limb pain. Generally, the reports for all of these were positive, in the sense that a sufferer was given a dose of ketamine and acutely indicated that pain intensity lessened. There is no indication from this literature of superior efficacy for ketamine for any particular type of chronic pain syndrome.

Randomized, Controlled Studies

Almost all of the IV studies comparing ketamine to placebo or another analgesic found ketamine to cause acute reductions in pain of a greater intensity than placebo and at least equal reduction as active control (sometimes greater). The main questions concern how long the analgesic effects last and whether they translate into functional improvement, and few studies broached these two questions. A few of the representative controlled trials of ketamine for chronic pain are reviewed next.

Eide et al. (1994) studied eight patients with postherpetic neuralgia in a crossover study comparing ketamine, morphine, and placebo. Ketamine was administered at 0.15 mg/kg over 10 minutes, a very low dose, but interestingly with good analgesic effect—better than with the other two groups. No follow-up was undertaken beyond acute assessments of pain reduction at the time of infusion.

Backonja et al. (1994), in a randomized, crossover trial, compared ketamine 0.25 mg/kg IV push to placebo injections in six patients with chronic neuropathic pain. Five of the six had an acute pain reduction with ketamine and not with placebo.

Eide et al. (1995a) treated nine patients with post–spinal cord injury pain in randomized, crossover fashion with ketamine bolus of 0.06 mg/kg followed by 0.006 mg/kg/min for 17–21 minutes, saline, or alfentanil. Ketamine with these very low doses did offer acute pain reduction, but there was no follow-up.

Sörensen et al. (1995) randomized 31 patients with fibromyalgia to ketamine 0.3 mg/kg over 10 minutes ($n=11$), lidocaine ($n=11$), or morphine ($n=9$), with each group having one injection of active drug and one with placebo in randomized, crossover manner. Ketamine bested placebo for up to 90 minutes post-injection.

Max et al. (1995) treated eight patients with chronic posttraumatic pain once each with placebo, alfentanil, and ketamine infused over 2 hours with a mean dose of 58 mg. Analgesia occurred with ketamine only after onset of unpleasant side effects, the latter of which outlasted the analgesia and included visual distortion, sedation, and distorted bodily sensations (e.g., of a limb not belonging). Thus, the authors were not sanguine about the role of ketamine in treating chronic pain.

Nikolajsen et al. (1996) treated 11 patients with phantom limb pain, in randomized crossover fashion, with ketamine 0.415 mg/kg over 45 minutes versus placebo infusion. Pain relief was superior with ketamine and lasted up to 24 hours in a few of the patients.

Persson et al. (1998) used IV ketamine in eight patients with chronic ischemic limb pain and randomly compared it to morphine. Ketamine was given at 0.15, 0.30, or 0.45 mg/kg over 10 minutes. All doses of ketamine helped pain acutely in a dose-dependent manner, and better than morphine, but the effects lasted only about an hour.

Graven-Nielsen et al. (2000) studied 29 patients with fibromyalgia in crossover manner, each patient receiving one session of ketamine 0.3 mg/kg over 30 minutes and one session with placebo. Seventeen of the 29 patients responded acutely to ketamine in terms of pain reduction, better than with placebo, but there was no follow-up.

Leung et al. (2001) studied 12 patients with chronic pain (6 with Type I CRPS, 1 with Type II CRPS, 4 with postherpetic neuralgia, and 1 with post–spinal cord injury pain). Each subject received three infusions at different sessions in randomized, crossover fashion: ketamine, alfentanil, and diphenhydramine (an anticholinergic used as active placebo). Ketamine doses were not specified, but they were designed to achieve blood levels of 50, 100, and 150 ng/mL at different times during the ketamine session based on previously published data on dose–blood level relationships. Both ketamine and alfentanil caused acute reductions in pain. No follow-up data were obtained.

Mitchell and Fallon (2002) treated 35 patients with ischemic limb pain with either ketamine plus opioids (*n*=18) or placebo plus opioids (*n*=17). Ketamine was administered as a single infusion of 0.6 mg/kg over 4 hours. Assessments of pain were undertaken 1 and 5 days later. Ketamine's analgesic effects were sustained over this time. Of note, anxiety and depression ratings, something rarely measured in chronic pain studies, improved with ketamine but not placebo.

Kvarnström et al. (2003) compared ketamine, lidocaine, and placebo in 12 patients with neuropathic pain in a randomized, crossover trial. Ketamine was given at 0.4 mg/kg over 40 minutes. Ketamine's benefit was present at 40 minutes but lost at 60 minutes, indicating only short-term efficacy. Notably, placebo infusions were associated with 22% drops in pain scores, highlighting the high placebo responsivity of chronic pain.

Jørum et al. (2003) studied 12 patients with neuropathic pain. Each patient, in randomized crossover manner, received one session each of 20 minutes of ketamine, alfentanil, or placebo solution. The ketamine dose was a 0.06 mg/kg bolus followed by 20 minutes of 0.006 mg/kg/min. This is a very small dose of ketamine. At any rate, ketamine and alfentanil caused equal reductions in pain acutely, greater than did placebo, but no follow-up was undertaken.

Kvarnström et al. (2004) treated 10 patients with post–spinal cord injury pain with 0.4 mg/kg ketamine over 40 minutes versus placebo and lidocaine in randomized crossover manner. The analgesic effect acutely (over 2.5 hours) was greater with ketamine than with the other two treatments. No further follow-up was undertaken. Side effects were common and included somnolence, dizziness, out-of-body experiences, and visual disturbances.

Lemming et al. (2005) randomized, in crossover manner, 33 patients with chronic whiplash-related pain to infusions of ketamine 0.3 mg/kg over 30 minutes compared to lidocaine, morphine, and placebo—thus, each patient had four sessions. All three active groups beat placebo for acute pain reduction, but no follow-up was obtained.

Gottrup et al. (2006) treated 20 patients with nerve injury pain with lidocaine or 0.24 mg/kg ketamine over 30 minutes and found acutely reduced pain in both groups. No follow-up was undertaken.

Eichenberger et al. (2008) studied 20 patients with phantom limb pain. Each received four infusions in randomized, crossover fashion: calcitonin, ketamine 0.4 mg/kg (10 patients), both calcitonin and ketamine, and placebo. Calcitonin is thought to have analgesic activity but did not in this study. Only patients receiving ketamine, which was infused over 1 hour, had analgesic effects on spontaneous pain. The effect lasted approximately 48 hours.

Noppers et al. (2011) randomized 24 patients with fibromyalgia to one 30-minute infusion of either 5 mg midazolam (a short-acting benzodiazepine) or 0.5 mg/kg esketamine. Fifteen minutes after infusion, there was a significantly greater drop in acute pain scores in the esketamine group, a difference lost at 8-week follow-up, at which time there was no longer an analgesic effect of either drug.

Niesters et al. (2014) randomized 10 patients with unspecified chronic pain syndromes in a crossover manner to one session each of placebo, morphine, and esketamine, the latter at 0.57 mg/kg over 60 minutes IV. Spontaneous pain relief was greatest with esketamine at 100 minutes, and the total duration of pain relief with that drug lasted 6–12 hours. Quantitative sensory testing, via pain threshold with a heat stimulus, was not differentially affected by the three treatment conditions.

Kim et al. (2015) randomized 30 patients with postherpetic neuralgia to ketamine 1.0 mg/kg IV over 60 minutes or magnesium infusions as a control, because some data had suggested that magnesium infusions might treat chronic pain. The infusions were administered every other day for a total of three infusions. Two weeks after the third infusion, 10 of 15 in the ketamine group had at least a 50% reduction in pain ratings, better than with magnesium. (No ratings were taken immediately after the infusions, interestingly, in spite of how easy it would have been.)

In summary, the studies virtually all show significant acute pain reductions with ketamine, and usually better than with placebo or other medications commonly used to treat pain such as opioids or lidocaine. Side effects are common and cluster into vestibular (dizziness, nausea) and psychotomimetic (dissociative states, hallucinations). The main questions concern how long the effects last, as most of the studies involve only short-term pain assessment (i.e., day of infusion), whether pain reductions translate into better daily function, and of course long-term safety. Additionally, it is interesting to speculate on the mechanism of pain reduction with ketamine. Is it a true primary analgesic effect mediated via the complex pain processing systems of the central nervous system? Or does ketamine simply cause patients to be more psychologically comfortable and relaxed (or on a drug high, if one prefers that term), an effect that in turn translates into reduced self-reported pain scores? For example, if patients in chronic pain take commonly abused drugs, such as alcohol, benzodiazepines, or marijuana, and get high enough, would they similarly report less pain for a while?

Route of Administration

IV administration of ketamine is the gold standard: it gives 100% bioavailability. However, it does have inconveniences, such as the pain and anxiety of establishing IV access (some people hate needles) and the cost of having to monitor patients' oxygenation and heart rate during and for a while after each infusion. Also, for patients requiring serial administrations of ketamine to sustain initial analgesic benefits, IV infusions are time-consuming. Thus, especially in the chronic pain literature where mostly outpatient care is offered, attempts have been made to use alternative routes of administration. In this section, we consider these and some salient points from the literature. As far as the IV route is concerned, dozens of reports show good acute pain reduction using typical doses of less than 1.0 mg/kg infused over a few minutes, up to an hour or so. More intensive regimens have been attempted and will be discussed a bit later in this chapter.

The IM route has been used to good advantage (Hoffmann et al. 1994; Klepstad and Borchgrevink 1997; Øye et al. 1996) and should probably be explored more aggressively in the pain medicine community. It involves much less time commitment on the part of patient and practitioner (one shot as opposed to long-lasting IV infusions), guarantees good bioavailability (greater than 90%), can be used serially, is administered under controlled circumstances in the clinic (patients do not have their own supply), and is cheaper than IV use.

Topical ketamine (applied to the skin) appears to be popular among pain physicians, probably owing to its ease of application and the absence of needles. Medications applied to the skin work in one of two ways: either they are absorbed systemically into the bloodstream (examples of this include nicotine patches for cigarette withdrawal or fentanyl patches for pain) or they work at the level of the skin (lidocaine being an excellent example). Studies of topical ketamine for chronic pain syndromes have reported varying levels of success (see Sawynok 2014 for a review). As one example, Mahoney et al. (2012) randomly assigned 17 patients with painful diabetic neuropathy to 1 month of placebo cream or 5% ketamine cream daily and found no difference in results, although both groups had reductions in pain, once again illustrating the prominent placebo responsiveness of chronic pain syndromes.

In topical ketamine studies in which blood levels were obtained, levels were undetectable (Finch et al. 2009; Lynch et al. 2005), indicating that no significant systemic absorption occurs with topically applied ketamine. Thus, if there is a plausible mechanism for this application of ketamine, it must work at the level of the peripheral nerve ending, which is highly suspect given the central mechanisms of chronic pain. There are four ways it could possibly work on pain if no blood levels could be detected: 1) placebo; 2) a different component of the ointment is really causing the analgesia and ketamine is doing nothing; 3) ketamine works at the level of the peripheral nerve ending; or 4) ketamine is absorbed into neurons at the level of the peripheral nerve ending and travels up the axon to the level of the spine. The fourth of these was mentioned in passing by Poterucha et al. (2012) but seems unlikely as a plausible mechanism.

Sawynok (2014), in a review of the use of ketamine as a topical agent, provided possible explanations for why ketamine would confer analgesia intradermally: blockade of NMDA receptors on peripheral nerve terminals as well as other receptor actions (e.g., monoamine and opioid receptors) and anti-inflammatory activity. Sawynok did acknowledge that all these are speculative and admitted that more research is needed if topical application of ketamine is to be taken seriously. She pointed out that several of the randomized, controlled studies of topically applied ketamine in chronic pain show no difference in efficacy between ketamine and placebo.

The oral/sublingual route is obviously attractive in that no needles are needed and patients could potentially take ketamine at home, if that is deemed safe from a compliance/abuse standpoint. Oral refers to swallowing ketamine into the digestive tract, where it is absorbed in the intestines and goes straight to the liver, where it undergoes first-pass metabolism to its main metabolite, which is norketamine. The sublingual route refers to placing ketamine under the tongue for absorption there into the bloodstream. Investigators have attempted to use oral ketamine in one of two ways. The first is simply taking liquid ketamine in vials meant for IV use and swallowing it (it reportedly tastes quite bad). The other is to formulate special ketamine lozenges that can be sucked on or swallowed (and which do not taste so bad). Using the latter method, for example, Chong et al. (2009) administered 25 mg ketamine lozenges formulated in the hospital pharmacy in six patients with neuropathic pain and then followed blood levels of ketamine and norketamine. Patients either swallowed the lozenge (oral route) or had it placed under the tongue for sublingual absorption. Bioavailability (the proportion of a dose of ketamine that reaches systemic circulation, with the IV route being defined as 100% bioavailable) was identical for both routes at 24%, which is quite low. Thus, most of an oral or sublingual dose is either not absorbed or is rapidly metabolized to norketamine. Unfortunately, no pain outcome data were obtained in the Chong et al. (2009) study, which was a real missed opportunity.

Blonk et al. (2010) reviewed the oral ketamine for chronic pain literature (22 reports) and noted that it consists mostly of open-label case series describing what appear to be good results in some patients. In summary, several reports indicated that oral ketamine can be well tolerated if used in daily doses, and a significant number of patients reported good pain control. Most of the data are nonrandomized and noncontrolled, so placebo mechanisms are probably at work to a significant degree. Also, again, the bioavailability of ketamine is quite low when administered orally. Whether the main metabolite of ketamine, norketamine, has any analgesic efficacy is unknown.

An outstanding question is whether daily administration of ketamine increases risk of ulcerative cystitis. Its use must be viewed with caution, in my opinion. Also, of course, if patients use their own supply of ketamine, the chances of abuse and addiction go way up. Daily use of ketamine, for weeks or months, might have significant cognitive effects, and this issue has not been sufficiently explored. Thus, again, much more work needs to be done to establish the safety, efficacy, and need for daily oral ketamine use. Good controlled research with large sample sizes and monitoring for toxicity must be conducted before this route of administration can be recommended for routine use.

Some investigative groups have attempted to insert a needle or catheter into subcutaneous fat (usually in the abdominal wall area) as a way of giving one-time or prolonged infusions of ketamine in a manner more convenient than IV. Cohen et al. (2018) reported 75%–95% bioavailability with this route. In most of the reports, patients with chronic pain experienced analgesic benefit, but in some cases the infusions had to be stopped after a few days or so because of inflammation or induration (hardening of tissues) around the catheter site (Eide et al. 1995b; Hoffmann et al. 1994; Mitchell 2001).

Two reports involved intranasally applied ketamine in chronic pain (Carr et al. 2004; Huge et al. 2010) with apparent analgesic efficacy. Intranasal ketamine has the advantages of not involving needles, potentially being used at home if that is deemed appropriate, lack of first-pass metabolism to norketamine, and quick absorption into the brain circulation from nasal mucosa (Kushwaha et al. 2011). Yanagihara et al. (2003) found a bioavailability of ~45% with intranasal ketamine, obviously much lower than for IV use. If chronic pain demanded higher-intensity doses and more intense, essentially continuous administration methods, that is probably not possible intranasally: intense regimens would not be absorbed well, and much of the drug would simply be sneezed out or swallowed. There is a patented intranasal esketamine formulation (Spravato) approved for major depression, but it remains to be seen whether it will be used for chronic pain as well.

Studies Using Intense Ketamine Dosing Schemes

One of the frustrations of trying to summarize the ketamine for chronic pain literature is the vast heterogeneity of dosing schemes used—the doses are all over the map! In some studies, some fraction of a milligram of ketamine per kilogram of body weight is used (say 0.10 to 0.5 mg/kg or thereabouts) and is administered over 30 minutes or so, whereas other studies use continuous infusions going on for days or longer. There seems to be a signal indicating that stronger dosing schemes for ketamine may yield better acute outcomes as well as longer-lasting results. Although the word "intense" is arbitrary, a working definition for ketamine would include a continuous infusion beyond 4 hours or so, or a closely spaced set of serial daily infusions, for some days (rather than one infusion on one day only). Using this admittedly rather loose definition, studies using intense dosing schemes are listed in Table 6–2. Not included in this table are long-term, intense oral ketamine regimens, which I do not consider a realistic or advisable way to prescribe ketamine, at least at this time. Also not included are topical ketamine studies, and no intense dosing schemes using intramuscular ketamine. That leaves mostly IV and a few subcutaneous studies.

In Table 6–2, basic data are provided about dosing schemes. Good analgesia was reported with ketamine in general. In some reports, the duration of the infusion was fixed; in others, the infusions were individualized for each patient to achieve optimal analgesia. Side effects were common, including dissociation and dizziness. Rates of infusion could be adjusted accordingly. In some cases, infusions did not last beyond a few hours each but were repeated daily for some days and thus are considered intense for our purposes.

In this discussion on intense ketamine dosing schemes, special mention goes to the report by Kiefer et al. (2008a), in which a series of 20 patients with CRPS were actually admitted to an intensive care unit and anesthetized with up to 7 mg/kg/hour ketamine continuously (while being mechanically ventilated)—for 5 days! All patients were said to be completely remitted at 1 month, and at 3 and 6 months only a few (3 or 4) had relapsed. If valid, this study suggests that a highly intense exposure to ketamine can cause lasting beneficial neuroplastic changes in chronic pain patients.

Scrutiny of the outcomes seems to indicate greater acute pain relief and also possibly longer-lasting duration with these intense regimens, but desperately needed are studies in which patients are randomized into two or more dosing schedules of ketamine (intense versus non-intense) to confirm this impression.

Follow-Up Period

Several studies followed patients to see how long the initial analgesic benefit of ketamine lasted. Table 6–3 presents studies in which some type of follow-up outcome was presented. The dosing schemes of ketamine, as has

TABLE 6–2.   Intense dosing regimens of ketamine for chronic pain

Nicolodi and Sicuteri 1995	SQ injections 3/day for 3 weeks; 0.08 mg/kg per injection
Correll et al. 2004	Continuous infusions averaging 4.7 days; 10–30 mg/h
Good et al. 2005	Continuous infusions (median of 5 days, range 3–17); 100–700 mg/day
Goldberg et al. 2005	10 daily 4-h infusions; 40–80 mg/infusion
Webster and Walker 2006	Continuous infusions of 5–55 days; 0.12 mg/kg/h
Guedj et al. 2007	10-day continuous SQ infusion; up to 100 mg/day
Kiefer et al. 2008b	10-day continuous esketamine infusions; 50–500 mg/day
Kiefer et al. 2008a	5-day continuous general anesthesia with esketamine; up to 7 mg/kg/h
Sigtermans et al. 2009	4.2-day continuous infusion; mean dosing of 0.32 mg/kg/h
Schwartzman et al. 2009	10 daily infusions of 4 h/day at 0.35 mg/kg/h
Goldberg et al. 2010/2011	5-day continuous infusions; 10–40 mg/h
Amr 2010	Daily 5-h infusions for 1 week; 80 mg IV per infusion
Dahan et al. 2011	100-hour continuous infusion (esketamine); 0.0072–0.0432 mg/kg/h
Quinlan 2012	5-day continuous infusions; dose per day not specified
Salas et al. 2012	2-day continuous infusions; 0.5 mg/kg on day 1, 1.0 mg/kg on day 2
Polomano et al. 2013	3-day continuous infusions; up to 0.12 mg/kg/h
Douglas et al. 2015	5-day continuous infusions; 10–40 mg/h
Goebel et al. 2015	4.5-day continuous infusions; 0.15–0.9 mg/kg/h
Sheehy et al. 2015	0.1–0.3 mg/kg/h for 4–8 h on each of 3 consecutive days
Pomeroy et al. 2017	Continuous infusions mean of 4.8 days; mean rate of 0.53 mg/kg/h
Zekry et al. 2016	3–7-day continuous SQ infusions; mean = 6.1 days; 4–32 mg/h
Crumb et al. 2018	4-hour infusions up to 140 mg/h, administered 4 times over several weeks
Schwenk et al. 2018b	5-day continuous infusions, up to 1 mg/kg/h (mean 43.7 mg/h)

IV=intravenous; SQ=subcutaneous.

been emphasized, were quite variable, as was the period of follow-up. For example, if a particular study had a follow-up assessment at 2 weeks but nothing further, then we cannot infer any benefit beyond that time point. However, taking into account the massive heterogeneity of studies, the reports in Table 6–3 indicate that in some cases there is substantial analgesia lasting days, weeks, or even months after initial ketamine administration, mostly in studies that used what we have defined as intensive ketamine dosing. Outcome data are almost exclusively patient-reported pain and not functional capacity in activities of daily living, so we don't know whether patients reporting long-term analgesia actually experienced increased functionality in day-to-day life.

Studies Using Longitudinal Ketamine Dosing Schemes to Prevent Relapse

A number of investigators have attempted to prolong the period of analgesia after an initial ketamine administration by using ongoing dosing schemes. Most consist of daily oral ketamine strategies; a few groups used serial IV dosing schemes (Crumb et al. 2018; Kapural et al. 2010; Kim et al. 2015; Patil and Anitescu 2012). It is not clear from the reports whether the serial dosing maintains initial analgesic gains over and above the benefits of only the initial dose. In other words, randomized studies are needed in which chronic pain patients initially receive some type of ketamine dosing (preferably IV), and then half the patients receive intermittent placebo infusions and the other half receive an equal frequency of ketamine infusions. Additionally, given the uncertainty about duration of action of a ketamine infusion, the optimal frequency of serial infusions needs to be investigated. Should the infusions be every week? Every 2 weeks? Longer intervals? Finally, tolerability and safety issues with serial dosing are understudied. Such complications as liver toxicity, ulcerative cystitis, and cognitive decrement need to be monitored.

Regarding the latter, two ketamine data sets did examine cognitive testing. Koffler et al. (2007) reported neuropsychological testing from the study by Kiefer et al. (2008a), whereby chronic pain patients were anesthetized for 5 consecutive days with ketamine. Nine of the patients had cognitive testing before the 5-day therapy and 6 weeks later. Thorough testing revealed no changes induced by the aggressive anesthetic therapy, although two patients did experience flashbacks requiring treatment with the benzodiazepine lorazepam. Kim et al. (2016) divided 30 patients with CRPS into two groups: those who had a large number of ketamine infusions in the past 6 months ($n=14$, mean of 41.7 infusions) versus those who had only a few such infusions during the same time period ($n=16$, mean of 2.9 infusions).

TABLE 6–3.   Follow-up studies of the analgesic benefit of ketamine

Nicolodi and Sicuteri 1995	Four of 17 acute ketamine responders had sustained analgesia at 3 weeks
Sator-Katzenschlager et al. 2001	After intensive intrathecal ketamine, analgesia lasted up to 6 weeks
Mitchell and Fallon 2002	After one ketamine infusion, analgesia lasted ≤5 days
Correll et al. 2004	Several patients given multiday infusions had several months pain free
Webster and Walker 2006	Initial analgesia with ketamine lasted at least a month in about half the patients
Kiefer et al. 2008a	20 patients given anesthetic doses of ketamine for 5 days: complete remission in all patients at 1 month, 17 at 3 months, and 16 at 6 months
Sigtermans et al. 2009	Difference between esketamine and placebo at 1 week lost by 12 weeks
Schwartzman et al. 2009	Difference between ketamine and placebo was sustained over more than 12 weeks
Amr 2010	Difference between ketamine and placebo sustained at 2 weeks but not after
Kapural et al. 2010	A series of ketamine infusions induced analgesia that did not last beyond the immediate aftermath of each infusion; pain no different at 6 months
Noppers et al. 2011	After one 30-min infusion, significant difference with placebo only at 15 min; no difference at 8 weeks
Dahan et al. 2011	Up to 7 weeks of analgesia after one 100-hour esketamine infusion
Patil and Anitescu 2012	Half of those given one infusion had relief of ≤3 weeks
Quinlan 2012	3 of 11 initial ketamine responders had sustained benefit at 6 months
Kim et al. 2015	10 of 15 acute ketamine responders had sustained benefit at 2 weeks
Pomeroy et al. 2017	15 of 55 acute ketamine responders had sustained relief at 1 month
Granata et al. 2016	Ketamine-induced analgesia lasted 3–18 months in 29 patients
Schwenk et al. 2018b	40% of initial responders had a sustained benefit at 30 days

Note.   Only studies without ongoing ketamine administration.

Neuropsychological testing, focused on tests of sustained and divided attention and freedom from distraction, was conducted on all patients. The frequent infusion group performed less well than did the infrequent infusion group, although no patients demonstrated frank cognitive impairment. The authors cautioned that frequent, closely spaced ketamine infusions may have some effects on cognition, though no baseline testing was done to see whether indeed there was a change induced by ketamine.

Ketamine abuse and dependence are always concerns, especially with daily oral regimens. For ketamine to be considered standard of care in chronic pain medicine, much work needs to be done to elaborate the safest and most effective combination of dosing parameters. An interesting question regarding ketamine for pain is whether treatment of an acute pain syndrome with ketamine prevents the pain from becoming chronic. Three data sets indicated that this does not happen (Dualé et al. 2009; Mendola et al. 2012; Wilson et al. 2008).

Commentaries, Reviews, and Meta-Analyses

Cohen et al. (2018), on behalf of three large professional organizations (the American Society of Regional Anesthesia and Pain Medicine, the American Academy of Pain Medicine, and the American Society of Anesthesiologists), published a set of consensus guidelines on ketamine for chronic pain. This very thoughtful and well-referenced document takes a conservative approach, as most consensus statements do. The authors support using ketamine for chronic pain syndromes but with conservative (i.e., nonintensive) dosing regimens using IV therapy in refractory cases, again with low certainty and the strong need for more homogeneous and controlled data sets. Azari et al. (2012) wrote a systematic review with similar caution about whether ketamine was ready for routine use. Pickering and McCabe (2014) wrote a commentary essentially agreeing with the others that the data so far are interesting but that safety in chronic pain, especially with intense and serial regimens, is not yet established. Connolly et al. (2015) wrote a systematic review saying the evidence was of low quality. Zhao et al. (2018) published a meta-analysis and said the evidence for short-term efficacy was good but that higher quality studies were needed. Aiyer et al. (2018) reviewed NMDA antagonists and found moderate evidence for short-term efficacy of ketamine. O'Connell et al. (2013), in a Cochrane review (known for being very picky methodologically), found the evidence for ketamine in CRPS to be low. Niesters et al. (2014), in one of the more balanced reviews, indicated good evidence that ketamine can cause at least short-term significant analgesia but emphasized various risks and side effects and cautioned that close monitoring is needed when using ketamine for chronic pain. Michelet et al. (2018) published a meta-analysis concluding moderate evidence of at least short-term efficacy but concluded that the evidence supporting routine use in chronic pain was low.

Thus, in sum, the authors who have published reviews of ketamine in chronic pain have almost uniformly expressed the following: caution that the evidence thus far is of low to medium quality, with methodological limitations and large heterogeneity of patient groups and dosing schemes for ketamine, and concluding that ketamine cannot as yet be recommended for routine use in chronic pain; further caution that ketamine's tolerability and safety are in question and not yet established; and finally, that further work is needed of better scientific quality and standardized methodology.

Ketamine for Depression

Of all the roads traveled by ketamine, the use of this fascinating drug for depression has been the most stunning and game-changing. Ketamine clinics to treat depression have popped up all over the world. The clinical use of ketamine for depression has outpaced the scientific basis for doing so, in part because of the desperation the field of psychiatry has for new antidepressant treatments, but also the relative ease of using ketamine (and of course the profit-making potential these ketamine clinics have).

Review of Depression

The psychiatric profession defines depression by DSM-5-TR (American Psychiatric Association 2023). The nine criteria for a depressive episode are depressed mood, *anhedonia* (loss of ability to experience pleasure), low self-esteem, abnormal guilty thoughts, fatigue, poor sleep, poor appetite (sometimes increased appetite), troubles with concentration, and suicidal thinking. Having five of the nine symptoms—one of which must be anhedonia or depressed mood—for at least 2 weeks constitutes a *major depressive episode*. The symptoms must cause substantial functional impairment or emotional distress and cannot be accounted for by medical or neurological illnesses (e.g., hypothyroidism or obstructive sleep apnea) or a substance (e.g., reserpine or alcohol). Depression by this definition has become a massive public health problem worldwide, affecting some 10% of the population at some point in their lives. Compounding this situation is a high rate of treatment refractoriness to such interventions as psychotherapy, oral antidepressant medications, electroconvulsive therapy (ECT), and transcranial magnetic stimulation. The psychiatric profession, and indeed the human race, are hungry for other options.

Broadly speaking, major depressive episodes are classified as either bipolar or unipolar. If a patient has a history of mania, hypomania, or a mixed state, then the episode of major depression is said to be *bipolar*. On the other hand, if the episode of depression is not preceded by one of these states, then it is said to be *unipolar*. Psychiatric researchers have sought diligently over the decades to figure out whether bipolar and unipolar depressive episodes differ in terms of psychopathological features, treatment response, or neurobiology. In modern research settings, whether patients have bipolar or unipolar episodes is usually specified, and this is the case in much of the ketamine-for-depression literature.

Depressive episodes are also subdivided into psychotic and nonpsychotic. Some depressions feature delusional thinking or hallucinations: these are particularly severe and disabling states, with high associations with suicide, and are termed *psychotic*. If psychotic features are not present (which is the majority of depressive episodes), then it is termed *nonpsychotic*. Both bipolar and unipolar depressive episodes can be psychotic or nonpsychotic. Recall that ketamine has been used as a model for psychosis (see Chapter 5); thus, when it comes to psychotic depression, researchers have been quite hesitant to administer ketamine, and virtually all depressed patients who have been given ketamine have been nonpsychotic.

Another concept pertinent to depression, and that has received attention in the ketamine literature, is *treatment-resistant depression*, which refers to episodes that have been treated with one or more standard antidepressant treatments without success. As will be seen later, ketamine has succeeded most commonly for depressive episodes that are *refractory* (i.e., resistant) to one or more antidepressant medications.

Quantification of depressive severity must be undertaken for research. For this, depression rating scales are used. The most commonly used such scales are the Hamilton Depression Rating Scale (HDRS) and the Montgomery-Åsberg Depression Rating Scale (MADRS). These two scales are quite similar and consist of a set of questions pertaining to depressive symptoms: each item is rated such that a higher score on that item (e.g., suicidal thinking) indicates higher severity. The scores on each item are summed to yield the total score. Typical scores for these scales are >20 to indicate at least moderately severe depression and single digits to indicate remission from depression. The scales are conducted before any treatment is commenced and serially over time to assess degree of response. If the score falls by at least 50%, it is considered *response*; *remission* is less than ~10, depending on the study. Thus, a patient can have clinical response but still be quite symptomatic, whereas the definition of remission is essentially absence of depression. Of note, only severely depressed patients are enrolled in most trials, so even a 50% reduction in score can occur without concomitant remission. For example, a patient starting with a score of 26 who ends treatment with a 13 is said to be a *responder* but is not a *remitter* unless the score goes below a predefined level, usually 10 but sometimes 12 in some studies. Throughout this chapter, the terms response/responder and remission/remitter will be used in this manner.

The Road to a New Antidepressant

PCP for Depression

Repeating the PCP-to-ketamine pattern we have seen so often, depressive symptoms were seen in the mid-twentieth century as an opportunity to try PCP. A trial with PCP for psychiatric patients was undertaken at Hahnemann Medical College in Philadelphia (Bodi et al. 1959). According to the journal authors, unpublished observations by Parke-Davis pharmacologist Graham Chen led to this trial, in which 32 "psychoneurotic" outpatients were recruited to try PCP for therapeutic purposes. It was used by mouth daily. The authors thought that PCP seemed to be good for the patients, but that side effects were a limiting factor, as most patients who improved also had bothersome side effects at the therapeutic dose.

Meanwhile, across the pond, British psychiatrist Dr. Brian Davies, working at the Bethlem Royal and Maudsley hospitals in London, became quite fascinated with the newly discovered PCP (which he referred to by its proprietary name, Sernyl). Deriving information from the use of this drug in schizophrenia patients and in general anesthesia, he wondered if it would be a useful abreactive agent for psychotherapy. *Abreaction* is an old psychoanalytic term referring to times in psychotherapy when the patient recalls, in an emotionally charged manner, some previously blocked trauma or interpersonal conflict. It was felt to be helpful for therapy, and any medicinal agent that could facilitate it was thought to be worth pursuing. In his first report, Davies (1960) described his experience giving PCP to five patients, ages 21 to 40, with diagnoses such as personality disorder/neurosis, affective disorder, obsessional disorder (in three), and anorexia (in one, along with obsessional disorder). Patients reported being "back to normal" after about half an hour but had feelings of at least mild intoxication for several hours. Noted was temporary improvement in the obsessional symptoms (e.g., rituals such as hand washing), presaging the decades-later use of ketamine for OCD.

Intrigued by the surprising finding of an even brief anti-obsessional effect in this series, Davies (1961) followed up with a new series of five patients with obsessional disorders, each one receiving 10–20 oral administrations of PCP 5–15 mg. Two of the five had what was described as temporary abatement of compulsive behaviors with PCP. Based on the descriptions Davies gave of his patients' experiences with this drug, PCP is much more stimulating to people than is ketamine, which in part accounts for why it never really caught on in human medicine and why, when used recreationally, it can result in such toxic, highly agitated, and violent behavior.

Ketamine for Depression

The first report of a psychotropic benefit of ketamine came from Khorramzadeh and Lotfy (1973). Working in a teaching hospital in Shiraz, Iran, the authors reported on a series of 100 psychiatric inpatients given ketamine, age range 16–66 years. Other than mentioning that none of the patients had psychosis or an organic brain syndrome, no diagnostic information was given. One might assume that the patients probably had nonpsychotic depression and anxiety disorders. All had symptomatic relief and abreactive responses at varying doses of IV ketamine. Most patients in the entire cohort were said to be doing well at 1 year of follow-up.

Even more esoteric yet is the report, published in Spanish from Argentina, of Fontana and Loschi (1974). Like the one from Iran, it appears that these authors conceptualized ketamine as an abreactive agent that facilitated psychotherapy, rather than as a direct-acting antidepressant without any intervening psychotherapy. Their description, which is quite lacking in detail of pharmacological or patient characteristics, is that ketamine facilitated "regression" to aid in psychodynamic therapy. These two 1970s reports were essentially ignored and seem to have had no influence on later clinical developments related to ketamine, but they are of historical interest.

The early 1970s included an animal model study of ketamine as possible antidepressant (Sofia and Harakal 1975). That era featured rodent models testing putative antidepressant compounds. The authors submitted ketamine to the tests and found that, indeed, it blocked various effects that were thought to predict antidepressant activity in humans. They recommended that clinical use of ketamine for depression be studied, although there is really no evidence from the literature that this suggestion influenced any later events. Thus, this report also appears to be of historical interest only.

For about 30 years, beginning in the late 1950s, antidepressant pharmacotherapy was dominated by the tricyclics and monoamine oxidase inhibitors (MAOIs)—hard to tolerate, hard to take. A period of stagnation had set in. Then, interest and excitement in the treatment of depression was re-ignited, both within the field of psychiatry and in the public at large, by the introduction of Prozac in 1986 by Eli Lilly pharmaceutical company. Within a short time period, Prozac (a selective serotonin reuptake inhibitor, or SSRI) became a household name. A picture of the by-then-famous green and white capsule even appeared on the cover of *Newsweek* magazine on March 26, 1990, and in 1994, Elizabeth Wurtzel published her best-selling memoir *Prozac Nation*. A spate of "me too" serotonin reuptake inhibitors were spawned: paroxetine, sertraline, and fluvoxamine, to name a few of the early ones. These drugs became so well known that patients would request an SSRI in their appointments with doctors. But something was still missing. Even though these drugs on the whole were easier for doctors to prescribe and patients to tolerate than tricyclics and MAOIs, a revolution in depression care did not materialize. A lot of people took these pills, and a lot of them got no or little benefit from them. The world of psychiatry still hungered for something better.

Meanwhile, in the neuropharmacology laboratory literature, a new idea had been brewing. Drs. Ramon Trullas and Phil Skolnick of the U.S. National Institutes of Health published a now oft-cited paper (Trullas and Skolnick 1990) outlining the animal literature pointing to NMDA receptor blockade as a possible mechanism to target depression. The notion that NMDA receptor antagonism might treat depression took hold in the basic science neuropharmacological literature. Later, these authors with more colleagues (Skolnick et al. 1996) reviewed animal data suggesting that then-currently available antidepressant medications and ECT in rodents all caused adaptive changes in NMDA receptors. This was a new notion to psychiatry, which had for decades focused on monoamines and their receptors (dopamine, serotonin, and norepinephrine) as molecules of interest for depression. However, in neither of these influential papers was ketamine mentioned. At that time (the late 1990s), ketamine was still mostly an anesthesiologist's drug in clinical practice as well as a neuropharmacological probe in the laboratory.

What came next changed it all. A psychiatric research group at Yale University, led by John Krystal, already had experience with ketamine in their studies using it as a model for schizophrenia (as we saw in Chapter 5). This well-read group of scientists were aware of the Skolnick et al. (1996) paper outlining the rationale for NMDA receptor blockers as possible antidepressants. This, combined with their knowledge that ketamine indeed blocks these receptors and their by-then extensive experience using the ketamine paradigm (0.5 mg/kg over 40 minutes) in humans, led them to reason that ketamine should be tested in humans for depression.

Ketamine had added advantages for them: it was already available on the market, so they did not need special FDA approval to undertake the study, and on top of that, it was cheap and easy to obtain. They performed a small trial (Berman et al. 2000). The rest, as it is often said, is history. The years since that publication have seen a torrent of studies using ketamine as an antidepressant. This story thus represents a fabulous success of translation from bench to bedside in modern psychiatry.

So what did Berman et al. (2000) do in their seminal study? They undertook a cautious, preliminary trial of ketamine for depression, using modern concepts of diagnosis, quantification of depressive severity, and the scientific method. Seven patients with unipolar depression received, in randomized crossover manner, one intravenous infusion each of racemic ketamine 0.5 mg/kg over 40 minutes (mimicking how they used it in their schizophrenia model studies) and saline placebo. In the 72 hours of follow-up with depression ratings, there was a 14-point reduction on HDRS with ketamine (a substantial drop on that scale) and none with saline. There was a 50% response rate, meaning at least a 50% reduction in rating scale scores, for ketamine and 0% for saline. Changes in Brief Psychiatric Rating Scale (BPRS) scores, a measure of psychotomimetic effects during the ketamine infusions, did not correlate with ultimate reduction in depression ratings. The authors pointed out that the study was functionally nonblind, as patients could easily distinguish between ketamine and saline, a problem that has dogged trials such as this. Importantly, there was no pharmacokinetic or pharmacodynamic rationale given for the dosing schedule for ketamine; they appear to have used it simply because they were experienced giving this dose to normal control participants in their other studies. For good or for bad, researchers and clinicians in the field of ketamine for depression have largely persevered with this dosing scheme in subsequent studies and in clinical care.

Many years later, the Berman et al. (2000) study is cited often and is considered a paradigm-changing publication of historical significance. However, at the time of its publication, it caused nary a ripple. Perhaps the reason it sparked so little immediate interest is that psychiatrists had already become jaded by the innumerable compounds implicated as potential antidepressants. In addition, it probably seemed strange that an anesthetic drug could be considered an antidepressant.

It did not go completely ignored, actually. Another study of ketamine for depression was undertaken at the U.S. National Institute of Mental Health, headed by Dr. Carlos Zarate Jr., who in subsequent years became a prominent ketamine researcher. In this randomized crossover trial (Zarate et al. 2006), 18 patients with unipolar depression were given one infusion each, separated by at least a week, of racemic ketamine 0.5 mg/kg over 40 minutes or saline. One day after infusion, MADRS scores showed a 71% response rate for ketamine and a 0% response rate for saline. The rise in BPRS scores with the ketamine infusions almost correlated with degree of reduction in MADRS (the *P* value, an indicator of statistical significance, barely missed the 0.05 level at 0.06). Again the immediate dissociative and psychotomimetic effects of ketamine caused a break in blinding, and resultant possible placebo effect. But placebo or not, an eye-popping 71% versus 0% response rate for ketamine versus saline caused the field to take notice.

Diazgranados et al. (2010) and Zarate et al. (2012a) replicated the findings in patients with bipolar depression. They also noted a rapid reduction of the MADRS item for suicidal thinking, an effect that has proven quite robust in ketamine research in the ensuing years. The highest reduction in MADRS scores was noted 40 minutes after infusion, thus reinforcing the exciting rapidity of ketamine's antidepressant effects.

Murrough et al. (2013a) randomized 47 depressed patients to a single infusion of racemic ketamine 0.5 mg/kg over 40 minutes and 25 to midazolam (an anxiolytic/sedative) 0.045 mg/kg over 40 minutes. They found 24-hour response rates of 64% and 28%, respectively. Midazolam, a short-acting IV benzodiazepine, was used as an active control to make it harder for patients to differentiate from ketamine than saline, thus preserving the blinding.

Some well-conducted meta-analyses around that time all concluded that ketamine showed rapid, robust antidepressant effects vis-à-vis placebo. McGirr et al. (2015), Romeo et al. (2015), and Xu et al. (2016), all more or less simultaneously, reviewing essentially the same set of papers, reached this conclusion, but also that the effects of ketamine were largely gone by a week after the single administration.

As of this writing, the latest, and one of the largest, randomized controlled trial of ketamine for depression is that of Loo et al. (2023), in which subcutaneous ketamine 0.5 mg/kg and subcutaneous midazolam 0.025 mg/kg were compared using twice-a-week injections for 4 weeks in each group. The first cohort of patients (*n*=68) showed no significant difference in remission rates between the two groups (6.3% for ketamine and 8.8% for midazolam). Reasoning that the dosage of ketamine may have been too small, and considering that the later-published data showing 66% bioavailability of subcutaneous ketamine were not available at the time, the investigators started another cohort ($n=106$) in which the dosage of each medication was progressively increased for patients not showing clinical response. For ketamine, the stepwise dosages used were 0.5, 0.6, 0.75, and 0.9 mg/kg, going up to the next dosage level every other treatment for those not responding. A large percentage of this new cohort of ketamine-treated patients did in fact end up receiving the final dosage strength, and the remission rate in this cohort ended up being 19.6% versus 2.0% for midazolam. The population in this study was resistant to antidepressant medication and chronically depressed, so this seemingly small remission rate was actually pretty good for a highly refractory population. The take-home message from this study was that if subcutaneous ketamine is used (a convenient way to administer ketamine), the dosage has to be larger for most patients than the usual IV dose of 0.5 mg/kg.

Grunebaum et al. (2019) assessed the relationship between blood levels of ketamine and its metabolites drawn immediately post-infusion and 24 hours later in a trial comparing 0.5 mg/kg racemic ketamine over 40 minutes versus midazolam. Ketamine, norketamine, and dehydronorketamine levels did not correlate with reductions in depression rating scales. Interestingly, levels of (2R,6R)-hydroxynorketamine bore an inverse relationship with clinical response: the higher the levels of this metabolite, the less the reductions in depression scores. This hardly implicates this metabolite of ketamine as responsible for the antidepressant effect. A similar finding was that of Farmer et al. (2020), who used a randomized crossover design to treat depression patients once with 0.5 mg/kg over 40 minutes and once with saline infusions. Total hydroxynorketamine levels [(2R,6R)- plus (2S,6S)-hydroxynorketamine] inversely correlated with clinical response to ketamine infusions; (2R,6R)-hydroxynorketamine itself did not correlate with response.

A common question concerns potential predictors of good response among depression patients to ketamine. Niciu et al. (2014), pooling data from four studies, concluded that higher body mass index, family history of alcoholism, and absence of a prior suicide attempt all predicted somewhat better ketamine responsivity. These factors were not strong enough to exclude patients lacking them from receiving ketamine, however. Niciu et al. (2013b) concluded there was no evidence that ketamine causes depressed patients to become manic, which of course is very good news (traditional oral antidepressants can cause mania in bipolar patients).

Another issue in the ketamine-for-depression literature is a seeming independent antisuicidal effect of ketamine. Domany et al. (2020), Grunebaum et al. (2017), and Grunebaum et al. (2018) all conducted controlled ketamine studies in suicidality and found robust antisuicidal effects. Reductions in depression scores accounted for only about one-third of the variance in reduced suicidal ratings in the Grunebaum et al. (2018) study, indicating that ketamine's antisuicidal effect may be partially independent of an antidepressant effect.

Note should be made of the important question of whether ketamine is helpful and safe for adolescents with depression—the world is in crisis mode at this time with regard to teen depression and suicide. Di Vincenzo et al. (2021) reviewed five open-label case series of ketamine for teen depression. In general, favorable results were reported, but obviously much more data are needed in this important area. In an editorial on this topic, Parikh and Walkup (2021) distinguished between the possibility that ketamine is a "true" antidepressant versus being a sort of drug high that spills over into better-looking depression rating scale scores in adolescents—a question just as relevant in the adult literature.

Thus, in sum, it is now well established that a single administration of ketamine to depressed patients diagnosed according to modern criteria and followed with validated depression rating scales leads to rapid, robust antidepressant responses vis-à-vis various control groups. These single-administration racemic ketamine studies, mostly intravenous and randomized crossover in design, represent the initial cohort of ketamine-for-depression studies of the modern era. They established that this fascinating drug, heretofore considered an anesthetic, a recreational drug, or an esoteric laboratory probe, could actually rapidly treat depression—a genuine breath of fresh air for the stagnant field of depression treatment.

So the field of psychiatry at large seemed to believe it—ketamine could treat depression—but there were concerns. Is it safe? Does it lead to addictive behaviors? Does it impair cognition? Can its rapid effects last longer than just a few days? In addition to these clinical questions about the usefulness of ketamine in everyday practice, the findings increased activity in the field of laboratory neuropharmacology and led to psychiatry's getting over its almost-half-century obsession with monoamines and finding a new obsession: glutamate. What was the mechanism of ketamine's antidepressant effect? What lessons could ketamine teach about the underlying neurobiology of depression? Could pursuing this pathway lead to further, more definitive treatments? It is to these issues we now turn. We begin with some of the clinically relevant questions and end with the mechanistic ones.

Refining Ketamine's Use for Depression

What Is the Optimal Dose of Ketamine for Depression?

The single-administration studies established in principle that ketamine could have rapid antidepressant effects. Most of the studies used IV racemic ketamine at a dose of 0.5 mg/kg over 40 minutes or so, which has become something of a standard dose of ketamine for depression. However, that dose was arbitrary, and other investigators have wondered whether other doses could be better.

Li et al. (2016) randomized depressed patients to one of two doses of ketamine (0.2 or 0.5 mg/kg) or saline placebo with 16 patients per group. Depression ratings were followed only for about 4 hours after each infusion. There were more responders in both ketamine groups than saline, and each dose was associated with the same response rate. However, at 40 minutes post-infusion, the 0.5 mg/kg group did have lower depression rating scale scores than the 0.2 mg/kg group.

The same research group (Su et al. 2017) compared saline placebo, 0.2 mg/kg IV ketamine, and 0.5 mg/kg IV ketamine (racemic) in a parallel group design, single infusion, with 71 total patients. The infusions were over 40 minutes. In the group with relatively low baseline depression ratings, the two ketamine groups did not separate from placebo in antidepressant efficacy. In the groups with medium and high baseline depression ratings, the 0.5 mg/kg dose separated from the others in the first days following the infusion. By 28 days, there was no difference between the groups.

Fava et al. (2020) randomized 99 depressed patients to one infusion of midazolam 0.045 mg/kg or ketamine at a dose of 0.1, 0.2, 0.5, or 1.0 mg/kg, all infusions being over 40 minutes. Primary outcome was depression ratings on day 3 post-infusion. The two higher doses of ketamine (0.5 and 1.0 mg/kg) separated from midazolam, but the two lower doses (0.1 and 0.2 mg/kg) did not.

Regarding the trend in depression ratings over the days after infusion, it is noteworthy how unimpressive the dose response was. For example, on day 3 post-infusion, the ratings for the 0.1 mg/kg group were identical to those of the 1.0 mg/kg group. The 0.2 mg/kg group did the same as the midazolam group. Thus, this study was not terribly impressive, in my opinion, for a dose-response relationship with the antidepressant effects of ketamine, and quite frankly, the ratings for midazolam were not that bad (and it did not have an elevation in CADSS ratings). Of most practical significance, the 1.0 mg/kg dose clearly was no better than the 0.5 mg/kg dose, which is indeed helpful information for clinical practice.

Milak et al. (2020) randomized 37 depression patients to one infusion of ketamine at 0.1, 0.2, 0.3, 0.4, or 0.5 mg/kg or placebo, over 40 minutes. Depression ratings 24 hours post-infusion decreased in a dose-related manner, being highest at 0.5 mg/kg, which had a mean 50% drop in depressive severity. The placebo group had an approximately 14% drop in scores. Finally, as mentioned earlier, Loo et al. (2023) found a dose-response relationship with subcutaneous racemic ketamine in which doses of 0.6–0.9 mg/kg seemed to show better efficacy than 0.5 mg/kg. However, because the infusions were subcutaneous, with its lower bioavailability than the IV route, it is probably not proper to compare this study's results with the larger IV literature on ketamine dosing.

Overall, the dose-response literature for ketamine in depression is frustratingly vague and inconclusive. There is no clear signal that "more is better" with racemic ketamine infusions. The typical dose of 0.5 mg/kg, delivered over 40 minutes, is still the gold standard for IV use of racemic ketamine, more than 20 years after Berman et al. (2000) introduced it.

Two other studies of ketamine deserve mention for the innovative dosing schedules used. As recounted earlier, in Chapter 6, some groups used prolonged infusion times for ketamine in patients with chronic pain. Lenze et al. (2016), from Washington University in Saint Louis (including the legendary John Olney as a co-author), admitted 20 patients to an inpatient research unit for 96-hour infusions. Ten of the patients were randomized to receive ketamine the entire 96 hours, and the other 10 were randomized to receive 95 hours and 20 minutes of saline infusion followed by a final 40 minutes of racemic ketamine 0.5 mg/kg (thus mimicking the usual dosing method for ketamine). The dosing schedule for the 10 patients receiving ketamine the entire 96 hours was 0.15 mg/kg/hour to start with, titrating as tolerated up to 0.6 mg/kg/hour. Each group was followed for 8 weeks thereafter, with MADRS ratings at 2-week intervals. There was no difference between the two groups in MADRS ratings at any time point.

A few years later, the same group (without Dr. Olney, who had died in the interim) used the same technique only with an open-label design, without a control group (Siegel et al. 2021). Twenty-three depression patients received the 96-hour ketamine infusions at the same rate as in the randomized study described above. Nausea and anxiety were the main reported side effects. Psychotomimetic side effects were said to be low. Mean ketamine concentrations were targeted to be around 400 ng/mL. Mean MADRS scores averaged about 29 at baseline (indicating severe depression) and about 9 a day after infusion. At 8 weeks, mean scores were 15. Response at 2 weeks was not correlated with ketamine or norketamine blood concentrations. These outcomes are much better than in the randomized study, in which 8-week MADRS scores were around 22 in the intense ketamine dosing group.

This is a common finding in psychiatric pharmacology research: open-label case series show excellent response to a drug, whereas subsequent randomized controlled studies fail to show the same effects. In this case, the sequence was reversed (randomized trial first, open-label series second), but the ultimate findings the same: there is no basis for using the prolonged infusion technique based on this group's work, but perhaps further study is warranted.

Do Multiple Ketamine Administrations Help More Than Just One?

It became clear from the single-infusion studies that the impressive antidepressant gains with ketamine were transient. The next logical step in developing ketamine as a viable, clinically available antidepressant medication, and not just a laboratory probe used to study basic science mechanisms in rodents, was to see whether repeated sets of infusions were associated with either better acute responses or longer-lasting ones. In fact, I had such curiosity, and along with some of my colleagues at the Mayo Clinic, I undertook a small open-label study of up to four twice-a-week racemic ketamine infusions in 10 depression patients (Rasmussen et al. 2013). The dose of ketamine was 0.5 mg/kg given over 100 minutes. Based on MADRS scores, five patients remitted: one with one infusion, three with two infusions, and one with four infusions. Follow-up at 4 weeks revealed relapse in two of the remitters. In this small study, there seemed to be a signal that continued ketamine administrations can yield higher acute remission rates than a single infusion.

In the same year, Murrough et al. (2013b) also published an open-label study of ketamine in a larger sample (*n*=24 patients). They were given racemic ketamine 0.5 mg/kg over 40 minutes three times a week for 2 weeks. There was a 70.8% response rate, higher than those published in single-infusion studies. Additionally, median time to relapse in the follow-up phase was 18 days, longer than in the single-infusion studies. Thus, in these two early serial ketamine studies, a signal emerged of perhaps better acute and longer-lasting response.

In an early open-label report from a ketamine clinic, Diamond et al. (2014) gave 28 patients racemic ketamine for depression, 0.5 mg/kg over 40 minutes either weekly (*n*=15) or twice a week (*n*=13) for 3 weeks. The primary outcome was the Beck Depression Inventory (BDI). There was no apparent benefit of the twice-a-week frequency. Among the 8 of 28 patients who responded to ketamine, there was a 70-day median sustained response.

Singh et al. (2016a) published the first randomized, controlled trial of serial ketamine. Sixty-seven depressed patients were randomized to four groups: two- versus three-times-a-week infusions of racemic ketamine 0.5 mg/kg or placebo for up to 4 weeks. In the saline placebo groups, there was little change in MADRS scores, perhaps 3- to 5-point reductions over the 4 weeks. In the two ketamine groups (two and three times a week), there were much more substantial, and equal, reductions in scores (averaging 17-

to 18-point reductions). In the ketamine groups, responses were nicely sustained for up to 2 weeks on follow-up without further ketamine. Thus, this study implies excellent acute and sustained efficacy of serial ketamine, although the control group did not involve a single ketamine infusion (rather, six placebo infusions).

Ionescu et al. (2019) published a randomized study of repeat ketamine dosing for depression. Twenty-six patients were randomized to six infusions of racemic ketamine 0.5 mg/kg over 45 minutes or placebo, over 3 weeks (twice a week). There were no differences between the two groups in depression scores not only at the end of the 3 weeks, but, curiously, not after the first treatment either, in stark contrast to the extensive single-infusion literature. Scores barely went down in either group. The authors postulated that the dose of 0.5 mg/kg for ketamine was too low to be effective, but of course that is the same dose most other groups used.

Calabrese (2019), reporting on experience in a large private psychiatric ketamine practice, described results in 219 patients given six racemic ketamine infusions over 2–3 weeks, 0.5–1.2 mg/kg per dose over 40–50 minutes IV. The outcome focus was on suicidal thoughts in depressed patients, age range 14–86 years. Median dosing of ketamine achieved 0.75 mg/kg, a bit higher than what the formal randomized studies used. Suicidal ideations decreased incrementally with each treatment in the series, implying greater reductions than would have occurred with just one infusion. However, the case series was open label, without randomization to a control group or double-blinding of outcome assessment.

Phillips et al. (2019) approached the one-versus-several ketamine infusions issue creatively. Forty-one depressed patients participated in a three-phase study. In the first phase, all patients received in randomized crossover manner one infusion of ketamine 0.5 mg/kg and one of midazolam 0.03 mg/kg. Not surprisingly, response rates on MADRS were higher for ketamine 24 hours after infusion (27% for ketamine versus 0% for midazolam). All patients in this phase of the study eventually relapsed, at which time point they were entered (n=39) into an open-label phase of six ketamine infusions over 2 weeks. After a median of three such infusions, there was a doubling of response rate to ketamine (vis-à-vis the single-infusion phase) to 57%. This implies that, using patients as their own controls, serial ketamine infusions are better than one, although the second phase was open label and not randomized or double-blind. The third phase of the study consisted of weekly ketamine infusions to second-phase responders. MADRS scores were sustained, implying that maintenance ketamine can help sustain the initial acute-phase responses.

Sharma et al. (2020) conducted another randomized, controlled study of repeat ketamine infusions with an interesting design. Fifty-four depressed patients were randomized to receive either six racemic ketamine IV infusions at 0.5 mg/kg over 40 minutes in 2 weeks or five midazolam infusions at 0.045 mg/kg over 40 minutes followed by one ketamine infusion at 0.5 mg/kg as the sixth infusion. What was being tested, essentially, was whether six ketamine infusions is better than one. The day after the sixth infusion in both groups, MADRS scores were equal, indicating that one ketamine infusion is just as good as six. Along the 2-week time period, after the fourth and fifth treatments, there was a few-point difference in depression scores favoring the ketamine group. Interestingly, the day after the first infusion, essentially testing one ketamine versus one midazolam infusion, the MADRS scores were down considerably and equally in both groups. If the study had stopped there, it would have led to the conclusion that midazolam equals ketamine in rapid antidepressant efficacy. In the 6-month post-infusion follow-up period, relapse rates for initial responders were lower for the serial- than the single-infusion ketamine group, but the difference was not statistically significant.

A good summary statement about serial ketamine infusions, versus just one, is that in clinical practices these days, serial infusions are used to induce what seems like maximal induction phase improvement for depressed patients. According to the literature from large ketamine practices, it seems to take a few infusions, perhaps up to six, to achieve this.

The data set from the Janssen group of investigators of intranasal esketamine is discussed in a later section. A large number of patients were randomized to placebo versus serial intranasal esketamine, constituting the largest database yet of serial ketamine administrations. Note, however, that these studies did not compare one intranasal esketamine administration to more than one, just serial esketamine versus serial placebo, so the fundamental question of greater efficacy of more than one versus one is not answered in that data set.

Does Maintenance Ketamine Administration Prevent Relapse?

In general, researchers have been hesitant to continue the acute-phase schedule of ketamine into the maintenance phase. If a patient has received two- or three-a-week infusions of ketamine for 2–3 weeks, can they continue at that pace for many more weeks or months? This has not been tested, so the maintenance ketamine literature usually consists of a tapered frequency schedule.

McMullen et al. (2021) reviewed 22 studies investigating some type of post–ketamine-induction-phase maintenance treatment, such as psychotherapy, various pharmacotherapies, and ketamine itself. Of note is that supposed orally available NMDA receptor blocking agents, such as riluzole, were ineffective. In the review, it was concluded that maintenance ketamine was better than maintenance treatment with other agents in sustaining the initial ketamine-associated improvement in depression.

It is with keen interest that the field of clinical psychiatry has watched the data over the past few years broaching the question of whether the dramatic, rapid gains achieved with one or a few ketamine administrations can be sustained over time. The largest data set in this regard has been from the Janssen group in their pursuit of regulatory approval to market intranasal esketamine. Singh et al. (2020), representing this group, provided a nice review of maintenance ketamine studies up to that time. There were seven studies in the literature, all with racemic ketamine, and all with variable methodologies, dosing regimens, and durations of follow-up. There were non-uniform doses and frequencies of dosing, and no clear conclusions could be drawn, although a signal of sustained efficacy was evident in some samples over at least a few weeks after acute-phase treatment. For example, after an acute series of infusions given two or three times a week, weekly infusions could be efficacious in sustaining the original benefit. However, Singh et al. (2020) went on to review their experience in the Janssen group studies of several hundred patients who received ongoing weekly or every-other-week esketamine. Overall, good initial induction-phase improvement was maintained for up to a year of treatment, which was well tolerated, with side effects on days of treatment for up to 2 hours after administration being dizziness, dissociation, headache, nausea, and vertigo. Dropouts were relatively scarce.

A review of maintenance ketamine reports is provided by Smith-Apeldoorn et al. (2022). It is surprising how many such reports involved routes of administration other than intravenous. Overall, there were 17 IV racemic ketamine maintenance papers involving 222 patients, 8 intranasal esketamine reports involving 997 patients, and a few reports with other routes of administration. The general conclusion in this large review is that maintenance ketamine seems to be associated with the ability to sustain original, induction-phase gains in a manner that is well tolerated and accepted by patients.

Interdosing intervals have been widely variable and tend toward once a week to once every few weeks. Total duration of maintenance ketamine is also quite variable and could be weeks, months, or even years in some cases. These variables are individualized on a case-by-case basis, taking into account the severity of prior depressive episodes, degree of improvement with ketamine, tolerance of side effects, cost of care, and time needed to obtain the infusions. Patients often self-select when they will stop maintenance therapy, taking into account those factors. There is extensive clinical experience relayed in these reports but not much hard science. It is difficult to conduct randomized, controlled months-long maintenance studies. The intranasal esketamine data reviewed in Smith-Apeldoorn et al. (2022) were mainly that of the Janssen group data, which we discuss later in the section devoted to esketamine.

Is Ketamine Safe for Those With Psychosis or a History Thereof?

Ketamine causes psychotomimetic effects and has been used as a model for schizophrenia (see Chapter 5). Thus, clinicians and researchers have been hesitant to use it in those depressed patients who have concomitant psychotic features. However, those patients are the most severely debilitated, and it would be good to know whether ketamine can help them. Thus, some cautious case series in such patients have been undertaken.

Veraart et al. (2021) and Le et al. (2021) reviewed nine articles with a total of 41 patients, not that many in the greater scheme of things. Patients had either depression with psychosis or previous psychosis (e.g., schizophrenia) with current depression. A few patients with psychotic depression got better on ketamine, without psychotic exacerbation. A few patients with depression and psychosis got better at least temporarily, with no apparent psychotic exacerbation, either at the time of the infusion or later.

Souza-Marques et al. (2022) used a single dose of esketamine 0.5 mg/kg IV over 40 minutes, or occasionally subcutaneously, to treat depression patients. Those routes of administration are routinely available in Brazil, where the study was conducted. Fifteen patients with psychotic depression were compared to 30 patients with nonpsychotic depression (nonrandomized samples). In the psychotic depression sample, there was a 33% 24-hour response, and a 40% response rate at 24 hours in the nonpsychotic sample. Probably because of the small sample sizes, there was no statistically significant difference between groups, but the important point is that the psychotic depression patients seemed to do well and sustained no exacerbation in psychosis—yet more data encouraging further exploration of ketamine and its enantiomers for treatment of the very important and disabling syndrome of psychotic depression.

Gałuszko-Węgielnik et al. (2023) reported a series of four patients with treatment-resistant psychotic depression whose psychoses improved with ketamine and were not worsened at all.

Probably the best data yet on the efficacy of ketamine for psychotic depression come from the study of Ekstrand et al. (2022), the so-called KetECT study comparing the efficacy of ketamine and ECT. In the ketamine group, 9 of 18 psychotically depressed patients sustained remission with a series of ketamine infusions at 0.5 mg/kg over 40 minutes each, given three times a week (it took an average of six such infusions for remission, which was defined as a MADRS score ≤10 on two successive ratings). None of the psychotic patients had increases in psychosis with ketamine. A remission rate of 50% for the severe syndrome of psychotic depression is quite impressive, and if replicated, would open up a new treatment for such patients.

What About Esketamine?

As discussed in Chapter 4, what we commonly refer to as "ketamine" (racemic ketamine) is a half-and-half mixture of two enantiomers: esketamine and arketamine. Starting with a batch of racemic ketamine, different enantiomers of tartaric acid can be added, which bind to one of the two ketamine enantiomers (depending on which tartaric acid enantiomer is added in), leaving a batch of the other enantiomer of ketamine. Thus, using different enantiomers of tartaric acid, the chemist can produce batches of pure esketamine or pure arketamine. It is a relatively easy thing to do, so industrial quantities of both ketamine enantiomers can be produced for mass distribution.

Esketamine has been commercially available in some European countries (such as Germany and the Netherlands) and Brazil for a long time, typically for anesthesia. It is much more potent at blocking NMDA receptors than arketamine (by a factor of about 4) and racemic ketamine (by a factor of about 2). Thus, smaller doses of esketamine than racemic ketamine typically have been given for anesthesia situations. (Arketamine, which is discussed for depression in the next section, is not available anywhere yet for clinical use.)

The biggest impetus in the effort to develop esketamine as an antidepressant has been brought about by the Johnson & Johnson pharmaceutical company, via their subsidiary Janssen Research and Development, which has funded several large trials of esketamine for depression in their efforts to obtain regulatory approval to market esketamine for depression. Although the details of this pharmaceutical giant's decision to pursue esketamine approval are obviously confidential, one can reasonably assume that, since racemic ketamine is already cheap and not patentable, there would be no reason to spend the mega-millions of dollars needed to obtain regulatory approval for a drug any other company could use. Thus, they have pursued esketamine, probably because it is known to be four times more potent as an NMDA blocker than arketamine. This mechanism for the most part has been fundamentally assumed to be the basis for the antidepressant effects of racemic ketamine.

Further, Janssen added another proprietary element to their pursuit of approval for esketamine: a patented intranasal formulation, as opposed to intravenous use. From reading their papers from the clinical studies of es-ketamine, it is apparent a great deal of money was spent on the large sample sizes and complex designs. It paid off: esketamine was approved in the spring of 2019 in the United States and later that year in the European Union. In the U.S.A., the FDA approved esketamine nasal spray for major depressive disorder with either acute suicidal ideation or behavior or treatment resistance, in combination with an oral antidepressant medication. Janssen did not provide any rationale for why esketamine was studied or what proposed neurobiological mechanism they sought—they simply chose it and studied it. It should be noted that the Janssen group deserves credit for including patients in their studies from a diverse set of cultural and ethnic backgrounds. In particular, several of their studies were conducted in Asian countries, and there is also a substantial data set of esketamine work from South America.

In the Janssen group studies of esketamine, the first was not with intranasal administration but rather IV administration (Singh et al. 2016b, study name PERSEVERE). Thirty treatment-resistant unipolar depression patients each received one infusion of saline, 0.2 mg/kg esketamine, or 0.4 mg/kg esketamine, all over 40 minutes. Placebo nonresponders were then randomized to one of the two doses of esketamine. Decreases in MADRS scores 24 hours after infusions averaged 3.6 points for placebo, 16.8 points for 0.2 mg/kg esketamine, and 16.9 points for 0.4 mg/kg. Efficacy of esketamine was evident by about 2 hours after infusions—so, very quickly.

After the double-blind phase was a 2-week open-label phase, in which responders to initial treatment received the same thing as on day 1 on day 4. Nonresponders to initial placebo on day 4 got 0.2 or 0.4 mg/kg esketamine, and nonresponders to initial esketamine got 0.4 mg/kg on day 4. On days 7, 10, 14, and 17, there were four more optional treatments. During the open-label phase, there were more dramatic decreases in MADRS scores than during the randomized placebo-controlled phase. The majority of decreases in scores occurred after the first treatment. This was an initial, small, essentially proof-of-concept study from which the drug company could design larger trials.

In the study called SYNAPSE, Daly et al. (2018) conducted a 14-site, multicenter, acute-phase randomized study of intranasal esketamine versus placebo nasal spray (saline solution, biologically inert), in addition to an oral antidepressant, for unipolar depression patients who had been refractory to at least two oral antidepressants. The patients were nonpsychotic, nonbipolar. At the end of the acute placebo-controlled phases, those receiving 84 mg esketamine had 20%–25% remission rates, whereas only 3% of placebo-treated patients remitted. During the open-label phase (mean

MADRS score about 20), scores drifted down over the weeks to a mean at the end of about 15, which were sustained well during non-esketamine treatment follow-up for 8 weeks. This study, in addition to providing good data on the acute response of depression to esketamine, also provided good data on maintenance esketamine, albeit in a fairly small sample.

In the TRANSFORM 1 study, Fedgchin et al. (2019) randomized 346 treatment-resistant, nonpsychotic, unipolar depressed patients to placebo spray versus 56 or 84 mg esketamine nasal spray, all in addition to starting a new oral antidepressant for each patient. Alas, there was minimal improvement in the 84-mg group over placebo, so this was a negative study that was submitted to the FDA for esketamine approval.

In the TRANSFORM 2 study, Popova et al. (2019) conducted a 28-day double-blind evaluation of acute-phase esketamine for treatment-resistant depression in 39 centers. There was a 4-point difference on MADRS favoring esketamine over placebo on day 28. There were 114 patients in the esketamine group and 109 in the placebo group. This TRANSFORM 2 study was considered a positive study for the Janssen group in their submission to the FDA. (Two such studies are needed for approval.)

Ochs-Ross et al. (2020) reported the TRANSFORM 3 study in those at least 65 years of age. TRANSFORM 3 was considered a negative study for FDA approval purposes, as the main outcome variable of MADRS score differences at the end of 4 weeks was not statistically significantly different between esketamine and placebo.

The three TRANSFORM studies were acute-phase studies. Next, the Janssen group turned its attention to maintenance-phase studies. In study SUSTAIN I, Daly et al. (2019) tested whether ketamine discontinuation in stable remitters and responders resulted in higher relapse rates. After acute-phase esketamine treatment, those with stable response or remission over 16 weeks of treatment were randomized to continuation versus discontinuation of esketamine. Those randomized to discontinuation received placebo nasal spray. Of the 176 esketamine stable remitters who were randomized to continuation versus discontinuation, 26.7% in the esketamine group and 45.3% in the placebo group relapsed in the weeks after randomization. This study was accepted by the FDA as a second positive efficacy study for esketamine and helped win approval of this drug for use in the United States.

Wajs et al. (2020) presented the Janssen study known as SUSTAIN 2, in which induction-phase responders received open-label esketamine for up to a year, starting at twice-a-week frequency for 4 weeks, going to weekly for 4 weeks, and then either staying at weekly or going to every other week. Over the months, treatment frequency could be changed back and forth from weekly to every other week depending on how the patient was doing. By study end, total response rate was reported as 76.5% and remission rate 58.2%.

Williamson et al. (2022) pooled together the safety data on the Janssen group esketamine studies, examining 928 patients' experiences with esketamine. In the first week of treatment, incidences of various side effects were as follows: dizziness 20.6%, dissociation 16.7%, elevated blood pressure 4.3%, nausea 14.0%, vertigo 12.1%, and sedation 3.8%. Generally, these effects became milder over time. If any of the effects occurred at both sessions during the first week, they were more likely to recur at later sessions (than if they occurred only once or not at all). Thus, if a patient tolerates esketamine during the first two sessions, it is unlikely that new-onset side effects will occur later, unless the dose is increased.

Turkoz et al. (2022) performed a post hoc analysis of data from the two ASPIRE studies in suicidally depressed patients. They wanted to know what happened to patients who did not respond early to esketamine (182 esketamine and 180 placebo patients). For those who did not respond to esketamine 24 hours after first inhalation, at day 25 there was a 63.1% response rate, versus 48% for placebo patients (statistically significant). For 1-week nonresponders to esketamine (that is, after two inhalation sessions), at day 25 there was a 48.4% response rate versus 34.5% for the 1-week placebo nonresponders, a difference that was not significantly different. At day 25 for the entire samples of both groups, there was a 74.6% versus 58.3% difference between esketamine and placebo, respectively, which was a highly significant difference. (Again, it is interesting how well the placebo-treated patients did.)

Providing perspective on the Janssen group studies, Canuso et al. (2018) noted that the FDA considered these data for approval of esketamine (marketed under the name Spravato) intranasal under "fast track" and "breakthrough" designations, meaning the process was expedited due to a perceived urgent public health need. For efficacy, TRANSFORM 2 and SUSTAIN I were considered positive; TRANSFORM 1 and TRANSFORM 3 were not. A Risk Evaluation and Mitigation System is required as part of FDA approval, meaning special monitoring must be undertaken. In the case of esketamine, this means 2 hours of monitoring after each dose, which must be administered under the auspices of a health provider, and each patient must be entered into a registry.

The approval of esketamine was not met with universal enthusiasm. Horowitz and Moncrieff (2021) mentioned that in the SUSTAIN I trial (Daly et al. 2019), one site in Poland accounted for the positive findings (essentially all relapses after discontinuation of esketamine). All other sites in the trial showed no difference between the continuation versus discontinuation groups. This is of course suspicious. When patients were receiving ongoing maintenance esketamine inhalations, it was probably pretty easy for patients who were discontinued to know that they weren't getting the real thing anymore. Thus, functional unblinding was probably at play. Regarding safety, Horowitz and Moncrieff (2021) mentioned that there were no deaths in 486 placebo patients and 6 in 1,861 esketamine patients (three suicides, one motor vehicle accident 26 hours after an esketamine administration, one acute respiratory/cardiac failure, and one myocardial infarction). There were five nonfatal motor vehicle accidents in the esketamine group and one cerebral hemorrhage (nonfatal). The suicides were 4, 12, and 20 days after last esketamine administration. The question of whether there was an esketamine withdrawal effect was broached. Finally, a host of other side effects were more common in the esketamine groups: increased depression, dissociation, and dizziness, for example.

Turner (2019) cited seven concerns about the FDA approval of esketamine: 1) treatment resistance was defined as refractoriness to any two antidepressants (Turner considered this an inaccurate definition); 2) one of the two nonsignificant trials involved those older than 65; 3) there was only a 4-point difference in depression scores between placebo and esketamine in one of the positive trials (TRANSFORM 2); 4) the discontinuation trial involved an enriched sample of those who responded to esketamine, leading to a possibly biased outcome; 5) the same trial was heavily influenced by the one site in Poland; 6) the overall effect size of esketamine is consonant with olanzapine, quetiapine, or aripiprazole augmentation of antidepressants, the latter drugs being cheaper and much better studied; and 7) rapid onset of response was not formally demonstrated.

Another harsh criticism of the FDA approval of esketamine was provided by Cristea and Naudet (2019). They decried weak acute efficacy of esketamine and lack of long-term efficacy, especially considering the patient population studied (chronically ill). They also were not convinced of long-term safety, and they criticized the use of inert placebo as a comparator group and not a well-established antidepressant treatment. Finally, they were not pleased with the outcome being only scores on a depression rating scale (as opposed to functional outcome assessments, which are probably more meaningful to patients who are chronically ill). They believed the FDA should hold future submissions for approval for depression to a higher standard.

Another post-approval disapproval opinion piece was registered by Dr. William Lugg (Lugg 2023), who hails from Melbourne, Australia. Dr. Lugg described the regulatory process in that country, overseen by the Therapeutic Goods Administration (TGA). After two go-rounds rejected esketamine for approval by the TGA, the drug company appealed the decision by going straight to the office of the Ministry of Health. Five weeks later, on March 5, 2021, approval was granted! Dr. Lugg also noted substantial donations by the Janssen-Cilag company (one was $166,955 to the Liberals/Nationals Party, the other $197,400 to the Labor Party) in the years right before esketamine approval was requested. (It's good to have money.)

Like it or not, esketamine was approved and has been in clinical use as of this writing for almost 5 years. The use of esketamine is regulated, and doctors must register with Janssen to prescribe it. It is present on the clinical landscape, but it does not seem to have been a game changer in the field of ketamine for depression; most use still involves intravenous racemic ketamine, which is cheap and easier to obtain and use.

Speaking of racemic ketamine, how does its efficacy compare to esketamine's? Bahji et al. (2021) compared the antidepressant efficacy of esketamine and racemic ketamine, reviewing 24 trials representing 1,877 participants, 97.8% with unipolar depression. Overall, racemic ketamine was associated with better antidepressant and antisuicidal benefits than esketamine, although in the one head-to-head comparison of the two (Correia-Melo et al. 2020), there was no difference in acute outcomes. All racemic ketamine trials in this analysis involved IV administration, whereas most esketamine trials involved intranasal administration (indeed, the only IV esketamine trial involved a comparison to racemic), so it is possible the results reflect less antidepressant efficacy of esketamine in a pharmacodynamic way and more that the pharmacokinetics of the intranasal route of administration resulted in lesser benefits. The bioavailability of intranasal ketamine preparations is about 50% that of IV administration.

What About Arketamine?

Arketamine might be called "the forgotten ketamine enantiomer." In this section, we consider what's going on with arketamine, starting first with discussion of basic science data that are driving this interest and following with clinical data in humans.

Animal Studies of Arketamine

A most fascinating series of publications emanated from the lab of Dr. Kenji Hashimoto, a neuropharmacologist at Chiba University in Japan. Hashimoto and his team have dominated the animal-based arketamine literature. Several of their papers strongly advocated arketamine as a longer-lasting antidepressant (in rodents), without esketamine's side effects. Hashimoto disclosed in his papers that he has a patent on the use of arketamine as an antidepressant in humans. In an early letter, he advocated for further study of arketamine as a possible antidepressant alternative to either racemic ketamine or esketamine (Hashimoto 2014). Zhang et al. (2014a) and Yang et al. (2015), two teams led by Hashimoto, used a mouse model of depression involving neonatal exposure to dexamethasone (which presumably causes at least some mice to show later signs analogous to depression in humans). Both arketamine and esketamine (compared with saline) reduced "depressive features" in the tests immediately, but only arketamine resulted in extended benefit several days later, thus leading the authors to proclaim arketamine to have longer-lasting antidepressant benefits in mice.

Some recent attention has also been focused on the possible antidepressant efficacy of a metabolite of arketamine, namely (2R,6R)-hydroxynorketamine (see Chapter 4 for the molecular structure of this compound). Yang et al. (2017) tested the metabolite in male adult mice. Depression (or at least its rodent analog) was induced with either lipopolysaccharide injection or social defeat stress. Mice received arketamine, esketamine, or (2R,6R)-hydroxynorketamine and were tested for depression-like behavior. The two ketamine enantiomers prevented this, but the hydroxy metabolite was only weak at best, thus contradicting other results showing it has antidepressant effect in rodents.

Human Studies of Arketamine

In the first human report with arketamine, White et al. (1980) randomized surgical patients to anesthesia induction with 2 mg/kg racemic ketamine, 1 mg/kg esketamine, or 3 mg/kg arketamine. (The dosing was based on the higher potency of esketamine than arketamine at NMDA receptor blockade.) Adequacy of anesthesia, emergence restlessness, postprocedural amnesia, pain scores, unpleasant dreaming, and patient self-reports of overall acceptability all favored esketamine over arketamine. The field of anesthesiology pretty much lost interest in arketamine. In the decades since the study was published, there is virtually nothing in the anesthesiology literature about arketamine. In a later report with normal volunteers, White et al. (1985) confirmed the superiority of esketamine over arketamine as a general anesthetic. Øye et al. (1992) and Mathisen et al. (1995) studied arketamine and esketamine in six healthy volunteers and pain patients and generally found better analgesic efficacy with the latter compound.

Vollenweider et al. (1997a)Vollenweider et al. (1997a)Vollenweider et al. (1997a) studied 10 volunteers, each receiving three infusions: one with saline, one with arketamine, and one with esketamine. With esketamine, strong dissociative, visual, and mood effects occurred (the latter being described as dysphoric to flat). Arketamine, on the other hand, produced none of these effects but rather a state of relaxation. This study is important because of the comparisons of ketamine's two enantiomers at equal doses, showing how dramatically different their effects are.

Persson et al. (2002) administered 7 mg intravenously over 30 minutes of esketamine and arketamine, on separate occasions, to 10 healthy male volunteers (24–62 years old). The volunteers performed a working memory task and reported subjective effects while under the influence of each enantiomer. Side effects including drowsiness, dizziness, inebriation, dreamlike experiences, floating sensations, distorted body image, and distorted vision or hearing (subjectively rated by the volunteer) were present for esketamine but virtually absent for arketamine at this dosage. Working memory task performance was equal between the two enantiomers. This study showed that at equal doses, arketamine is better tolerated in terms of dissociative effects than esketamine.

Pfenninger et al. (2002) followed cognitive and mood assessments for 1 hour after infusions of racemic ketamine (0.5 mg/kg), esketamine (0.25 mg/kg), and arketamine (1.0 mg/kg) over 30 seconds in randomized, crossover fashion to 24 healthy volunteers. About 20%–25% had dreams with the three compounds, equal among them. Overall mood and cognitive outcomes were also similar for the three compounds. About half the patients had unusual dreams while sleeping the night of the infusions (which were done in the daytime), indicating some carryover effect beyond the presence of the compound in the brain. The point of this paper was that if the dose of arketamine is high enough, its clinical effects are similar to those of esketamine.

A recent review of this topic was provided by Hashimoto's team at Chiba University (Zhang et al. 2022). This paper cited pharmaceutical companies known to be pursuing arketamine as an antidepressant in humans: Perception Neurosciences, a subsidiary of Atai Life Sciences (U.S.); Otsuka Pharmaceutical Co. (Japan); Jiangsu HengRui Medicine Co. (China); and Jiangsu Enhua Pharmaceutical Co. (China). (It appears the race is on!) Hashimoto mentioned that the drug company that owns the patent on MK-801 (dizocilpine) had some data on it in humans as an antidepressant, unpublished, but it failed (it was successful in rodents). This would be another piece of evidence that NMDA receptor blockade is unrelated to ketamine's mechanism of action because its *inhibitory constant* (K_i, the concentration of the inhibitor required to decrease the maximal rate of the reaction by half) is extremely low. From Wei et al. (2022), its $K_i = 0.0019$ μM (compared with phencyclidine's, $K_i = 0.06$ μM, and esketamine's, 0.3 μM). MK-801 is the mother of all NMDA receptor blockers: if it fails to effect some human outcome variable, then that variable is probably unrelated to NMDA blockade. Alternatively, there may be a potency of NMDA receptor blockade that is antidepressant in humans (and ketamine may have that potency), whereas higher potencies (such as are achieved with PCP and dizocilpine) may yield effects that either are not antidepressant or are too toxic to be tolerated.

With all the exhaustive attention accorded to arketamine in the animal literature, and quite frankly the hype that has gone along with that, the time certainly has come for human data. Is arketamine really a good human antidepressant, better tolerated than esketamine or racemic ketamine, and perhaps associated with less abuse liability? As of this writing, the jury is still out.

Fortunately, there are some data thus far. Leal et al. (2021) provided the first-ever data on the use of arketamine in human depression. Seven patients with depression were treated with arketamine in an open-label manner (i.e., no placebo group, no blinding), 0.5 mg/kg over 40 minutes. Each patient was said to be refractory in the current depressive episode to at least two conventional antidepressant medications. Average MADRS depression rating scale scores decreased an eye-popping 20 points in just 24 hours—thus, the average patient went from "severely" depressed (i.e., score ~30) to "remitted" (a score of 10) with this one low arketamine dose. No psychotomimetic side effects were noted. Good results indeed—but perhaps too good to be true? Alas, a follow-up study, this one properly controlled with a placebo group and blinded administration and outcome assessment, was negative (Leal et al. 2023). Ten depression patients were randomized to first receive arketamine 0.5 mg/kg IV over 40 minutes or saline, with a crossover to the other infusion a week later. Results showed that at no time point did depression rating scale scores (MADRS) differ between the two infusions. Importantly, scores went down only a few points with arketamine, in marked contrast to the dramatic 20-point drop in the open-label study just cited. This is another disappointing example, quite frequent in antidepressant medication research, in which an open-label trial shows great-looking efficacy but a follow-up controlled trial is a failure.

As of this writing, Perception Neuroscience has studied potential antidepressant properties in humans of arketamine (which this company has codified PCN-101). Early 2023 results were posted on its website of a phase 2a trial of PCN-101 for treatment-resistant depression in 102 participants. In the 2-week trial, participants received in randomized fashion one injection of saline placebo, 30 mg PCN-101, or 60 mg PCN-101. (Note that the doses were not weight based.) The main outcome was change in MADRS scores 24 hours after the infusion, but participants were followed for 2 weeks. Mean reductions on the scale were an impressive 15.3 points for PCN-101 60 mg and 13.7 for saline placebo, the difference not being statistically different. (Another victory for placebo!)

Unfazed by these negative results, Perception Neuroscience announced on April 13, 2023, that the first patient had been enrolled in their next study of PCN-101, a phase 1 study comparing the safety and tolerability in normal, nondepressed participants (projected sample size = 16) of 60 mg intravenous PCN-101 versus 60 mg, 90 mg, and 120 mg subcutaneous

PCN-101. It was a crossover design in which each participant will receive each of these four administrations/dosages. The results of the study were posted to their website on August 8, 2023. They found that the highest dose of subcutaneous delivery, 120 mg, was well tolerated, with minimal sedation or dissociation, and resulted in the same peak blood concentration as 60 mg IV (Perception Neuroscience 2023). Thus, Perception Neuroscience believes this formulation may ultimately be suitable for at-home use.

So that is what Perception Neuroscience is up to! If they want a return on the inevitable millions of dollars needed to obtain FDA approval for their product, they need something to patent that no other drug company can use, and something that will attract potential patients away from the two other currently available ketamine products: racemic ketamine (which is available everywhere but only in a clinic situation) and esketamine, which is also available only in a clinic setting. So Perception Neuroscience is looking to pursue at-home use of its product as an attractive alternative. But it must actually work (not just be well tolerated), and so far the data on that score seem discouraging. Perhaps with further study, there will be a dose of arketamine (PCN-101) that works acceptably for depression but still maintains a tolerability advantage over other ketamine products. Time will tell.

What Are the Risks of Ketamine for Depression?

Thus far, the main adverse outcomes mentioned in the literature of ongoing ketamine administration are possible cognitive toxicity, ulcerative cystitis, and abuse liability.

Cognitive Impairment

A review article by Gill et al. (2021) of five studies indicated no initial signal indicating cognitive toxicity of ketamine beyond the immediate time period of administration. Araújo-de-Freitas et al. (2021) compared cognitive testing between esketamine and racemic ketamine, single infusions, and found mostly improved cognition on day 7 after infusion, with no differences between the two groups. Thus far, there is no signal of cognitive toxicity of serial ketamine administrations over time in medically controlled circumstances.

Ulcerative Cystitis

As we discussed earlier in Chapter 3 on recreational use of ketamine, long-standing, regular, high-dose ketamine use results in ulcerative cystitis, sometimes to a crippling degree. So far in the ketamine-for-depression literature, no such effect has emerged. The key to minimizing this effect probably lies in letting ketamine and its metabolites clear from the urine in between administrations to minimize the toxic effect they have on the inner bladder lining.

Abuse Liability

Le et al. (2022) provided a nice clinical and preclinical review of the abuse liability of ketamine. Ten human studies were reviewed; none showed a propensity for medically supervised ketamine administration to cause cravings or addictive behavior. However, there are occasional reports of patients abusing ketamine when they are able to obtain their own supplies. This leads to the common recommendation that ketamine be administered only under medical supervision and that patients not be given prescriptions for their own supplies to be taken at will.

Even if patients in a ketamine clinic are unable to obtain their own supplies of ketamine, it is possible that they may still crave ketamine in between administrations. Clinicians must be vigilant for such an effect if operating a ketamine clinic.

Is Ketamine a True Antidepressant or Just a Feel-Good Drug?

What does it mean for a treatment to be antidepressant? Reductions in depression rating scales? A neurobiological change that is currently unidentified? In much biomedical clinical research, the main outcome measure pertains to a physiological mechanism, whereas patients' subjective feelings of well-being are secondary outcomes. For example, in research on new treatments for congestive heart failure, the primary outcome is echocardiographic evidence of improved cardiac pump function (not how well the patient is feeling). In depression research, however, the primary outcome is depression rating scales, which are almost exclusively patient-reported answers to questions on how well they are feeling, and not some neurobiological indicator of brain function. Thus, any intervention that makes people feel good can be construed as an antidepressant. The usual treatments for depression—oral antidepressants and ECT—do not make nondepressed people feel better and are therefore considered true antidepressants.

So why does ketamine make people feel better? Is the mechanism the same as for oral antidepressants or ECT, or as for opiates, alcohol, stimulants, benzodiazepines, or marijuana products? Drugs of abuse and recreational drugs are not considered true antidepressants. If depressed patients, naive to these types of compounds, were administered any one of them in proper dosage, their depression rating scores would undoubtedly go down for a while, but they are not antidepressants because of their addictive potential. So why is ketamine considered an antidepressant, when it too has addictive potential?

Ketamine seems to straddle the boundary between true antidepressants and drugs of abuse that just make people feel good. What is the difference? There is no clear answer, but the question is a worthy one to consider.

Does Ketamine Work by the Placebo Effect?

The concept of placebo has been extensively studied. When the expectation of an outcome causes that outcome, then a placebo effect is said to occur. For example, if a patient in acute severe pain is told they are receiving morphine, but are actually given an inert sugar pill instead, many patients still report pain reduction. The placebo effect has been implicated as a mediator of response with oral antidepressants as well. One of the factors of a good placebo is that the patient must believe the treatment is real. And one factor that helps patients believe is if the substance has a discernible effect, such as dissociation with ketamine.

Mathai et al. (2020) reviewed eight studies in which an attempt was made to correlate degree of induced dissociation at ketamine infusion with subsequent antidepressant efficacy. In five of the studies, no association was found. Two studies found an association between the rise in CADSS post-infusion and later reduction in depression rating scale scores. Thus it appears that overall, the antidepressant response to ketamine is not mediated, at least not strongly, by the sensation of dissociation immediately induced by the infusion.

That doesn't mean ketamine lacks a placebo effect. It is worth noting that in the studies comparing ketamine with saline placebo, saline is associated with virtually no antidepressant efficacy at all (not surprising, since saline solution causes no discernible changes or feelings that would make patients believe it is "real"). On the other hand, some of the studies comparing ketamine to midazolam showed impressive responses with midazolam (which is not known to be an antidepressant but has anxiolytic and sedative effects). In a review of ketamine-versus-saline and ketamine-versus-midazolam studies, Wilkinson et al. (2019) found that ketamine had greater effect sizes compared with saline than with midazolam, and that the reason for this was higher efficacy with midazolam. For example, Murrough et al. (2013a) found 24-hour response rates (at least 50% reductions in depression rating scale scores) of 28% with just one small infusion of midazolam. Sharma et al. (2020) found 24-hour reductions in the same scale of about 14 points on average with midazolam, which happened to be identical to the reductions with ketamine. Furthermore, those 1-day reductions in scores were largely sustained in the midazolam group, with four additional midazolam infusions over the next couple of weeks. In the latest ketamine-versus-midazolam study, cited earlier (Loo et al. 2023), the 1-day reductions in MADRS scores were virtually identical between the ketamine and midazolam groups.

Why would a short-acting benzodiazepine be associated with such impressive outcomes of depression? Could midazolam itself be a true antidepressant, or is it merely a good placebo? If the latter, then is ketamine simply a better placebo? Again, these questions are important but as yet unanswered.

What Are the Proposed Neurobiological Mechanisms of Action of Ketamine for Depression?

We begin this section with two fundamental questions regarding ketamine for depression: what does it do, and where does it do it? We need to know about the receptors it binds to, the neuromolecular cascades it initiates, and the cellular neuroplastic and cerebral circuitry changes it ultimately causes, and we need to know where in the brain these essential changes take place.

Both questions are inordinately complex, and after decades of intensive search, neither is definitively answered. We lack fundamental understanding of how the human brain works in the normal state, and we lack the technology to study the living human brain at the levels of molecules, cells, and circuits. Finding the neurobiological basis of any psychiatric disorder or treatment has been the holy grail of biological psychiatric research for decades.

Some recent reviews have attempted to pinpoint ketamine's mechanism of action for depression. Widman and McMahon (2020) noted that in animal models of depression, neuronal abnormalities such as dendritic spine loss and circuit dysfunction occurred. They claimed that ketamine reverses these things and reviewed the rodent data, focusing on excitatory/inhibitory balance in the medial prefrontal cortex and hippocampus, two regions commonly implicated in depression and treatment thereof. They pointed to strong findings that ketamine's antidepressant effect in rodent models requires activation of AMPA receptors, increased BDNF release, increased synthesis of synaptic proteins, and stimulation of the mTOR type 1 complex. All these steps in the cascade of actions of ketamine presumably begin with NMDA receptor blockade. They gave two hypotheses to explain this process.

The disinhibition hypothesis is the most commonly cited in recent years. In this hypothesis, NMDA receptors on GABA-ergic interneurons, in the cortex and hippocampus most prominently, are blocked by ketamine. This causes decreased activity of the GABA-ergic interneurons, which normally inhibit glutamatergic pyramidal cells. The latter are thus disinhibited, and their extra activity causes stimulation of postsynaptic AMPA receptors with the accompanying cascade of neuromolecular events, ultimately leading to neuroplastic changes that presumably restore synaptic homeostasis, the predepression equilibrium.

In contrast, the direct inhibition hypothesis posits that NMDA receptors on pyramidal cells are blocked by ketamine, particularly those with GluN2B subunits. This causes desuppression of protein synthesis that normally occurs with eEF2 kinase, with resultant insertion of more AMPA receptors at excitatory synapses and thus more AMPA-mediated neuronal activity. Normally, eEF2 kinase suppresses protein synthesis.

These two mechanisms are not necessarily mutually exclusive—both may be at play with ketamine. One implication of this theory is that selective GluN2B antagonists might be antidepressant, but alas they have not yet been effective in humans. It is also noted that in rodents, the ketamine metabolite (2R,6R)-hydroxynorketamine does seem to stimulate AMPA receptors without first causing NMDA receptor blockade. Thus, perhaps it will turn out to be a good human antidepressant without the two problems associated with NMDA receptor blockade, namely, dissociation and abuse potential. In rodent models, ketamine is noted to increase dendritic spine density in the hippocampal CA1 region and the medial prefrontal cortex. These effects persist after ketamine is cleared from the system, suggesting a mechanism for its prolonged clinical effects.

In another review of the possible mechanism of action of ketamine for depression, Kang et al. (2022) cited no fewer than 139 studies on cell cultures, animal models, and humans pertinent to ketamine antidepressant mechanisms. Overall evidence according to these authors supported rapid increases by ketamine in intracellular signaling molecules that modulate neuroplasticity and correlate with antidepressant efficacy. Molecules and receptors of interest (to give an idea of how expansive this whole neuroplasticity topic has become) include glutamate, AMPA receptors, mTOR, BDNF, tropomyosin-related kinase B, VGF nerve growth factor, eEF2 kinase, P70 ribosomal S6 kinase, glycogen synthase kinase 3, insulin-like growth factor 2, extracellular signal-related kinase, and *microRNAs* (small molecules involved in protein synthesis). Over the coming years, undoubtedly many more neuromolecules of interest will be added.

In a landmark study of this topic in the journal *Science*, Li et al. (2010) studied rat brain preparations after rats had been given ketamine and found evidence of increased activation of mTOR, which as discussed earlier is a protein complex involved in many neurometabolic actions. Ketamine caused robust activation of this pathway, as exemplified in several complex neuromolecular assays. Activation of mTOR led to increased dendritic spine density, evidence of synaptogenesis (which is postulated to be involved in the mechanism of all successful antidepressant treatments, especially ketamine). Ketamine led to increases in a variety of proteins involved in synaptogenesis. Administration of an AMPA receptor blocker prevented the ketamine-induced activation of mTOR, indicating more evidence for AMPA receptor activation in the mechanism of action of ketamine for depression. Rapamycin, an mTOR inhibitor, prevented the antidepressant effects of ketamine in rodent models. These and other complex neuromolecular aspects of this landmark study essentially started the fascination with the mTOR pathway as ketamine's mechanism of action in modern biological psychiatry.

In an important, elegant, and highly cited paper, Zanos et al. (2016) performed a series of studies whose main objective was to show that in rodents, the mechanism of action of ketamine or its metabolites is independent of NMDA receptor activation. We review four main aspects of this complex series of studies. First, replicating findings of the Hashimoto group in Japan, arketamine in mice performed better than esketamine. Arketamine does not potently block NMDA receptors and esketamine does, providing evidence of NMDA receptor blockade's independence of the antidepressant mechanism of ketamine. In addition, MK-801 (dizocilpine), an extremely potent and selective NMDA receptor blocker, did not induce sustained antidepressant effects in these mouse depression models.

Second, a specially formulated ketamine molecule, 6,6-dideuteroketamine, which binds to NMDA receptors but is not metabolized to other compounds (in particular, hydroxynorketamines), was found not to be antidepressant in animals, the implication being that a metabolite of ketamine is the active effector. Third, the authors compared the esketamine metabolite (2S,6S)-hydroxynorketamine and the arketamine metabolite (2R,6R)-hydroxynorketamine and found the latter to be the better antidepressant compound in rodents. These findings have led to intense speculation that (2R,6R)-hydroxynorketamine is the main effector of ketamine's antidepressant activity. This compound does not block NMDA receptors (in the study, it did not displace radiolabeled [3H]MK-801, a potent NMDA receptor blocker). It was shown to enhance AMPA receptor activity, and blockade of AMPA receptors prevented its antidepressant effects in the rodents.

Finally, the Zanos et al. (2016) study found that (2R,6R)-hydroxynorketamine did not affect prepulse inhibition, coordination, or locomotor activity. Neither did it display cross-drug substitution for ketamine in rodent models of abuse liability. Taken together, these last findings suggest better tolerability of this compound—but do any of these rodent findings extend to humans? The field awaits a clinical trial.

One study in humans is informative in this regard. Zarate et al. (2012b) studied 67 depressed patients given single ketamine infusions and drew blood for multiple ketamine metabolites, including 6-hydroxynorketamines, at serial time points after infusion and 24 hours later. The most substantial metabolites beyond norketamine were (2S,6S)- and (2R,6R)-hydroxynorketamine, but levels of these were quite low (they peaked at less than 50 ng/mL). Their levels bore no correlation with antidepressant efficacy, suggesting that the 6-hydroxynorketamines are not involved in the antidepressant mechanism of ketamine. Furthermore, for the most part, these metabolites were measurable only several hours after the infusion and after many patients started to feel better. If the hydroxynorketamines are supposed to be therapeutic, then these results refute that supposition. Yet again, human results do not necessarily align with rodent data.

When it comes to discussions of the neurobiological mechanism of action of ketamine's antidepressant effects, human data are more important than animal data, of course. In this regard, it is worth mentioning that for all the attention focused in the last few years on mTOR activation as the mechanism of action of ketamine for depression in animal models, an effect that is blocked by rapamycin, a recent clinical study in humans showed that administration of rapamycin actually extended the antidepressant benefits of a single infusion of ketamine rather than blocking it (Abdallah et al. 2020). This went totally against the a priori hypothesis. Twenty depressed patients were included, all of whom had one infusion of ketamine plus saline and one of ketamine plus rapamycin. There were no differences in remission rates 24 hours after infusion, but 2 weeks later, the ketamine-plus-rapamycin infusions were associated with a significantly higher sustained remission rate. What to make of this? Probably that we simply cannot extrapolate from rodent data to humans. Perhaps the former can be used for now in the absence of the ability to study neuromolecular signaling in humans and for the reason to search for alternate molecular targets for newer therapies.

Wei et al. (2022), representing Hashimoto's group, articulated an argument against NMDA receptor blockade as arketamine's antidepressant action (at least in rodents, but probably in humans as well). The authors pointed out the utter failure of orally available and tested known NMDA receptor blockers in humans with depression: some of these are commercially available for other indications (e.g., memantine for Alzheimer disease) and others are still in development (e.g., rapastinel, lanicemine, traxoprodil, and AV-101).

As indicated earlier, (2R,6R)-hydroxynorketamine has attracted attention as a possible antidepressant. Bonaventura et al. (2022) attempted to find out where in the brain this compound binds once it crosses the blood–brain barrier. It does not bind to NMDA receptors, μ opioid receptors, κ opioid receptors, or δ opioid receptors. It has no binding at σ-receptors or metabotropic glutamate receptors. In another technique, a radiolabeled version of the compound, [³H](2R,6R)-hydroxynorketamine, was tested to see whether it displaced numerous protein targets in commercially available assays (HuProt has >16,000 gene product proteins in its assay, Protoarray has >9,000 proteins, and Retrogenix has >6,000 cell-surface and secreted human proteins). In all these massive assays, there were no hits for (2R,6R)-hydroxynorketamine; the compound appears to be neurobiologically inert. The only places in rodent bodies where radiolabeled product was found was the liver, where it is metabolized, and the kidney, where it is excreted. It is quite difficult to conceive of this molecule's being a potent, rapidly active antidepressant when it binds to nothing in the brain and is present after ketamine administration at a delay and then at only tiny concentrations. Obviously, however, the field awaits human data in a clinical trial.

One paper that led to a flurry of letters to the editor was published by Williams et al. (2019). In the tiny study, 12 depressed patients were each treated in crossover fashion with one infusion of ketamine preceded 45 minutes earlier by a placebo or 50 mg naltrexone, a potent opioid receptor antagonist (similar to the intravenously available naloxone). Ketamine infusions after the naltrexone were virtually void of any antidepressant effects, whereas those preceded by placebo had the usual efficacy associated with a single 0.5 mg/kg ketamine infusion over 40 minutes. There was no difference in dissociation induced by the two infusions, indicating that naltrexone did not block NMDA receptors (which are believed to mediate dissociation induced by ketamine). The original intent of the investigators was to have a larger sample size, but an interim analysis showed such a dramatic difference—and the depressed people were simply not getting better when the infusion was preceded by naltrexone—that the trial was terminated early so that no more depressed people would be denied efficacy. The implication was simple: the antidepressant efficacy of ketamine is mediated not by NMDA receptor blockade but rather by opiate receptor agonism.

Yoon et al. (2019) studied five people with both depression and alcohol use disorder who each received one long-acting naltrexone injection (380 mg) 2–6 days before a ketamine infusion (0.5 mg/kg over 40 minutes), in a total of four weekly infusions. All participants had abstained from alcohol for a few days or more. One patient left the protocol after two infusions resulted in dramatic improvement of depression. The other four patients ended up with low depression rating scale scores a few hours after the fourth infusion, with a lot of scatter in scores along the way. These results contradict those of Williams et al. (2019). Thus, it remains for future research to determine whether NMDA receptor blockade, opiate agonism, or perhaps another as-yet-unknown mechanism helps ketamine treat those with depression.

Ketamine and Electroconvulsive Therapy

ECT is a procedure commonly used in modern psychiatry to treat patients with depression, mania, catatonia, and exacerbations of schizophrenic psychoses. It involves a series of electrically induced seizures performed under anesthesia. A typical course of treatments for depression is 6–12 sessions three times a week. (To know more about ECT, please consult my earlier book, *Principles and Practice of Electroconvulsive Therapy* [Rasmussen 2019].) ECT is often considered the gold standard for antidepressant efficacy— new treatments that come along are often compared to it.

Ketamine and ECT interact in three ways. First, ketamine has been used as the anesthetic for ECT in numerous studies. However, it has not caught on for this purpose, because it is not well tolerated (it causes a lot of headaches, nausea, dizziness, and out-of-body experiences upon awakening). Also, ketamine has been used to augment a course of ECT, usually in the form of a dose along with the first ECT treatment. This use of ketamine also has not caught on either, because there is sparse evidence that it adds any significant efficacy to the already highly efficacious treatment. Third, ketamine efficacy has been compared to that of ECT. ECT causes memory impairment as a side effect, is expensive, is sometimes hard to find, and can be inconvenient for patient and caregiver (as time taken away from usual activities to get a treatment can be substantial). Ketamine, on the other hand, is relatively easy to administer and is cheaper. But fundamental to this comparison is, how does ketamine's efficacy compare to that of ECT?

Ghasemi et al. (2014) compared three ECT sessions (which is an unusually small number for that modality) versus three ketamine sessions (0.5 mg/kg IV over 45 minutes) in depressed patients. There were only nine patients per group. Depression rating scores decreased to a greater extent with ketamine, particularly after the first treatment.

Kheirabadi et al. (2019) compared IV ketamine 0.5 mg/kg twice a week versus ECT twice a week in inpatients with depression ($n = 16$ in both groups). There was no difference in HDRS scores at any time along the course of treatments. Scores went from 24–26 at baseline to 14–16 at end of treatment. During 3 months of naturalistic follow-up, scores were nonsignificantly lower in the ECT group, probably owing to the small sample size (i.e., an underpowered study). Each group had only six treatments, which may have been too few, especially in the ECT group.

In a later study from the same group, Kheirabadi et al. (2020) randomized 45 patients who were referred for ECT to receive 0.5 mg/kg intramuscular ketamine, 1.0 mg/kg oral ketamine, or ECT (n=15 in each group), with each modality administered in 6–9 sessions over 3 weeks. After the first session, depression ratings were equal in the three groups. Ratings of suicidality were lower for the two ketamine groups at 1 day and during the second week, but not during the rest of the first week. At 1-week and 1-month follow-ups, there were no differences among the three groups on ratings of depression or suicidality. This study seems to show that a few sessions of intramuscular or oral ketamine are equivalent to ECT. Note that psychotic patients were excluded from the study.

Sharma et al. (2020) randomly assigned 13 depressed patients to ECT and 12 to ketamine 0.5 mg/kg over 45 minutes IV, both given in six sessions over 2 weeks. There was a 92.3% remission rate with ECT versus 50% for ketamine. Three of the ketamine patients dropped out before completing six sessions: two for inefficacy and one for side effects.

In the Ekstrand et al. (2022) study mentioned earlier, KetECT, depressed patients were randomized to receive either ketamine (n=95) or ECT (n=91). Ketamine was dosed at 0.5 mg/kg over 40 minutes IV and given three times a week, as was ECT. The ECT remission rate was 63%, and that for ketamine was 46%, a statistically significant advantage for ECT. Older age was associated with better response for ECT (and lesser response for ketamine). There was no statistically significant difference in remission rate between the treatments for those 50 and younger. For psychotic patients, ketamine resulted in an impressive 50% remission rate, and ECT resulted in a 79% remission rate. Because of the small sample size of those with psychosis, that difference was not statistically significant (but probably real, as it is well known that ECT is especially effective for psychotic depression). In the 12-month follow-up phase, there was a 64% relapse rate in the ECT group and a 70% relapse rate for ketamine, not statistically different. There was no difference in average time to relapse. It is impressive that in this large sample of ketamine patients, all severely depressed and hospitalized and even some psychotic, there was a 46% remission rate.

Anand et al. (2023), in the ELEKT-D study, randomized patients to IV racemic ketamine versus ECT. In contrast to the KetECT study (Ekstrand et al. 2022), ELEKT-D involved almost all (~90%), outpatients, a less severely ill population. In addition, the patients had a mean current episode duration of 2 years, average age in the mid-40s, average age of onset of depression of age 19, and a median of five previous depressive episodes. None of the patients were psychotic, and many had comorbid psychiatric disorders and prior medication trials. This was a less severely ill but very chronically depressed group of patients. Two hundred patients were randomized to ket-amine and 203 to ECT, but 31 patients dropped out of the ECT group once they knew that would be their treatment; four in the ketamine group dropped out. (Thus, a lot of patients dropped out because they did not want ECT.) ECT was administered three times a week; ketamine, at 0.5 mg/kg, was administered twice a week, both for 3 weeks. Responders (those who had at least 50% reduction in depression rating scale scores) were followed nat-uralistically for 6 months. Response rate was 55.4% with ketamine and a low 41.2% with ECT. Remission rates (a virtual complete abatement of depres-sive symptoms) were 32.3% with ketamine and 20% with ECT, the latter being extremely low for an ECT sample. More memory complaints oc-curred with ECT. On follow-up, 34.5% of ketamine patients and 56.3% of ECT patients relapsed during the 6-month period. There was one suicide attempt in the ketamine group. The authors concluded that for nonpsy-chotic depression, ketamine is at least as effective as ECT.

Whether ketamine truly matches the well-known historical efficacy of ECT for depression continues to be debated. However, these comparative studies, the last two very large ones, do provide some of the best-documented efficacy data for ketamine to date.

Chapter 8

Other Uses of Ketamine in Psychiatry: Anxiety Disorders, Substance Use, and Psychotherapy Augmentation

---

KEY POINTS IN THIS CHAPTER:

- Ketamine has had limited success as treatment for PTSD and OCD.

- Ketamine has shown interesting efficacy for some substance use disorders.

- The dissociative and psychedelic effects of ketamine have been used to augment psychotherapy for anxiety and depression.

Since its success in treating depression was discovered, ketamine has been used as a treatment for posttraumatic stress disorder (PTSD), obsessive compulsive disorder (OCD), eating disorders, autism, generalized anxiety disorder, social anxiety disorder, and a variety of substance use disorders. Ketamine is relatively easy to use, cheap, and profitable, and those in the psychiatric profession and their patients are desperate for something that will alleviate the pain of these conditions. The use of ketamine for this broad array of disorders broaches the mechanistic question of whether there is some type of general action of ketamine that nonspecifically lowers emotional distress. (Oral antidepressant medications are used for these other conditions as well.)

Ketamine for Anxiety and Eating Disorders and Autism

Posttraumatic Stress Disorder

Feder et al. (2014) undertook a randomized crossover trial of ketamine compared to the active placebo midazolam. The study interventions in those with PTSD consisted of one infusion of 0.5 mg/kg IV ketamine over 40 minutes and one infusion of 0.045 mg/kg IV midazolam over 40 minutes. The two infusions were separated by at least a week. The outcome assessments 1 day after each infusion showed a 50% reduction (approximately) in PTSD severity with midazolam and a 75% reduction with ketamine. For the subsequent 6 days of assessment, scores tended to go back up for both groups but not quite to baseline, with final 1-week scores a bit lower for ketamine than midazolam. What is really interesting about this study is how good midazolam was for PTSD regardless of how it compared to ketamine. Depression scores were also obtained (because a lot of PTSD patients have ongoing significant depressive symptoms), and those scores went down with both infusions equally; ketamine was no better an antidepressant in this study than midazolam.

In two separately published data sets, Pradhan et al. (2017; 2018) studied 30 patients diagnosed with PTSD. A special psychotherapy termed Trauma Interventions using Mindfulness Based Extinction and Reconsolidation (TIMBER) was given to all patients, half of whom got randomized to a concurrent ketamine infusion of 0.5 mg/kg over 40 minutes and the other half to placebo saline infusion. There were 12 sessions of TIMBER therapy, the elements of which are described in Pradhan et al. (2015). The infusions were administered the day of the first therapy session. A predefined criterion of response was based on a PTSD rating scale, and it lasted on average 33–35 days with ketamine and 16–25 days with saline, indicating that ketamine may have positively augmented the psychotherapy.

Hart et al. (1972) undertook a retrospective chart review study of 37 patients with depression, 15 of whom had PTSD as well. They received oral ketamine in an ongoing manner, weekly to every 2 months, dosed at 0.5–7.0 mg/kg for 6–36 months (median 31 months of treatment). Hospitalizations were reduced during this period in comparison to before initiation of ketamine in this highly recurrent, chronic population.

Albott et al. (2018), in an open-label study, treated 15 patients with PTSD and depression with six infusions of ketamine 0.5 mg/kg over

40 minutes spread out over 2 weeks; they were then followed weekly for 8 weeks. Criteria for remission of PTSD, based on rating scale scores, was reached in 80% by the end of the six infusions. There was a 60% remission of depressive symptoms. Median time to PTSD relapse was 41 days. Half of the PTSD remitters remained so for the whole 8 weeks. Thus, this data set is rather sanguine in its portrayal of ketamine efficacy.

Duek et al. (2019), in a data set published as an abstract, randomized 17 PTSD patients to IV ketamine 0.5 mg/kg or midazolam over 40 minutes, once, following a first session of *prolonged exposure therapy* (a type of therapy that teaches the patient to gradually approach trauma-related memories, feelings, and situations that they have been avoiding since the trauma). After 90 days, the PTSD symptoms were better in the ketamine than the midazolam group, although detailed data were not provided in the abstract. Considering that benzodiazepines are well known to impair memory consolidation, one question is, did ketamine enhance the psychotherapy efficacy, or did midazolam (a benzodiazepine) worsen it? The infusions in this study were given after a psychotherapy session, and it is prudent to assume no mental health expert would want to give a benzodiazepine right after a psychotherapy session.

Ross et al. (2019) treated 30 male combat veterans who had PTSD with six 1-hour ketamine infusions over 2–3 weeks, each dose 1.94 mg/kg on average (the first dose was 1.0 mg/kg). Depression and PTSD symptoms, but not self-reported substance use, decreased during the acute-phase study. These are relatively high doses of ketamine, which the authors of the study used to induce a "transpersonal" experience (i.e., a psychedelic effect).

Keizer et al. (2020) treated 11 inpatients who had comorbid chronic neuropathic pain and PTSD with continuous ketamine infusions for about 5 days. The ketamine doses were started at 2 µg/kg/min and increased by 1–2 µg/kg/min every 3–4 hours, targeting a final dose of 11–15 µg/kg/min, which was continued for 96 hours. Daily bedside psychotherapy was conducted for 90 minutes per session. Acute reductions in PTSD were substantial, but long-term outcomes were not provided.

Dadabayev et al. (2020) treated chronic pain patients, with and without concomitant PTSD, with one infusion of either ketamine 0.5 mg/kg or the nonsteroidal anti-inflammatory agent ketorolac 15 mg IV over 40 minutes in randomized fashion. Quite interestingly, the two drugs had equal good efficacy for pain (no surprise there) but also PTSD symptoms (big surprise: why would a drug similar to aspirin help PTSD?). The total sample was 41 patients in four groups (with and without PTSD, taking ketamine or ketorolac, about 10 patients per group). Another interesting finding was that dissociative symptoms as assessed by CADSS occurred even with ketorolac, a drug that normally would not be considered psychopharmacologically active.

Shiroma et al. (2020a) treated nine patients with chronic PTSD with prolonged exposure therapy along with three weekly ketamine infusions of 0.5 mg/kg 24 hours before psychotherapy sessions. PTSD rating scale scores were said to be much improved with this regimen, at least acutely.

Halstead et al. (2021), in a case report of a patient with PTSD, over a 13-day span administered ketamine four times in an oral lozenge formulation of 150 mg per lozenge. That combined with intensive psychotherapy was said to result in excellent resolution of PTSD symptoms that lasted 4 months. It is difficult to tell if it was the intensive therapy, the ketamine, or the combination that led to the improvement.

Feder et al. (2021) randomized 30 people with chronic PTSD to either six infusions of ketamine 0.5 mg/kg over 40 minutes or midazolam 0.045 mg/kg over 40 minutes, both groups having three sessions per week over 2 weeks. Predefined PTSD response rates (via rating scale) were 67% for the ketamine group and 20% for the midazolam group. It is interesting that in a group of chronic PTSD patients, 20% had response to midazolam, a short-acting benzodiazepine. In the ketamine responders, median time to relapse during follow-up was 27.5 days after the last infusion.

Abdallah et al. (2019; 2022) conducted a randomized study of patients with PTSD in three groups: saline placebo, 0.2 mg/kg IV ketamine, or 0.5 mg/kg IV ketamine over 40 minutes. The infusions were administered twice a week for 4 weeks (eight total). A total of 158 patients were randomized, 54 to saline, 53 to 0.2 mg/kg ketamine, and 51 to 0.5 mg/kg ketamine. All three types of infusion resulted in sharp reductions in PTSD symptoms 1 day after the first infusion, with continued small reductions over the next 4 weeks. Interestingly, there was no beneficial effect of ketamine over saline. Thus, this study, which is the largest randomized study of ketamine for PTSD to date, was negative for a specific ketamine effect on PTSD symptoms, although there was a benefit of the 0.5 mg/kg dose on depressive symptoms.

Bentley et al. (2022) reported on 15 military veterans with PTSD and depression who did not obtain significant relief with intranasal esketamine but, with subsequent switch to IV racemic ketamine, had much better results.

In an interesting offshoot of the ketamine-for-PTSD literature, a few investigators have approached the subject creatively by assessing whether ketamine administered as part of anesthetic/surgical care in wounded people helps or hurts chances of subsequent development of PTSD. Winter and Irle (2004) assessed 15 burn patients who did develop subsequent PTSD and 21 burn patients who did not. Having received ketamine as part of initial burn care was correlated with stronger PTSD symptoms, suggesting, somewhat disconcertingly, that ketamine actually may cause or at least predispose to PTSD. McGhee et al. (2008) studied Iraq War veterans burned during combat. Of those who received ketamine as part of initial burn care, 27% had PTSD according to a checklist rating scale, and 46% of those not receiving ketamine had PTSD. This implies a protective effect of ketamine regarding subsequent development of PTSD when used at the time of initial accident or burn care. In a follow-up report by the same group (McGhee et al. 2014) with a larger sample size of burned soldiers from Iraq ($n = 289$), there was no difference in rates of PTSD positivity by checklist screening at least 30 days after injury. The ketamine patients had longer hospital stays and more surgeries, but still did not have higher rates of PTSD.

Schönenberg et al. (2005) studied 56 victims of moderate-severity accidents for peritraumatic and current (i.e., 1 year later) symptoms of dissociation and PTSD. Controlling for accident severity and degree of subsequent disability, the investigators found that peritraumatic and current symptoms were correlated with having received esketamine, but racemic ketamine not so much, at the time of initial trauma care.

The same group (Schönenberg et al. 2008) assessed 50 accident victims for acute stress disorder (which is essentially a precursor of PTSD) 3 days after their accidents. Thirteen of these accident victims happened to have gotten ketamine as part of the initial sedation during their emergency care; 24 received opioids (and no ketamine); and 13 got non-opioid, nonketamine sedation. The three groups were matched to severity of accident and degree of injury. Symptoms of re-experiencing, hyperarousal, and avoidance (the hallmarks of posttraumatic stress) were greater in the group that received ketamine, which had more dissociative symptoms as well. The question is whether the ketamine or the accident caused the symptoms, which were assessed just 3 days after the use of ketamine. It could be that the symptoms simply represented some type of carryover ketamine side effect, rather than a true acute stress disorder. Indeed, the injuries were relatively minor (such as fractures, contusions, minor burns, and cuts) and not usually associated with severe psychological distress. All subjects were treated as outpatients and did not need hospitalization.

Following up on this literature, Zeng et al. (2013) reviewed three randomized saline-controlled ketamine-for-depression studies to see whether those with PTSD may have gotten worse with ketamine. The combined data set contained 10 depressed patients with comorbid PTSD, 12 with a history of sexual abuse, and 8 with a history of physical abuse. There was no signal indicating that any of these three groups had higher CADSS scores during ketamine infusions or worsened outcomes after their ketamine infusions, thus weighing against the notion that ketamine worsens chances of PTSD.

Mion et al. (2017) studied 274 Afghanistan war veterans who had been wounded in combat, 36% of whom carried a clinical diagnosis of PTSD. As part of their initial trauma care, 55% of the PTSD patients and 20% of non-PTSD patients had received ketamine. The results seemed to indicate that ketamine may have predisposed to subsequent development of PTSD, but after statistically controlling for injury severity, ketamine as an independent predictor of PTSD was eliminated.

Glavonic et al. (2022), in a theory paper attempting to explain why ketamine and other hallucinogens might help PTSD, elaborated the concept that such agents accelerate fear extinction, which is the basis of therapies for phobias and PTSD. The authors speculated that ketamine may facilitate fear extinction by either direct effect on the brain or making the patient more amenable to exposure therapies.

So the results from this surprisingly large literature on ketamine for PTSD, as in depression, tend to be short term, and it bears repeating that the largest randomized study (Abdallah et al. 2022) was negative.

Obsessive-Compulsive Disorder

Some investigators have tried treating OCD with ketamine, presumably on the theory of glutamatergic dysfunction, but probably because ketamine is available and and easy to use. Bloch et al. (2012), in an open-label case series, treated 10 OCD patients with one infusion of ketamine 0.5 mg/kg over 40 minutes and found essentially no benefit to OCD symptoms, although there was a decent but short-lived antidepressant benefit. Niciu et al. (2013a) described in detail two patients from that study who had increased depression and suicidality 1 day after their ketamine infusions. The authors cautioned against using ketamine for OCD except in research.

Rodriguez et al. (2013) conducted a randomized, crossover trial in which 15 patients with OCD each received, in random order, two infusions at least a week apart; one infusion was ketamine 0.5 mg/kg over 40 minutes, and the other was saline. One week after infusion, 50% of ketamine- and 0% of saline-treated patients had at least a 35% reduction in OCD symptom severity on a commonly accepted measure of significant clinical response in OCD studies. There was a lot of heterogeneity in response, however; for example, in 5 of 15 ketamine cases, OCD severity actually went up after infusion. The decrease on obsessionality scores right after the infusions was greater with ketamine than with saline. Over the subsequent week, mean scores trended back up but not to baseline, much as for single-infusion ketamine studies of depression. Reporting on MRS scans performed during the trial, Rodriguez et al. (2015) found that changes in prefrontal GABA correlated with reduction in obsessionality during the infusion.

Rodriguez et al. (2017) conducted an intranasal ketamine study in which patients were randomized to one intranasal administration of racemic ketamine 50 mg and another of intranasal midazolam 4 mg, in counterbalanced order. Fifteen of 20 eligible patients refused to participate because they disliked the intranasal route of administration. Of the remaining five, two completed both infusions, neither of whom liked the intranasal format and neither of whom got a good response to ketamine. The authors concluded that intranasal ketamine may not be acceptable to OCD patients.

In a follow-up to their randomized IV ketamine study, Rodriguez et al. (2016a) administered memantine, an orally available NMDA receptor blocker, to see whether it would help OCD symptoms. There was no placebo group. The initial ketamine responders ($n=4$) seemed to sustain their response while taking memantine, but none of the eight nonresponders to ketamine responded to memantine.

In an attempt to test whether exposure psychotherapy after ketamine for OCD may help sustain the initial benefits, Rodriguez et al. (2016b) treated eight OCD patients with open-label ketamine, one infusion of 0.5 mg/kg over 40 minutes followed by 2 weeks of 10 sessions of exposure therapy. One patient was said to be cured of OCD with this regimen, at least in the short term. Most patients had reductions in OCD severity in the first week after the infusion, with some drift upward over the next 3 weeks.

In an open-label case series, Shiroma et al. (2020b) treated 14 OCD patients with serial infusions of ketamine, with a mean of 5.4 infusions (range 2–10, two or three times a week). One patient got only two infusions (0.5 mg/kg over 40 minutes) because of poor tolerability. One patient got 10 infusions, with modest improvement. Eleven of the patients received no improvement in OCD symptoms, one showed virtually complete response, and two showed 25%–35% decreases in severity based on rating scales.

Thus far, the literature on ketamine for OCD is not terribly impressive. Most patients with OCD who receive ketamine get no substantial benefit, although occasionally a patient gets dramatic benefit. This is counterbalanced by a few patients who reportedly have gotten worse with ketamine. Over time, hopefully larger studies will be undertaken to see if ketamine does have a place in OCD treatment.

Eating Disorders

The same desperation for more effective treatments has applied to eating disorders. Mills et al. (1998) reported on a series of 15 patients with long histories of eating disorders, age range 23–42. The duration of the eating disorders was 5–21 years. Ketamine was administered at 20 mg/hour IV for 10 hours per session (a large dose). Patients were treated every 5 days to

3 weeks for two to nine sessions per patient. Nalmefene, an opiate receptor blocker, and amitriptyline, a tricyclic antidepressant, were also given to assist with weight gain. Outcome assessments focused on compulsiveness, interestingly. Anorexics tended to gain weight, whereas compulsive eaters such as bulimics tended to lose weight with the ketamine regimen. Of the nine patients classified as responders, the mean number of sessions with ketamine was 4.1; it was 8.3 in nonresponders. One female patient with anorexia gained enough weight to resume menstruating (which halts with weight loss) and even had a successful pregnancy. Several of the responders were noted to have substantial improvements in long-standing neurotic emotions and comportment.

Schwartz et al. (2021) treated four patients with comorbid depression and eating disorders. Case 1 was a 49-year-old woman with anorexia nervosa, depression, and PTSD. She received two intramuscular injections of 0.4 mg/kg ketamine 24 hours apart, followed by seven more injections spread out over half a year. She reportedly felt more comfortable and less obsessed by weight and eating issues, gained some weight, and went off disability status. Case 2 was a 30-year-old woman with anorexia who got an initial intramuscular ketamine shot of 0.5 mg/kg and four subsequent ketamine sessions over about half a year. Each one was 0.5 mg/kg in one arm and 0.4 mg/kg in the other. Her weight went up, and she began menstruating again, but her body image did not change much. Case 3 was a 33-year-old woman who got six intramuscular ketamine injections of 0.5 mg/kg each over about half a year. Her weight stabilized, with reductions in depression and anxiety. Case 4 was a 35-year-old woman whose initial ketamine dose was 0.5 mg/kg IV followed by 0.85 mg/kg doses for a total of nine ketamine sessions over half a year. There was no benefit to the eating disorder, although there was a variable benefit to mood.

Robison et al. (2022) treated five patients with eating disorders (four anorexia and one bulimia) with four weekly intramuscular ketamine injections of varying doses (typically 25–60 mg) in a group format as part of the residential program's therapy. No immediate rating scales were performed relevant to eating disorders, but a survey was sent out several months after participation. Three of the five patients returned the survey, two of whom felt the ketamine helped the eating disorder in some way.

Generalized Anxiety Disorder and Social Anxiety Disorder

A particularly well-designed randomized crossover trial was conducted by Taylor et al. (2018), in which 18 adults with social anxiety disorder each received two infusions, separated by 28 days, one of ketamine 0.5 mg/kg over

40 minutes and the other with saline placebo. Social anxiety symptom rating scales were obtained. Predefined clinical response 3 hours after infusion was about one-third in the ketamine group and none in the saline group.

Glue et al. (2017) treated 12 patients with either generalized anxiety disorder or social anxiety disorder with subcutaneous ketamine weekly for 3 weeks at escalating doses of 0.25, 0.5, and 1.0 mg/kg. Ten of the 12 patients were said to be acute responders, but they were followed for only a few hours after each dose.

In a follow-up to their earlier report, Glue et al. (2020) conducted a study with 12 patients with either generalized anxiety disorder or social anxiety disorder, giving serial 0.25, 0.5, and 1.0 mg/kg ketamine doses in random manner but with a randomly inserted dose of midazolam 0.01 mg/kg along the way without the patient knowing when that medication was given. All doses were subcutaneous. The 1.0 mg/kg dose of ketamine clearly had the best response in terms of anxiety ratings 1 week after the dose. Interestingly, the 0.25 mg/kg ketamine dose was bested by the midazolam dose for anxiety ratings until day 7. If the study comparison had been 0.25 mg/kg ketamine versus 0.01 mg/kg midazolam, and no other doses of ketamine had been used, then the conclusion would have been that midazolam is better for anxiety than ketamine. Glue et al. (2018) and Truppman Lattie et al. (2021) reported that most of the patients who responded to initial ketamine injections for anxiety received ongoing maintenance injections once or twice a week for 3 months. Most of the patients reportedly had better daily functioning with the ketamine in terms of their anxiety symptoms. Whittaker et al. (2021) reviewed the literature on randomized studies of ketamine in patients with anxiety disorder. There were only a few studies, but the general conclusion was that ketamine looked promising.

Autism

A few patients with autistic disorder have been given ketamine. Wink et al. (2021) gave 21 autistic patients two doses of intranasal ketamine 30 and 50 mg 1 week apart, followed by two placebo doses (or vice versa, the placebo doses preceding the real ketamine doses). There was no evidence for a change in aberrant behaviors or social functioning.

Ketamine for Substance Use Disorders

It would appear to be simply too ironic: a drug of addiction being used to treat addiction. Yet a surprisingly large literature has appeared for just this purpose, focusing on using ketamine in the treatment of alcohol, opiate, cocaine, and cannabis use disorders.

Alcohol Use Disorder

Krupitsky (1992) and Krupitsky et al. (1990; 1992) gave a group of 86 people with alcohol use disorder an *aversive pharmacotherapy regimen* (aethimizol-bemegride-ketamine); 100 were given control psychotherapy. There was a 69.8% 1-year abstinence rate in the pharmacological group and 24% in the psychotherapy-only control group, which sounds almost too good to be true.

Krupitsky and Grinenko (1997) reviewed 10 years of research into ketamine-assisted psychotherapy for alcohol use disorder, in which some type of psychotherapy was paired with ketamine treatments. Overall 1-year abstinence rates were 65.8% with ketamine therapy and 24% without. The authors described three stages to the therapy. The first stage was preparatory psychotherapy sessions, the second stage was aethimizol-bemegride-ketamine along with smelling of alcohol, and the third stage was group psychotherapy. There was no random assignment, importantly, because people volunteered for ketamine.

Kolp et al. (2006) indicated that as part of a private psychiatric practice, several dozen patients participated in various types of psychotherapy (individual and group) and had one or two ketamine administrations during that time. Unfortunately, specifics on ketamine dosage and administration were not provided. Abstinence rates over time seemed to correlate with the intensity of the psychotherapy. Further elaboration on the rationale for ketamine-enhanced psychotherapy for alcoholism is provided in Kolp et al. (2009).

Yoon et al. (2019) studied five patients with comorbid depression and alcohol use disorder. All got an intramuscular shot of long-acting naltrexone, an opiate receptor blocking agent. This was followed 2–6 days later by the first of four weekly ketamine infusions of 0.5 mg/kg over 40 minutes. All five patients were said to have an antidepressant response to the ketamine in spite of opiate blockade. Four of the five got reduced alcohol craving after ketamine (but note that naltrexone is also used in the treatment of alcohol use disorder). The results of this study (that naltrexone did not block the antidepressant effects of ketamine) rebuts the findings of Williams et al. (2019) on the same topic.

Das et al. (2019) theorized that people with alcohol use disorder have maladaptive reward memories that perpetuate drinking. If one could retrieve a maladaptive reward memory, then have its reconsolidation or reinforcement blocked via NMDA receptor blockade, then perhaps the maladaptive reward value of alcohol would decrease, and drinking as well (so the investigators postulated). To this end, they studied three groups. In one group, the participants (drinkers who were not seeking treatment) underwent an experimental maladaptive reward memory retrieval task and also got ketamine. The idea here is that ketamine disturbs reconsolidation of the memory, and this group was theorized to drink less. The second group had ketamine alone, that is, without any maladaptive reward memory retrieval task. The idea here is that if this group has the same reduction in drinking, then ketamine must work via some other mechanism than the postulated effect on reconsolidation of maladaptive reward memories. The third group got no ketamine but did have the maladaptive reward memory retrieval task. The total sample size was 90 participants ($n = 30$ in each group).

On day 1 of the study, the baseline assessments were done; on day 3, the interventions were done (ketamine dosing was designed to achieve a blood level of 35 ng/mL for 30 minutes, a relatively low level). A maladaptive reward memory was induced by giving the participant a beer to hold, assessing reactivity to alcohol visual cues, and then generating negative prediction error by unexpectedly telling the participant not to drink the beer (or orange juice, in the group with no maladaptive reward memory). Negative prediction error—that is, inducing an expectation in the participant and then making it not happen—is believed to be necessary for maladaptive reward memory destabilization. Craving measures and ethanol consumed, as assessed on day 10, decreased more in the memory-plus-ketamine group than in the other groups, the degree of which correlated with ketamine blood levels. The results were not dramatic. The memory-plus-ketamine group started out with greater alcohol usage at baseline and ended up at 9 months with the same as the other groups.

Dakwar et al. (2020) administered one infusion over 52 minutes, randomly assigned to either ketamine 0.71 mg/kg ($n = 17$) or midazolam 0.025 mg/kg ($n = 23$), to a group of people with alcohol use disorder enrolled in a 5-week outpatient therapy program. The infusion was during the second week. The patients were followed in person for 21 days, with a telephone follow-up at 6 months. During 3 weeks after infusion, 47.1% of the ketamine group used alcohol and 17.6% drank heavily. Of the midazolam group, the respective percentages were 59.1% and 40.9%, indicating better outcomes with ketamine. Acute dissociative symptoms during the infusions did not correlate with outcomes. At 6 months, of those who could be reached via telephone, 75% of the ketamine and 27% of the midazolam group reported abstinence. There was a longer time to first heavy drinking with ketamine, but not a longer time to first drink.

In a follow-up study, Rothberg et al. (2021) evaluated responses on a mysticism scale assessing such qualities as ego quality, unifying quality, inner subjective quality, temporal/spatial quality, *noetic* quality (mystical or spiritual quality), ineffability quality, positive affect, and religious quality to the experiences with either ketamine or midazolam. Interestingly, the significance of ketamine versus midazolam disappeared when the variable "induced mystical experiences" was entered into the statistical analysis. In other words, it was the amount of mystical experience induced by the drug, and not the drug itself, that predicted effects on alcohol drinking.

Grabski et al. (2022) randomized 96 people with alcohol use disorder to either mindfulness-based psychological therapy or alcohol education and to three infusions of either saline or ketamine 0.8 mg/kg over 40 minutes weekly. Follow up was at 6 months. There was no significant difference in relapse rates during that time, but there were 10.1% more days abstinent with ketamine than saline. There were 15.9% more days abstinent in the ketamine-plus-therapy group versus the saline-plus-alcohol-education group, indicating that mindfulness-based therapy adds something to the ketamine (or perhaps vice versa). The two therapies were delivered in seven sessions over about 3 weeks. The percentage of days abstinent at baseline tended toward 72%–80% in the four groups but was 70%–88% at 6 months, indicating relatively small effect sizes.

In sum, the data so far on the use of ketamine for alcohol use disorder are intriguing but hardly convincing. The idea that ketamine may become some type of standard part of treatment seems unlikely.

Opiate Use Disorder

Krupitsky et al. (2002) randomized 70 recently detoxified heroin addicts to either 2.0 or 0.2 mg/kg intramuscular ketamine before enrollment in a psychotherapeutic program. Beginning about a month after infusion, abstinence rates were 85% and 52% in the high- and low-dose groups, respectively. At 2 years, the rates were 18% and 3%. Thus, one injection of high-dose ketamine resulted in improved abstinence rates for heroin. The same group, Krupitsky et al. (2007), tested whether repeated ketamine infusions helped even more. Fifty-nine people who had recently undergone detoxification for heroin addiction received one intramuscular ketamine injection of 2.0 mg/kg right before discharge from the hospital, along with psychotherapy. One part of the group then received two more such injections with psychotherapy 1 and 2 months after discharge. The others received only the psychotherapy sessions at the same time points. At 1 year of follow-up, abstinence rates were 50% in the multiple-dose group and 22% in the single-dose group, implying that multiple doses enhance abstinence rates.

Jovaisa et al. (2006) used a radical approach, randomizing 50 opiate addicts to anesthesia with either ketamine or some other anesthetic drug and then administering naloxone or naltrexone during the anesthesia. There was no difference in proportion of patients free of opiate usage at 4-month follow-up.

Cocaine Use Disorder

The literature on ketamine for cocaine use disorder is dominated by one investigative group, led by Dr. Elias Dakwar and colleagues at Columbia University. Dakwar et al. (2014a) gave eight cocaine-dependent participants infusions on three separate occasions, in counterbalanced, randomized order, of lorazepam 2 mg, ketamine 0.41 mg/kg, and ketamine 0.71 mg/kg. Each infusion was 52 minutes. Ketamine but not lorazepam infusions resulted in increased motivation to quit cocaine and reduced cocaine craving in response to a cue. The visual cues for the craving task were pictures of cocaine usage paraphernalia, and ratings were conducted the day after the infusions. Dakwar et al. (2014b) reported more data on the same eight patients, this time consisting of mysticism experiences as possible predictors of the cocaine-craving outcome measure. A few items on the mysticism rating scale included "realizing the unity of all things," a feeling of awe, a new view of reality, a feeling of holiness, a feeling that all things seem alive, a peaceful state, an absorption with something greater than oneself, ineffability, and timelessness/spacelessness. All these are based on a published mysticism rating scale (Hood 1975). Mysticism experiences, but not dissociation, induced by ketamine correlated with the outcome assessments.

Dakwar et al. (2017) studied 20 cocaine-dependent participants, each receiving in counterbalanced order one infusion of ketamine 0.71 mg/kg or midazolam 0.025 mg/kg over 52 minutes. The day after each infusion, each participant had five "choice sessions" in which they could receive 25 mg cocaine or $11.00. Outcome was the total amount of cocaine chosen. Of the 10 participants who received ketamine at the first infusion, two of them maintained abstinence for the entire 2-week gap between infusions and thus did not receive another infusion so as to avoid obligatory test administrations of 25 mg of cocaine (obviously, if a participant has maintained abstinence for 2 weeks, one would not want to spoil this with further cocaine exposure). None of the 10 participants who got midazolam for the first infusion maintained 2 weeks of abstinence from cocaine, and thus all 10 received their ketamine infusions. For the outcome measure assessing choice between cocaine or money, the ketamine infusions resulted in a score of 1.61; the midazolam infusions led to a score of 4.33 (the higher the score, the more cocaine was chosen over money). Overall cocaine usage in the 2 weeks after infusion was much less after ketamine than after midazolam. The same was true for self-reported cocaine craving.

Dakwar et al. (2018) studied 18 cocaine users. Each participant received three infusions, each one during a 6-day hospitalization on a research unit. The first infusion was saline. The second and third infusions were counterbalanced: one ketamine 0.71 mg/kg and the other midazolam 0.025 mg/kg over 50 minutes. Each stay was separated by 2 weeks to check for acute abstinence rates. Measures of near-death experiences, mystical experiences, and dissociation were obtained after each infusion to see if these experiences correlated with abstinence. Outcome measures for cocaine included abstinence rates during the 2 weeks after infusion, cocaine craving during that time, and self-administered cocaine in the research setting after the infusion. Presumably, if the infusion decreased cocaine craving, the participant would choose money over cocaine. The percentage improvement composite score of all three of these measures constituted the main outcome measure. For ketamine, this composite (in which a higher score is a better outcome) was 56%; it was 20.7% for midazolam. Mystical experiences induced by the drug were the only significant mediator of the outcome measure other than the drug itself.

Dakwar et al. (2019) studied 55 cocaine-dependent participants enrolled in a 5-week mindfulness psychotherapy program. Each participant received one infusion during the first 5 days of the program: either ketamine 0.5 mg/kg or midazolam 0.025 mg/kg over 40 minutes. The participants were followed in person for the remainder of the 5-week program and again with a telephone interview at 6 months. Outcome measures included questionnaires assessing craving and use of cocaine. Abstinence in the last 2 weeks of the program was 48.2% for ketamine and 10.7% for midazolam. At 6 months, there was a 44% abstinence rate in the ketamine group and 0% in the midazolam group.

Cannabis Use Disorder

Azhari et al. (2021) conducted an open-label trial to test the feasibility of combining ketamine infusions with motivational enhancement therapy and mindfulness-based relapse prevention therapy of cannabis use disorder. Eight cannabis users got either one ($n=5$) or two ($n=3$) infusions of ketamine (0.71 mg/kg over 50 minutes for the first, 1.41 mg/kg over 90 minutes for the second, if given). The second one was offered to those participants who did not seem to get benefit with the first infusion after 2 weeks. The two therapy techniques were delivered the day before and the afternoon after an infusion. The mindfulness component was delivered twice a week for 4 weeks after the infusions. There was a sharp reduction in cannabis use during this open-label trial, indicating a need for controlled research to be done.

Ketamine-Assisted Psychotherapy

Ketamine-assisted psychotherapy is by no means mainstream in modern mental health practice. For it to be legal, at least in the United States, the physician must purchase ketamine from a pharmaceutical manufacturer, store it properly (under lock and key), and provide documentation, to be reviewed by the Drug Enforcement Agency, regarding where each milligram of purchased ketamine goes. Ketamine is a Schedule III controlled substance, and the physician must document that the purchased ketamine is actually being administered to patients under proper supervision and is not being diverted for recreational use.

As one might presume, undertaking this venture in one's private practice is time-consuming and involves a lot of paperwork. Nonetheless, at least a few practitioners have done it and wrote about their experiences. In a recent review of the concepts of ketamine-assisted psychotherapy, Mathai et al. (2022) divided the accounts into two groups: experience-based and non–experience-based protocols. In the former, it is the psychological experiences induced by ketamine that are considered therapeutic, whereas in the latter, ketamine is typically used at a subpsychedelic dose with the hope of causing neuroplastic brain changes that enhance the efficacy of subsequent psychotherapy. This is called neuroplasticity-based ketamine-assisted psychotherapy.

Experience-based ketamine-assisted psychotherapy is further divided into *psycholytic* and psychedelic. The former consists of lower doses with which the patient is still able to engage in conversation while the ketamine is administered; thus, it is a type of relational therapy. Psychedelic ketamine psychotherapy uses high enough doses that the person is not able to engage in verbal discourse; it is thus a nonrelational therapy. Psychedelic effects of high-dose ketamine are subjectively assessed by each person who experiences them. Cultural background is one of the key aspects of the *cognitive set* (introduced in Chapter 3 when we discussed psychedelic experiences) that each ketamine patient brings to the session. Thus, clinicians should be sensitive to patients' diverse backgrounds and explore their expectations before the sessions.

Recent reviews explore the theories behind ketamine-assisted psychotherapy and offer some unanswered questions. Reiff et al. (2020) expounded on the difference between psycholytic and psychedelic therapy. The former attempts to enhance psychoanalytic psychotherapy to facilitate bringing unconscious conflicts to the surface. The latter uses high doses to induce a transcendent state that itself is seen as therapeutic and that is combined with transpersonal psychotherapy to help the patient learn how to convert the psychedelic experience into long-lasting life change.

Questions include why these approaches might work—what is the mechanism of action? Is one form of psychotherapy combined with ketamine better than another? What promotes change, a direct effect of the drug—in which case the psychedelic experience may be epiphenomenal, essentially a side effect? Or does the psychedelic experience itself cause improvement? Is the psychotherapy necessary to obtain maximal improvement from the effects of the drug?

Schatzberg (2020) pointed out that what gets better with psychedelic-assisted therapy is not just symptoms such as better sleep or concentration, but also higher-level aspects of human well-being such as sense of serenity in life and feelings of enlightenment, and that outcome measures in studies of this modality should assess such things. The best candidates for this type of therapy seem to be chronically depressed or anxious patients, who are usually highly refractory to multiple modalities such as medications and psychotherapies, versus those with acute, fulminant psychiatric syndromes.

Krediet et al. (2020), in another review, pointed out with regard to anxiety such as in PTSD, that the glutamate system has been shown in rodent models to be involved in fear extinction and memory reconsolidation, two things that are targets in trauma-focused therapy. Additionally, in the animal models, ketamine has been shown to enhance fear extinction and block memory reconsolidation, which are two goals of trauma therapy. Thus, ketamine's neuroplastic effects may render the brain more receptive to psychotherapy. This raises the question of when ketamine should be administered—before the therapy, to give it time to have its necessary effects? Or during therapy, if those effects are maximal with ketamine in the central nervous system? The answer is unknown at this time.

Psychedelic (Experience-Based) Ketamine-Assisted Psychotherapy

In this type of ketamine-assisted psychotherapy, it is the psychological effects of ketamine that are considered crucial to the therapeutic action. The doses used are thus high enough to gain the expected dissociative, out-of-body experiences, visual hallucinations or illusions, and strong emotional reactions that are characteristic of ketamine. The first practitioner of this technique was Dr. Salvador Roquet from Mexico in the 1970s. Details of ketamine dosing (as well as numerous other psychedelic drugs he used in his practice), therapeutic technique, patient population, and outcomes are lacking. Mention of Roquet is thus relegated to historical interest only.

Several authors have described psychedelic experience-based ketamine therapies. Also from the 1970s came an esoteric report from South America (Fontana and Loschi 1974). This Spanish-language report lacked specifics of ketamine dosing or patient diagnosis (and thus is also just of historical interest), but ketamine was said to cause dreamlike states that allowed the therapist to influence the patient's psychodynamics and help effect change.

In a good review of psychedelic-assisted psychotherapy, Schenberg (2018) pointed out that in high-dose therapy, the peak or mystical experience may be therapeutic in and of itself without accompanying psychotherapy, which might simply be called psychedelic therapy. The three stages of psychedelic-assisted psychotherapy were nicely described by Majić et al. (2015). The first stage consists of an intense psychedelic experience when the drug is administered. This may lead to what is called a *peak experience* (if all goes well), so different from normal that the person is left with the second stage, the so-called *afterglow*, lasting days to weeks, which is a period of increased well-being and even elation. This is followed (again if things go well) by a residual phase, long lasting, consisting of an altered mindset and approach to life.

Probably the most extensive scientific work in this area has been conducted by Dr. Evgeny Krupitsky, from St. Petersburg, Russia. In a series of papers beginning in the 1990s and 2000s, Krupitsky presented the results of his technique using ketamine to help alcohol- and heroin-dependent patients overcome addiction. (We discussed some of these papers earlier in this chapter.) The authors (Krupitsky 1992; Krupitsky and Grinenko 1997) described that, as they became more familiar with the effects of ketamine on their patients, they realized that many patients had profoundly existential, spiritual reactions that seemed transformative in their lives. The group decided to abandon the aversive conditioning use of ketamine and adopted a transpersonal psychotherapeutic approach.

Transpersonal psychology and psychotherapy are based on efforts to facilitate a person's spiritual growth, essentially attempting to effect a transformation of people into newer, better versions of themselves, as opposed to merely focusing on symptom reduction. Krupitsky's transpersonal approach to ketamine psychedelic psychotherapy, particularly regarding treatment of alcohol use disorder, included a three-step process. The first step, preparation, involved several sessions educating the patient about the ketamine psychedelic experience and elaborating the goals of therapy. The second step was administration of ketamine, typically 2–3 mg/kg intramuscularly with a therapist in attendance to be supportive for the couple of hours or so under the influence of ketamine. The dose was purposefully high enough to induce a transcendental state, a *non-ordinary state of consciousness* (NOSC). These states, under proper attention to the patient's cognitive preparation (*set*) and the *setting* of administration, are believed to be transformative. The third step was integration, which consists of several psychotherapy sessions to process the experience under ketamine and articulate what effect it has had on the patient's desire to live a different life, preferably one free of alcohol. Krupitsky also used this technique for heroin addiction (Krupitsky et al. 2002; Krupitsky et al. 2007).

Dr. Eli Kolp has written on ketamine psychedelic psychotherapy as well. (Also originally from Russia, he immigrated to the United States to continue his psychiatric practice.) In an in-depth description of the technique used (Kolp et al. 2014), he enumerated four stages of ketamine-induced psychedelic experiences for psychotherapy:

1. *Empathogenic* dose: 0.25–0.5 mg/kg intramuscularly lasting up to an hour. Awareness of body is preserved. There are lessened ego defenses (i.e., the patient is more likely to talk about painful psychological issues) while the patient is still verbally interactive. The experience can be consciously recalled later.
2. *Out of body*: 0.75–1.5 mg/kg intramuscularly, also lasting an hour or so. Self-awareness is intact, but body and mind are dissociated. Disembodied consciousness results, consisting of dreamlike states with archetypal beings and various memories.
3. *Near death*: 2–3 mg/kg intramuscularly lasting about an hour. Loss of identity occurs. One's life may be reviewed. This dose may be transformational for the patient upon awakening and reflecting back on the experience.
4. *Ego dissolution*: 2–3 mg/kg intramuscularly lasting up to an hour. The patient achieves a feeling of total transcendence, "cosmic unity," with an ineffable aspect to it.

Kolp referred to all these stages as NOSCs. Like other practitioners of ketamine psychedelic psychotherapy, he stressed the importance of set and setting during these sessions, with particular attention to good preparation beforehand and integration afterward. Kolp described the various ways he has used ketamine in his practice: he first used it for alcoholism (Kolp et al. 2006), then for various other addictions (Kolp et al. 2007), and then for people looking for growth optimization (addictions, nonpsychotic depression, personality disorders) (Kolp et al. 2014). He believed that higher doses, in the near-death and ego-dissolution range, were optimal for transformative experiences. When the ketamine was given, intramuscularly, relaxing music was played, and the patient wore eyeshades. After return of ordinary consciousness, an hour or so after administration, they discussed the experience with a therapist and were instructed to write down everything they remembered. This was followed by the integration phase, later the same evening as the ketamine session, itself followed by weekly psychotherapy for 3 weeks after completing the residential phase.

Kolp wrote that he noticed his patients becoming more at ease, less tortured by ruminations and worries, more thoughtful, with fewer inner conflicts, more spiritual, and with broadening of world views—all these are the essence of the goals of transpersonal psychotherapy.

Another strong proponent of ketamine psychedelic psychotherapy is Dr. Phil Wolfson in San Francisco. He and colleagues described their approach in several publications, most notably *The Ketamine Papers: Science, Therapy, and Transformation* (Wolfson and Hartelius 2016). In this multiauthored book about ketamine, several psychiatrists described their practices using ketamine psychedelic psychotherapy.

Mollaahmetoglu et al. (2021) interviewed 12 participants from a study in which ketamine was paired with either alcohol education or mindfulness training (the full results were published in Grabski et al. 2022). In that trial, ketamine was used at a dose of 0.8 mg/kg IV over 40 minutes and was not intended to cause a psychedelic experience; the authors wanted to know whether it enhanced psychotherapy results. In the event, in-depth interviews with the 12 participants revealed that ketamine left some of them feeling indelibly changed; they felt they had gained deep, meaningful insights into their lives. Neither the mindfulness therapy nor alcohol education interventions were specifically tied to ketamine experiences. This study shows that even when no specific experience of ketamine is intended when that drug is used, there still may be one.

Dames et al. (2022) undertook a study at Vancouver Island University in Canada. Health care professionals self-identifying as having depression and PTSD enrolled in a 12-week intensive psychotherapy program (40 total hours of therapy) in a group format. There were also three 4-hour ketamine sessions with accompanying psychotherapy in a group format. For the first session, oral lozenges were used; at the other sessions, intramuscular injections were used. The oral dose of ketamine was not specified; the IM doses were 1.0–1.5 mg/kg, which is pretty high. Ninety minutes after the ketamine administrations, group sharing occurred. Thirty-seven of the participants were said to have PTSD (generalized anxiety and depression were other common diagnoses). Responses were said to be quite dramatic in this program, with several personal testimonials given. There was an eye-popping 86% "cure rate" for PTSD based on rating scales, which again seems simply too good to be true. I have to surmise that the participants were simply reporting how satisfied they were with this intensive, group, very personalized therapy program.

The essence of a program like this is, a group of people were given two interventions at once: intensive psychotherapy and ketamine therapy. Which one was responsible for the reported improvement? Did ketamine have anything to do with it? Or was it attributable to the high group cohesion that occurred? Because the study design was open label and not randomized, we'll never know.

Neuroplasticity (Non–Experience-Based) Ketamine-Assisted Psychotherapy

In this use of ketamine-assisted psychotherapy, the ketamine's presumed mechanism of action is neuroplastic changes that render the brain more responsive to subsequent psychotherapy. The psychotherapy techniques can be any of the usual types—cognitive, behavioral, mindfulness, trauma-focused, and so on. The idea is that ketamine's effect on the glutamate system ultimately impacts learning and memory processes that are the focus of psychotherapy. If ketamine enhances new learning, especially emotion-based learning, or enhances fear extinction, then these effects might be useful combined with psychotherapy.

Bottemanne and Arnould (2021) outlined a theoretical approach to augmenting *exposure and response prevention psychotherapy* for OCD with ketamine. They postulated that ketamine might enhance fear extinction, which underlies exposure and response prevention therapy (as well as prolonged exposure therapy for PTSD), by modulating NMDA and GABA functioning in the amygdala and prefrontal cortex. The idea is to administer ketamine in sub-anesthetic doses to produce the effects and undergo the psychotherapy while the effects are still in place. Presumably, ketamine-induced neuroplasticity in this manner renders the brain more responsive to the psychotherapy techniques.

Veen et al. (2018) postulated four time points in which ketamine may help PTSD: 1) pretrauma, to enhance resilience; 2) immediately after trauma, to prevent initial memory consolidation; 3) during exposure therapy, to block reconsolidation; and 4) also during exposure therapy, to enhance fear extinction. The authors argued that item 3 currently offers the best hope for ketamine-assisted therapy of PTSD. In moving forward with this hypothesis, researchers will need to elaborate the specifics of the psychotherapy (presumably some trauma-focused prolonged exposure therapy) and how and when to embed ketamine with it (dosage, timing). Thus, in summary, ketamine is being proposed to target memory processing—in therapy, we want the PTSD patient to retrieve the current memories, destabilize them (i.e., block reconsolidation), and replace them with a healthier emotional response. Future studies of ketamine augmentation of prolonged exposure therapy are called for.

Bottemanne and Arnould (2021) proposed using exposure and response prevention therapy for OCD during (as opposed to after) ketamine infusions. The theory here is that ketamine's neuroplastic effects occur rather quickly, so therapy must occur at the same time to get maximal results. The same group (Bottemanne et al. 2022) described their protocol, in France, for ketamine-assisted psychotherapy of mood disorders. The first stage was preparation, in which they reached a correct diagnosis, established rapport, educated the patient about ketamine's effects, and set patient expectations. The next stage was administration of ketamine at 0.5 mg/kg IV over 40 minutes or 28 mg (for over age 65) or 56 mg (if under 65) intranasal esketamine. This stage could include multiple sessions to achieve maximal improvement. The third stage was integration, which consisted of 30- to 60-minute therapy sessions 2–6 hours after each ketamine administration. Acceptance and commitment therapy included debriefing the patient about the experience. Finally, the amplification stage consisted of more therapy the day after the ketamine sessions, or a few days later. Of note, the Bottemanne et al. administration of ketamine for depression mirrors that of many practices today, but they have been careful to integrate a psychotherapy regimen into the practice, which is probably a great idea to maximize and consolidate the gains from the ketamine alone.

Wilkinson et al. (2021) conducted a randomized trial in which 28 depression patients who responded to 3 weeks of twice-a-week ketamine infusions were randomized to 14 weeks of *cognitive-behavioral therapy* (CBT) or 14 weeks of care as usual, which involved office visits to monitor progress without psychotherapy. Ketamine doses were 0.5 mg/kg IV over 40 minutes. The idea is that ketamine may enhance response to therapy. At the end of the trial, depression rating scale scores were indeed lower in the CBT group than the treatment-as-usual group. However, the design of this trial really tested whether CBT does better than treatment as usual in sustaining initial ketamine benefits, rather than whether ketamine augments CBT. If the latter issue is to be broached in a study, then there should be randomization of psychotherapy candidates to pretreatment with ketamine versus placebo; that design would address whether ketamine truly enhances response to CBT.

Shiroma et al. (2020a) treated nine PTSD patients with three ketamine infusions at weekly intervals paired with prolonged exposure therapy sessions, followed by weekly prolonged exposure therapy sessions for a maximum of 10 sessions. Ketamine dosing was 0.5 mg/kg IV over 40 minutes. Each postketamine prolonged exposure therapy session was 24 hours after the infusion. Scales assessing PTSD severity showed substantial improvement. For three patients, prolonged exposure therapy was stopped after seven sessions because goals were achieved. There was no control group.

Pradhan and Rossi (2020) treated three patients with opiate addiction with one session of ketamine 0.75 mg/kg IV over 40 minutes, a week later with 1–2 weeks of five sessions of transcranial magnetic stimulation, and then five TIMBER psychotherapy sessions over the same 1- to 2-week period. Opiate craving scores decreased. There was no control group.

Pradhan et al. (2017; 2018) treated 18 PTSD patients with TIMBER psychotherapy combined with either one ketamine infusion at 0.5 mg/kg IV over 40 minutes or a saline infusion. The first TIMBER session occurred during the infusion, the second one was the next day, and there were 10 more sessions at weekly intervals. (Note that the first psychotherapy session was during a ketamine infusion.) Results showed that PTSD severity scores dropped more with concomitant ketamine, indicating that ketamine bolstered the psychotherapy, which is in accordance with the theory that ketamine's neuroplastic changes may render therapy more effective.

The literature on ketamine-assisted psychotherapy is intriguing, particularly with regard to the neuroplasticity-based, nonpsychedelic uses that have been subject to scientific inquiry in recent years. If the types of studies just reviewed can be replicated, it would be fairly easy to incorporate low-dose ketamine into psychotherapy practice. These low-dosage studies are likely to be much more palatable to the larger psychiatric and mental health communities and easier to study than high-dosage, psychedelic-based ketamine protocols. The latter will probably continue to be used only in a small number of private practices with highly motivated, psychedelic-oriented clinicians.

Chapter 9

Is Ketamine a Neuroprotectant or a Neurotoxin?

KEY POINTS IN THIS CHAPTER:

- Ketamine has been shown to cause neurotoxicity in rodent models.

- Concerns have been raised about potential neurotoxicity in humans, especially in children undergoing surgery who are anesthetized with ketamine.

- Ketamine has shown promise as a neuroprotectant in some neurological syndromes, most notably status epilepticus.

John Olney, Excitotoxicity, and Ketamine as Neuroprotectant

The best place to start untangling ketamine's dual effects—neurotoxic and neuroprotective—is with the late icon of brain damage research, John Olney of Washington University in St. Louis.

Olney spent several decades conducting groundbreaking research into mechanisms of pharmacological neurotoxicity. In 1974, he coined the expression *excitotoxic*, which has become standard terminology to refer to neuronal damage induced by states of excessive levels of excitatory amino acids, most notably glutamate (Olney 1974). Olney and de Gubareff (1978) published a good early presentation of his excitotoxicity theory applied to a specific illness, Huntington disease, a neurodegenerative disease. He reviewed his 1970s work in the laboratory documenting excitatory amino acid–mediated nerve damage and theorized that drugs that somehow block its actions could be clinically effective. At that time he made no mention, of course, of ketamine, because it was not until the early 1980s that the discovery was made that ketamine blocks glutamate receptors.

Labruyere et al. (1986) (a group including Olney) induced prolonged seizures in rats with kainic acid (an excitatory amino acid), the damage from which was prevented by ketamine. This early report may be the first ever to document a neuroprotective effect of ketamine, albeit in rodents.

Olney provided a good review of the state of excitotoxicity research to the late 1980s (Olney 1990). This paper reviewed the 1980s data, from animal laboratory research, documenting the role of excitatory amino acids in causing neuronal damage and the potential for NMDA receptor blockade to prevent at least a part of it. The notion was put forward that NMDA-blocking drugs such as ketamine may have clinical utility for mitigating the brain-damaging effects of neurological conditions that were due to excitotoxicity from glutamate excess: anoxic brain injury, traumatic brain injury, stroke, hypoglycemic brain injury, status epilepticus, and maybe even neurodegenerative disorders such as Alzheimer or Huntington disease.

Thus, in the late 1980s, excitotoxicity created a lot of buzz, as it was believed that many acute neurological events such as traumatic brain injury and stroke caused damage through excitotoxicity, that glutamate was the main excitotoxic neurotransmitter, that NMDA receptors were the main vehicle by which glutamate did its harm, and that blockers of this receptor (most notably ketamine) showed promise as neuroprotectants in studies with lab animals. The field was poised to charge ahead and make the transition from the lab to the bedside (clinical practice) with human ketamine neuroprotection studies. But then something changed the whole picture.

But Wait ... Does Ketamine Actually Destroy Neurons?

It is the height of irony that the man most responsible for purveying the theory that ketamine can be neuroprotective, John Olney, is also the one most responsible for warning the world that ketamine may be neurotoxic.

In the late 1980s, the attitude for ketamine neuroprotection research was "full speed ahead"—until Olney et al. (1989) published a groundbreaking report suggesting that ketamine may kill neurons. In that study, which has been cited innumerable times in the decades since, adult rats were treated with MK-801, phencyclidine, ketamine, or tiletamine (another NMDA receptor blocker that is structurally similar to ketamine). Rats got these drugs at different dosages and schedules, and their brains were sectioned at different intervals after exposure. All drugs induced vacuoles (which were interpreted as brain damage) in neurons in the posterior cingulate cortex and retrosplenial cortex. (These vacuoles have been termed *Olney lesions.*) The order of potency was MK-801 → phencyclidine → tiletamine → ketamine, which corresponds with the drugs' binding to the PCP site of the NMDA receptor. This report has been profoundly influential, for the charge to develop ketamine as a clinically useful neuroprotectant was essentially diverted into asking whether ketamine can damage human brains, an investigation that continues today.

A clear finding, and a source of frustration for clinicians, in the ketamine-as-neurotoxin-versus-neuroprotectant literature is that in animals, both phenomena are unequivocally found depending on age and type of neurological condition (e.g., stroke or traumatic brain injury). But in humans, the data are murky and the conclusions are speculative. A little later, we survey papers dealing with reviews focusing on humans, but definitive conclusions await future neurodiagnostic technologies. Next we look at the data in animals, but just a few of the most informative, because the Olney et al. (1989) landmark paper set the stage for decades of ketamine-induced neurotoxicity research in animals.

Neurological Effects in Animals

A seminal paper in this literature was that of Ikonomidou et al. (1999), published in the journal *Science*. Postnatal rats were injected with various NMDA receptor blocking agents (dizocilpine, phencyclidine, or ketamine) (dizocilpine, aka MK-801, is perhaps the most potent noncompetitive NMDA receptor blocking agent available) at 0, 8, or 16 hours, and brains were sectioned at 24 hours. Staining to detect *apoptosis* (programmed cell death, some degree of which is normal in the brain) was undertaken in the histologic sections. Widespread apoptosis was seen with these drugs. Postnatal day 21 rats were given dizocilpine, and no apoptosis was seen. Dizocilpine given to pregnant rats caused apoptosis in the fetal brains. It was suggested that ketamine anesthesia should not be given to pregnant women or human infants. It was also suggested that users of ketamine, PCP, or ethanol (which also blocks NMDA receptors) who are pregnant could be harming their children's brains. This was a seminal paper in the NMDA receptor blockade–induced neurotoxicity literature, particularly regarding the age effect.

In an oft-cited study, Brambrink et al. (2012), led by Olney, studied ketamine-induced lesions in the brains of young macaques (rhesus monkeys), both fetal and neonatal. Apoptotic neurodegeneration (programmed cell death) was assessed by caspase-3 staining, a procedure sensitive to that neuropathological process. On postnatal day 6, 5-hour ketamine infusions were administered to the neonates, and on gestational day 120 (full term in this species is 165 days), 5-hour infusions were administered to the pregnant macaques, and the fetuses were extracted 3 hours later. Neuronal loss assessed via the staining technique was 2.2 times greater in the fetal brains than the neonatal brains, and both were greater for the ketamine-treated than nontreated brains. The time of exposure (5 hours) was chosen to mimic human anesthesia exposure time, although ketamine is rarely used for that long in neonatal or obstetrical anesthesia. The areas in the macaque brains showing excessive apoptosis were widespread. Because this report involves a species much closer to humans than rodents are, the concern about human ketamine-induced neurotoxicity in the young exposed to anesthesia was high.

Slikker et al. (2007) pointed out that it was already known that ketamine caused neurotoxicity in juvenile rodents. The time had come to test it in primates. Rhesus monkeys were exposed to ketamine via 24-hour infusions at anesthetic doses either in utero (gestational day 122, about 75% of that species' gestational duration), at postnatal day 5, or at postnatal day 35. Monkeys were then killed, and their brains were examined histologically. Neurotoxicity was seen in the fetal and early postnatal monkeys but not in the older (day 35) monkeys. In a separate group of postnatal day 5 monkeys, 3-hour infusions of ketamine did not cause neurotoxicity. This elegant study revealed the importance of age and duration of exposure to ketamine as important variables in neurotoxicity.

Paule et al. (2011) studied six macaques on postnatal day 5 or 6 who were given 24-hour infusions of ketamine and six non–ketamine-exposed controls. A test battery for cognitive functions specially designed for this species was administered to the two groups serially. Differences appeared around age 10 months and (at the time of the report) were extended to 3.5 years, showing a decrement in performance in the ketamine-exposed group. Extrapolating this to humans, it may mean that ketamine anesthesia delivered to a human infant would cause subtle neuronal damage that may not become clinically detectable until years later.

Morris et al. (2021) recently conducted a study in adult rats (age 11–15 weeks in Sprague-Dawley rats and 12–14 weeks in Wistar rats). Three compounds were administered to different groups of rats: ketamine, dizocilpine, and the ketamine metabolite (2R,6R)-hydroxynorketamine. According to histological analysis, IV ketamine did not cause Olney lesions in the posterior cingulate or retrosplenial cortex, necrosis of cells, or Iba-1 staining (which reacts to cell damage). Dizocilpine led to many Olney lesions and Iba-1 staining. (2R,6R)-hydroxynorketamine did not cause histopathological abnormalities. These results held for single doses as well as multiple doses. Thus, these authors were unable to replicate the classic finding of Olney et al. (1989), that ketamine causes the lesions that bear Dr. Olney's name.

Kalopita et al. (2021) offered a perspective on ketamine-induced neurotoxicity from a developmental standpoint. They reviewed animal studies, mostly in embryonic or newborn rodents and one in pregnant macaques, all showing toxic lesions caused by ketamine in the young of these species. They posit that ketamine first deregulates NMDA receptor expression, causing upregulation. This leads to excessive susceptibility to glutamate excitotoxicity, which in turn causes premature differentiation of neural progenitor cells. Intracellular calcium signaling is altered, as excitation of the NMDA receptor leads to influx of calcium from the extracellular space. This alters mitochondrial function, leading to a cascade ultimately resulting in damaged or dead neurons.

Nogo et al. (2022) reviewed the literature on possible neuropathological changes associated with ketamine. The answer to the basic question—Does repeat ketamine exposure in humans cause neurotoxicity?—seems to depend on whether the exposure is to a juvenile or an adult, based on animal data. It also depends on dose, frequency, and duration of exposure. The authors focused on three commonly invoked mechanisms of ketamine-induced neurotoxicity: diminished parvalbumin-containing cortical interneurons; tau hyperphosphorylation; and Olney lesions.

Parvalbumin-containing interneurons are GABA-ergic inhibitory neurons that regulate cortical pyramidal cell firing. Without them, there is excitatory/inhibitory imbalance. Deficits in humans with loss of such neurons include working memory, social function, and executive function. Parvalbumin-staining interneuronal function has been implicated in the ketamine model of schizophrenia. In animal models, ketamine in juveniles leads to loss of parvalbumin-staining cells (Jeevakumar et al. 2015). There is a fear, of course, that a similar phenomenon may occur in juvenile humans given ketamine in anesthesia.

The second pathological mechanism discussed by Nogo et al. (2022) is *hyperphosphorylation of tau protein*. Tau proteins are associated with microtubule function intracellularly. So-called tau-opathies are disorders of excessive tau accumulation (e.g., Alzheimer disease). The question is whether ketamine may cause accumulation of hyperphosphorylated tau proteins.

Last, they mention Olney lesions, the tiny vacuoles in the posterior cingulate and retrosplenial cortices of adult rats discovered by Olney et al. (1989) mentioned earlier. If they do occur in humans as well, how would we know? We cannot do biopsies. Neuroradiologic techniques, at the current level of technology, cannot detect findings at the microcellular level. The posterior cortical areas where Olney lesions occur in rats are critical, in humans, for information processing. Do acute disruptions in them caused by ketamine in humans correspond to Olney lesions, perhaps temporary ones? How long will it take before neuroscientists find a way to detect such lesions in the living human brain?

At any rate, the Nogo et al. (2022) ketamine neuropathology review is well referenced: there are 13 parvalbumin-staining interneuron studies, 5 hyperphosphorylated tau studies, and 8 Olney lesion studies in animals cited.

Thus, beginning in 1989 with Olney and colleagues' seminal paper describing the lesions in adult rat brains that bear his name, continuing research in lab animals seems to confirm that ketamine can indeed cause neurotoxicity. The big question is whether this happens in humans. Intense interest in this topic has been generated, and there are essentially three scenarios in which concern currently exists that ketamine may damage human brains: 1) use as an anesthetic agent in infants and children; 2) recreational use; and 3) serial ketamine administrations in modern medical practice (mostly for depression and chronic pain). Next we consider the evidence for these situations.

Anesthesia in Infants and Children

In the early 2000s or so, as the data on ketamine-induced neurotoxicity in juvenile rodents became clear, concern began to be raised about whether it translated to human children. It wasn't only ketamine that displayed neurotoxicity in animals—barbiturates, propofol, and inhalational agents did as well. Pediatric anesthesiologists faced a real dilemma. By that time, of course, the field had abandoned the old practice of operating on children without anesthesia, but the safety of the anesthetic agents used had to be above suspicion. This dilemma has led to a surge of research interest in the safety of anesthetic drugs in children, including ketamine. The field of anesthesiology has settled on the use of ketamine in adults for anesthesia induction and maintenance or procedural sedation and analgesia as safe—there is no concern for neurotoxicity for these uses of ketamine in adults.

Ramsay and Rappaport (2011), responding to the frightening possibility that anesthesia in young children may be neurotoxic, pointed out rightly that what started this whole process was not a clinically identifiable human problem but rather a laboratory rodent (and occasionally primate) problem. Confounding issues include the type of anesthetic, dose, duration of exposure, number of exposures, and age at time of exposure. Any effects are likely to be subtle, since decades of using modern anesthetics in children have failed to reveal any grossly identifiable problems. Also, follow-up would need to extend years to decades, since it may take that long for subtle effects to be detectable, and even then only with detailed testing and clinical assessment. It would be virtually impossible to conduct controlled research with outcome measures 10–15 years later. Thus, retrospective studies are likely to be the best source of clinical guidance. Since we cannot do brain biopsies on people in clinical research, and neuroradiological studies are too insensitive and far too expensive, the sample sizes would have to number in the hundreds or even thousands, and the main outcome measures would be neurocognitive function, school performance records, and usage of mental health services.

Warner et al. (2018) conducted what is probably the best retrospective study to date of whether anesthetic exposure to young children is associated with later developmental differences: the Mayo Anesthesia Safety in Kids (MASK) study. Several hundred children were studied in late childhood or adolescence in three groups: unexposed to anesthesia as children; exposed to one anesthetic administration as children; and exposed to more than one anesthetic administration as children. The exposures in question were when the child was younger than 3, with testing done in late childhood or adolescence.

The primary outcome measure of general intelligence did not differ in the three groups, which was reassuring. Processing speed and fine motor abilities were a bit worse in the multiply exposed group than the others, but the singly exposed group did not differ from the never-exposed group. Parental reports of neurobehavioral function were also worse in the multiply exposed group. The anesthetics were not broken down into specific agents (ketamine versus others). Most of the anesthetic exposures involved more than one agent; for example, induction with an intravenous agent such as ketamine followed by maintenance of anesthesia with an inhalational agent. In another report from the MASK study, Warner et al. (2019) tested older children and adolescents also exposed either never, once, or more than once to anesthetics in a neuropsychological battery. There was no evidence of a decrement in performance among 8–12- or 15–20-year-olds, reassuringly.

Guerra et al. (2011) studied 95 infants <6 weeks old undergoing heart surgery. The outcome was neurodevelopmental status at 18–24 months. There was no statistical association between any anesthetic variable, including ketamine, and outcome. This is a highly reassuring report given the very young age of the patients, although longer-term follow-up would probably be needed to confirm the results.

Probably the most ambitious review to date of the issue was provided by Lin et al. (2017), in which no fewer than 475 studies were reviewed (truly heroic!), 443 in animals. A majority found either neurostructural (85% of studies) or subsequent functional (77% of studies) abnormalities after anesthetic exposure in young, developing rats. There were also 32 human studies, a decent number, almost all of which were retrospective. Among them, 58% picked up on some signal of neurocognitive findings related to anesthesia. As with several other commentators, they rightly pointed out that the findings may not relate to anesthesia but other factors, such as severe pain, inflammation from the surgery, the psychological trauma to children of the whole process, and other illness-related factors. One conclusion from the vast animal literature was that no specific age emerges beyond which it is safe to provide anesthesia without neurotoxicity, a duration of administration below which is safe, or a specific type of anesthetic agent or regimen that is safer than the rest. This literature is on the one hand universally acknowledged to be very important (brain development in children), yet after all these years of intensive thought and study, no conclusions can be drawn.

Ketamine Abuse

The second area of concern for possible ketamine-induced neurotoxicity in humans is nonmedical, or recreational, use. As described in Chapter 3, there is currently a rather alarming epidemic of ketamine abuse among young people in Asian countries such as China, Taiwan, and Hong Kong. Much (if not most) of the world's pharmaceutical supply of ketamine originates in Asia, and undoubtedly there is diversion from the legal supply chain to recreational sale on the street. In contrast to the situation with pediatric anesthesia using ketamine, there is no controversy: nobody supports ketamine abuse. The literature in humans supports the contention that such use is neurotoxic. Outcome measures include neurocognitive testing, neuropsychiatric testing, and neuroradiological scanning.

Narendran et al. (2005) studied 14 chronic ketamine abusers and 14 age- and sex-matched non-users. Hair samples were taken and analyzed to confirm chronic ketamine use. Subjects were using for at least 2 years, at 200–300 mg ketamine per week over the previous 3 months. A special radioligand that binds to dopamine Type I receptors, [^{11}C] NNC 112, was injected and given time to disperse into the brain and bind to its receptors. Prefrontal binding was increased in the chronic ketamine users. Neurocognitive assessment revealed no differences between the two groups in an extensive battery.

What to make of these results? The dopamine binding clearly showed a finding in the ketamine users, but this did not extend to testing of cognitive abilities. Are we to say the dopamine binding results represent neurotoxicity from ketamine? It of course depends on how one defines neurotoxicity. One point of interest in this study is that ketamine at 200–300 mg per week is rather mild in comparison to other data samples for which users were ingesting far larger doses every day.

Liao et al. (2012) performed fMRI scans on 41 ketamine users and 44 non-users and found differences in the right anterior cingulate cortex and left precentral frontal gyrus, findings that, like so many in the fMRI literature, are impossible to interpret. Recruits were from a drug rehabilitation program and averaged just > 3 years of ketamine use. In another fMRI study, Chan et al. (2012) conducted scans on three ketamine users (1–2 g per day for a mean of 2 years) and three non-users. There was decreased cerebellar activity in the ketamine users, another finding with no explanation.

Wang et al. (2013) conducted structural MRI scans on 21 ketamine addicts. Duration of usage was 0.5–12 years, about 1 g a day with mostly daily use by nasal inhalation. Lesions appeared on the scans after 2–4 years of ketamine use. A wide variety of cortical and subcortical lesions were seen; nothing specific was found. White matter holes or degenerative patches were common. Most participants were < 30 years of age. Patches occurred in those with < 2 years of use, and more evident atrophy occurred later. This study is important because, with the wide range of durations of use, it gives an idea of the evolution of apparent ketamine-induced brain damage over time.

In another structural MRI study, Liao et al. (2011) studied the same group (41 ketamine abusers and 44 non-users) as discussed earlier in fMRI data (Liao et al. 2012). They found decreased gray matter in the ketamine abusers that negatively correlated with duration and estimated lifetime amount of ketamine use (i.e., the more the use or duration, the less gray matter was present). Mean age was late 20s, and use duration was about 3.5 years. Cognition was also assessed. The ketamine group performed worse on digit symbol, trail making test A, and Stroop Color-Word tests, which are all basically working memory tests.

Morgan et al. (2010) studied five groups: frequent ketamine users (at least four times a week); infrequent ketamine users (at least once a month but less than four times a week); abstinent, former ketamine users (no use for at least a month); polydrug, nonketamine users; and non-users. There were 20–27 subjects per group, tested cognitively 1 year after initial evaluation. Extensive neuropsychological testing in these patients (mean age 20s to 30s) showed worse performance in memory, attention, and problem solving in the frequent users of ketamine vis-à-vis the other groups. Ketamine use tended to stay constant for the year after initial testing until the follow-up evaluations. There seemed to be a trend of increasing use correlating with worsened cognitive performance. The abstinent ketamine users' initial cognitive performance did not differ from polydrug (nonketamine) or non-drug groups. This may indicate that ketamine abstinence may lead to improved performance, which is certainly good news if true. The authors did not have a group of initial frequent users who embraced abstinence over the subsequent year, however, which of course dilutes the results.

Morgan et al. (2014) studied 11 chronic ketamine users (at least three times a week for at least a year) and 15 ketamine non-users as controls. fMRI was performed during a spatial memory task. Ketamine use was a mean of 9.7 years, five times a week (this study was conducted before ketamine became highly regulated in England, so the drug was more available for such use at that time). These users also consumed multiple other drugs regularly, such as cocaine, MDMA, alcohol, tobacco, and cannabis, thus confounding the results. Ketamine users did less well on the spatial memory task than the nonketamine users (who also used the other drugs in equal quantity, providing some modicum of control). There were differences in medial temporal activation (less in the ketamine user group) on fMRI scanning. On neurocognitive testing, attention and working memory were worse in the ketamine user group. Mean time since last ketamine use was 1.6 days, providing some confidence that the results were not merely representative of acute ketamine toxicity.

The same group (Roberts et al. 2014) compared diffusion tensor imaging MRI of the head in 16 chronic ketamine users (mean duration 7.25 years, mean 26.25 days a month using ketamine, average 2.75 g/day) versus 16 polydrug (but not ketamine) users. Both groups had a lot of nonketamine drug use. In the ketamine user group, right-sided white matter microstructural abnormalities were seen that correlated with the degree of dissociation experienced with ketamine use.

In sum, there are hints from neuropsychological testing, neuroimaging, and neuropsychiatric testing that ketamine has a detrimental, neurotoxic effect in regular, heavy abusers. There is also a signal that with abstinence, improvement in cognition can be seen, but we have no data on whether neuroimaging, either structural or functional, returns to baseline. As indicated earlier, this is not a controversial matter. Nobody recommends heavy, daily, long-lasting ketamine use. Probably any neuroactive compound taken in sufficient quantities frequently enough and for long enough will cause lasting neurotoxicity.

Administration of Ketamine in Psychiatry and Pain Medicine

The third area of concern about whether ketamine causes neurotoxicity is the modern field of ketamine therapeutics in psychiatry and pain medicine. Recall that ketamine is administered serially to patients in an ongoing manner to prevent depression relapse. Some patients are being treated with weekly ketamine administrations for months or even years on end in these modern scenarios. Does ketamine cause anything that would be called neurotoxicity in these settings? As of this writing, not much study has been made of this question, which is a shame. It would be beneficial to take samples from patients who have been treated with, say, a year's worth of serial infusions and perform neuropsychological testing or neuroradiological scanning.

The worries with long-lasting, regular ketamine infusions include cognitive problems, as far as neurotoxicity goes. Some (meager) data are available in this regard. Studying ketamine for depression, Zhang and Ho (2016) summarized the cognitive outcome data available, and there was very little. A more modern review, Gill et al. (2021), included only five studies. Liu et al. (2019) had a sample size of 50 who received six IV infusions of 0.5 mg/kg over 40 minutes in an open-label (i.e., not randomized or blinded) study with cognitive testing 1 and 14 days after the final infusion. There were no decrements in performance. Chen et al. (2018) randomized 71 patients to one infusion of either 0.5 or 0.2 mg/kg ketamine or saline; cognitive improvements were seen in the higher-dose group on day 14, but no differences in any group on day 3. Murrough et al. (2013a) randomized 25 patients to single infusions of either ketamine 0.5 mg/kg or placebo and found impairments in memory recall at 24 hours with ketamine. (This would probably be considered an expected side effect, not neurotoxicity.) Murrough et al. (2015) randomized another sample, this time of 43 patients, to a single infusion of ketamine or placebo (midazolam) and found no differences between the groups 1 week after infusion; scores improved equally in both groups and, incidentally, did not correlate with change in depression severity scores.

Shiroma et al. (2014) studied 15 depressed patients treated six times with open-label ketamine and found improvements in cognitive function in multiple domains after the final infusion. Lara et al. (2013) studied 26 depressed patients given 10 mg racemic ketamine sublingually every 2–3 days, in most cases for up to several months, and found subjective improvement in cognition, but no objective testing was done. McIntyre et al. (2021) studied 68 adult outpatients with depression treated with 0.5–0.75 mg/kg ketamine infusions twice a week for 2 weeks. Neurocognitive testing was completed at baseline and after two infusions. Digit symbol substitution (working memory and processing speed), trail making test (same cognitive domains), and subjective reports of cognition all improved. Of course, this study involved only two subanesthetic infusions of ketamine, and few would predict neurotoxicity from such a minimal exposure.

Shiroma et al. (2022) provided a more comprehensive review of 13 ketamine-for-depression studies from 2014 to 2022. These studies looked at cognitive function beyond the time of infusions (weeks or months later) and found no signal of any decrement, even with repeated ketamine infusions. These were all short-term studies involving no ongoing, maintenance ketamine infusions lasting weeks or months or longer. Depression scores tended to improve along with cognition scores in domains such as attention, working memory, and executive function. Of course, these domains have long been known to be impaired in severe depression and to get better with improvement in depression.

The important point is that short courses of ketamine do not impair cognition beyond the time of the infusion and shortly thereafter (24 hours or so). Whether improvement in depression causes impairment (or probably more likely the inverse of that) is not settled. The literature is in need of cognitive outcome data in long-term maintenance ketamine regimens.

The Search for Neuroprotectant Properties of Ketamine Presses On

Circa 1990, ketamine researchers were simultaneously concerned about the possibility that ketamine kills neurons and excited about the neuroprotective potential shown in the animal studies. The neurological conditions in question are devastating: traumatic brain injury, prolonged status epilepticus, malignant ischemic stroke, subarachnoid hemorrhage, and cardiac arrest. In these conditions, the initial injury to the brain, the primary brain injury, is more or less permanent. Beyond the primary injury, over the subsequent hours, days, and weeks, secondary neurological processes occur that are very complex and can extend the initial damage substantially. This is referred to as secondary brain injury. The field of neuroprotection research seeks to prevent or at least minimize this secondary injury damage. Could ketamine be fit for this purpose? We'll start with some general reviews of overall mechanisms by which ketamine might be neuroprotective, followed by a consideration of the literature for each of the conditions.

Possible Neuroprotective Mechanisms

An early paper from the rodent literature is instructive. Simon et al. (1984) subjected rats to bilateral carotid artery occlusion, mimicking human stroke. The rat brains were reperfused later and cut out, and the hippocampi were sectioned. Ischemic microscopic damage was blocked on the side pretreated with a competitive NMDA receptor blocker, 2-amino-7-phosphonoheptanoic acid. This may be the first paper demonstrating that NMDA blockade protects against ischemic brain damage (in rodents). The literature from animals strongly supported the idea that in hypoxic-ischemic neuronal injury paradigms, excitotoxicity caused the damage.

Bell (2017) summarized the proposed mechanisms whereby acute neurological syndromes might cause brain damage in stroke, traumatic brain injury, subarachnoid hemorrhage, or status epilepticus and how ketamine might target these mechanisms. The theory is that glutamate spillage due to acute injury starts exciting extrasynaptic glutamate receptors, of which NMDA receptors are the most numerous. Typically, synaptic receptors are stimulated by normal glutamate amounts, but in glutamate excess, even the NMDA receptors at the periphery on the postsynaptic membrane (which usually do not get stimulated) become involved and cause toxic damage. From this article, we see that even after all these decades, the original excitotoxicity theory proposed by Olney persists.

The second mechanism of neurological damage proposed by Bell (2017) is neuroinflammation. Ketamine has some esoteric molecular actions in animal models documenting an anti-inflammatory effect, which may be involved in its neuroprotective effects, at least in animals.

A third mechanism is *apoptosis*, programmed cell death. Apoptosis is a normal process in the brain in which dysfunctional or no-longer-needed neurons die or are killed. Acute neurological events may accelerate apoptosis to a degree, causing normal neurons to die, and there is some evidence from animals that ketamine may inhibit this process.

Finally, *microthrombosis* (the formation of small clots) was proposed by Bell (2017) as a mechanism of neuronal death in acute neurological syndromes. Theoretically, ketamine may inhibit this process that mediates brain damage, especially in subarachnoid hemorrhage. Thus, the article certainly shows that the enthusiasm for ketamine having significant neuroprotection in humans is still present, although clinical evidence in humans is still lacking.

Ketamine in Neurosurgery and Neuro-Intensive Care Medicine

In neurosurgical and neuro-intensive care situations, increased intracranial pressure can reduce cerebral circulation and contribute to brain damage. In the early 1970s, some small case series implied that ketamine caused increased intracranial pressure when used as an anesthetic (Evans et al. 1971; Gardner et al. 1971; Gardner et al. 1972). This essentially halted the use of ketamine in those settings in which intracranial pressure was likely to go up, such as acute traumatic brain injury, subarachnoid hemorrhage, malignant stroke, or status epilepticus. For decades, it was considered an absolute contraindication in neurosurgery and neuro-intensive care units to use ketamine, which is a shame, since it's so good for sedation or anesthesia without disrupting cardiac output or respiration. One of the reasons so little progress has been made since ketamine was first proposed as a neuroprotectant is hesitancy to use it for fear of worsening cerebral perfusion.

That attitude changed with a landmark study by Mayberg et al. (1995). In 20 patients undergoing brain tumor or aneurysm clipping neurosurgery, induction of anesthesia was undertaken with thiopental and maintenance with isoflurane and nitrous oxide. Intracranial pressure was monitored. During the procedures, a 1.0 mg/kg intravenous dose of ketamine was administered, and intracranial pressures went down. The key was that, in contrast to the situations that led to the alarming reports of the 1970s, CO_2 levels were kept down with adequate mechanical ventilation (high levels of CO_2 in the blood, called *hypercapnia*, result in increased intracranial pressure).

Further studies have confirmed that ketamine appears to be a safe agent for neurosurgery and neuro-intensive care use in patients with brittle or high intracranial pressure (Bourgoin et al. 2003; Grathwohl et al. 2008; Kolenda et al. 1996). Indeed, one of the distinct advantages of ketamine vis-à-vis other sedatives and anesthetics is that it helps prevent systemic hypotension, which can further increase secondary brain damage after a neurological event.

Zeiler and West (2015) reviewed the animal and human data on ketamine's effect on the cerebrovascular system. They concluded that recent research refutes earlier concerns about ketamine's effect on intracranial pressure and arterial constriction, especially if proper attention is given to mechanical ventilation and CO_2 being sufficiently low. After they reviewed the animal and human data on cerebrovascular response to ketamine, they concluded that it increases cerebral perfusion, which made ketamine even more desirable than it already was. In another review, Jeffcote et al. (2023) also concluded from a literature review that ketamine is not associated with increased intracranial pressure when used for sedation in patients with moderate to severe traumatic brain injury.

Other neurosurgical and neuroanesthesia studies have documented safe use of ketamine. Growing optimism that ketamine is indeed safe in these settings has given clinicians confidence to pursue ketamine as a neuroprotectant in patients with acute neurological events. Next we review the literature for the various conditions of interest, focusing on clinical data in humans.

Ketamine and Cortical Spreading Depolarizations

In electroencephalography (EEG), electrodes are placed on the scalp, and electrical activity of the cerebral cortex is detected. A similar procedure is *electrocorticography* (ECoG), whereby a recording strip is placed directly on the surface of the brain. This allows recordings of electrical activity with very fine spatial resolution not possible with EEG. ECoG strips are typically placed during neurosurgery when the brain is exposed. Later on, in the neuro-intensive care unit, ECoG recordings can provide valuable information about brain function.

The output of an ECoG recording consists of a set of channels, each corresponding to an anatomic location under the electrode on the brain. Occasionally, depolarization on a channel is seen, and as time passes, depolarizations are seen in other channels nearby and appear to be spreading, thus the name *spreading depolarizations*. The rate of spread is typically a few millimeters a minute, a level of spatial resolution not possible with surface EEG recording. Spreading depolarizations are believed to represent losses of cellular transmembrane ionic gradients due to hypoxia. It takes energy to maintain the normal neuronal transmembrane ionic gradients, and because of the hypoxia accompanying such neurologic events as stroke, subarachnoid hemorrhage, and traumatic brain injury, spreading depolarizations can be appreciated in the neuro-intensive care unit on the ECoG recording. They presage secondary brain injury, and attempts have been made to suppress them in the hopes of preventing more damage.

Van Harreveld (1959) described spreading depolarizations in rabbit cortex after induction of anoxia. Later experiments proved that purified L-glutamate injected into rabbit brains caused the depolarizations. The author theorized that the initial brain injury causes excess glutamate or aspartate to be released, causing further neuronal damage. This was the first-ever report linking glutamate with a pathological brain process and thus constitutes a contribution to what John Olney later termed excitotoxicity and ultimately to the notion that ketamine may be neuroprotective. Thus, it stands as a landmark article. Gorelova et al. (1987) and Hernándéz-Cáceres et al. (1987) found that ketamine blocked intracerebrally injected potassium-induced spreading depolarizations in rats, the first report of such an effect of ketamine, albeit in rodents. Strong et al. (2002) provided the first ever report of cortical spreading depolarizations in humans, in 11 with traumatic intracranial hematoma, one with spontaneous intracranial hematoma, and two with intracranial aneurysms.

Hertle et al. (2012) studied patients after craniotomies (i.e., neurosurgery) for traumatic brain injuries, subarachnoid hemorrhage, or intracerebral hemorrhage who were residing in a neuro-intensive care unit. All patients had ECoG strips placed intra-operatively. Over time, the authors correlated the apparent effect of different sedative agents (benzodiazepines, barbiturates, opiates, ketamine) on cortical spreading depolarizations. Of 115 patients in the series, 76 showed spreading depolarizations. Ketamine was the only sedating agent associated with reduction of these phenomena.

This is the first report in humans providing data showing that ketamine can suppress cortical spreading depolarizations. It was theorized that NMDA receptor blockade may protect against the loss of normal ionic gradients that underlie spreading depolarizations. No outcome data were given, but this report brought some anticipation that perhaps ketamine may be neuroprotective for some conditions in the neuro-intensive care unit.

Schiefecker et al. (2015) published a case report that is instructive. A 66-year-old man after craniotomy for intracerebral hemorrhage evacuation had ECoG monitoring in the neuro-intensive care unit. Cortical spreading depolarizations occurred in clusters and disappeared when esketamine was administered, and then recurred when esketamine was withdrawn. Cerebral microdialysis measurements documented elevated extracellular glutamate, a finding that supports the glutamate excitotoxicity theory of secondary brain injury.

Carlson et al. (2018) described 10 patients after traumatic brain injury ($n = 8$) or subarachnoid hemorrhage ($n = 2$) who had ECoG strips placed during neurosurgery. In a randomized, crossover design, all patients received ketamine alternating with another agent in the neuro-intensive care unit. Spreading depolarizations were reduced with ketamine at a dose of 1.15 mg/kg/hour or higher during several days of recordings. No further outcome data were provided. This study stands as probably the best scientific evidence of a suppressive effect of ketamine on cortical spreading depolarizations.

Telles et al. (2021) reviewed the literature on ketamine for spreading depolarizations in animals and humans. Spreading depolarizations were demonstrated on ECoG in 14 animal studies (9 rat, 3 mice, 2 pigs) and 5 human studies. They concluded that the data were relatively robust in animals and humans that ketamine inhibits spreading depolarizations—but alas, there are no data to indicate whether this translates into better clinical function, such as better cognitive function.

Jeffcote et al. (2023), in another review, concluded that the evidence supports a reduction in spreading depolarizations for ketamine in the traumatic brain injury literature. Klass et al. (2018) reviewed no fewer than 114 substances that have been tried for spreading depolarizations in animals and humans, underscoring how seriously spreading depolarizations have been taken in the neuropharmacology literature. The authors acknowledged that ketamine reduces the phenomena in both humans and animals but lamented that translation into actual clinical benefits has not been studied.

An interesting perspective on this exciting area of research was provided by Helbok et al. (2020), in a commentary from a meeting of the Co-Operative Studies on Brain Depolarizations group, which was started in 2003 in response to basic science literature in mostly rodents. The authors cautioned against the notion that "all [spreading depolarizations] are bad and must be suppressed with ketamine" (p. 309), which is undoubtedly overly simplistic thinking. Overall, the tone of this commentary by well-educated, influential neuro-intensivists is that the so-called field of neuroprotection has been frustrating for the clinician (albeit wonderfully successful for those who study rodents). The finding that ketamine suppresses cortical spreading depolarizations is quite fascinating, but translation from the ECoG to ultimate neurological and cognitive function is desperately needed.

Cardiac Arrest/Cardiopulmonary Bypass

When a person suffers cardiac arrest or is placed on cardiopulmonary bypass during heart surgery, brain circulation is compromised. It is possible that addition of a neuroprotective agent may lessen the extent of brain damage, so there have been efforts to protect the brain during these scenarios. Hudetz and Pagel (2010) discussed the animal data on the effect of ketamine during low cardiac output and found ketamine to be neuroprotective.

In clinical data, Nagels et al. (2004) studied patients undergoing open-heart surgery with cardiopulmonary bypass and found that the addition of esketamine to propofol anesthesia did not result in improved neurocognitive performance. Bhutta et al. (2012) studied infants undergoing cardiopulmonary bypass during ventricular septal defect repair surgery and randomized about half to receive ketamine and half to saline before bypass. Neurodevelopmental testing 2–3 weeks after surgery did not differ. Thus, there was no evidence of neuroprotection with ketamine, but perhaps the authors did not wait long enough for a benefit to appear or did not conduct testing that was sufficiently sensitive to detect an effect. Hudetz et al. (2009a) induced anesthesia in adult heart surgery patients on cardiopulmonary bypass with fentanyl and etomidate, with 29 randomized to concomitant ketamine 0.5 mg/kg and 29 to saline. Incidence of postoperative delirium was 3% in the ketamine group and 31% in the saline group. Levels of C-reactive protein, a marker of inflammation, were lower in the ketamine group. The blood was drawn a day after surgery, and assessments for delirium were conducted up to 5 days after surgery. The question of whether ketamine's neuroprotective effect was due to blockade of excitotoxicity or an anti-inflammatory effect was discussed.

Published separately, but from the same data collection (Hudetz et al. 2009b), the group assessed postoperative cognitive dysfunction, a known risk for patients undergoing cardiopulmonary bypass. In a variety of cognitive domains, there were postoperative decrements in both groups but less in the ketamine group. These two reports probably constitute the best evidence to date of a clinically significant neuroprotective effect of ketamine in humans.

Regarding cardiac arrest, Ornowska et al. (2023) provided a nice review of proposed mechanisms of brain damage. Loss of blood flow to the brain causes a breakdown of ionic transmembrane gradients and an increase in intracellular calcium. This in turn causes an intracellular cascade, ultimately leading to cell death. Animal models of cardiac arrest clearly show a neuroprotective effect of ketamine (Giuliano et al. 2023). As of yet, there are no human data on ketamine in cardiac arrest. Conducting the appropriate studies would be enormously difficult to get approved by regulatory boards, as most people would probably hesitate to give a sedative drug like ketamine to a person who is acutely unconscious from a cardiac arrest.

Status Epilepticus

Ketamine has turned out to be a remarkably effective treatment for status epilepticus (SE). Whether it also prevents the brain damage caused by SE is unknown. *Status epilepticus*, with its rather stately-sounding Latin phrasing, is marked by seizure activity that lasts at least 5 minutes. If the patient is nonresponsive to two usually effective drug administrations and the condition lasts at least 30 minutes, it is referred to as *refractory status epilepticus* (RSE). RSE, once it is identified as such, calls for admission of the patient to a neuro-intensive care unit with induction of general anesthesia, intubation, and mechanical ventilation. If it persists for 24 hours despite the use of general anesthesia, it is called *superrefractory status epilepticus* (sRSE).

Algorithms exist for management of these states of SE, but in general, pharmacological management first usually entails benzodiazepine therapy (e.g., lorazepam, midazolam, or diazepam). If that does not work, the next step is usually an anti-epileptic drug, such as phenytoin (or fosphenytoin, which is a form of that drug more easily administered intravenously), levetiracetam, or valproic acid. Beyond this, the next step is usually induction and maintenance of general anesthesia with any of numerous medications such as midazolam (which at this point is given as an ongoing high-dose infusion rather than as a bolus as in the first step), barbiturates (such as pentobarbital or thiopental), propofol, or the drug of interest here, ketamine. sRSE can persist for days, weeks, or longer and is associated with high mortality and high neurological morbidity in those who survive. Given the prolonged state of anesthesia and mechanical ventilation, complications such as pneumonia, urinary tract infections, decubitus ulcers, sepsis, and numerous other medical issues are common. Cessation of the ongoing seizure activity is critical.

In the early 1980s, at Washington University in St. Louis, was a group headed by none other than John Olney (this was before the Olney lesion was coined). In one of this group's early studies (Labruyere et al. 1986), seizures were induced in rats with kainic acid, the ligand after which one of the three ligand-gated ion channel glutamate receptors is named. Ketamine and phencyclidine were theorized to block the brain damage induced by these seizures, as this group thought that glutamate excitotoxicity caused it, mediated via NMDA receptors. Indeed, ketamine and phencyclidine did prevent much of the kainic acid–induced seizure brain damage, but something else unexpected was noted: both drugs also stopped the seizures. Thus, the question arose whether the ultimate brain damage was lessened by these drugs because of mitigation of seizure-related brain damage (neuroprotection) or simply by stopping the seizures (these are two subtly different phenomena). Almost four decades later, the answer to this question is still not settled. In any case, excitement was caused by these data on two fronts: ketamine as possible neuroprotectant, and ketamine as possible antiepileptic.

In the 1990s, the attention turned to clinical evidence of ketamine for SE. The first-ever human report of ketamine for SE appears to be the single case of Walker et al. (1996), followed the next year by another case report (Kofke et al. 1997). Other case series followed.

Zeiler et al. (2014) reviewed the then-extant literature on NMDA receptor antagonists for status epilepticus, 23 articles with 162 patients. When ketamine was added to the regimens (which tended to be complex), there was a 56.5% response rate in adults and 63.5% response rate in children. A variety of dosage regimens was used, mostly starting with a bolus followed by an infusion.

In a thorough review of ketamine for RSE, Rosati et al. (2018) examined 27 case reports and 14 case series. Ketamine was used heterogeneously in this literature: latency from onset of SE to use of ketamine varied; dosing regimens ranged from 0.07 to 15 mg/kg/hour; duration of use was 6 hours to 29 days. Overall, 70.3% of RSEs were controlled by ketamine in adults. In the smaller literature on ketamine for children with RSE, there was a 61% response rate.

A curious finding in treatment of SE, RSE, and sRSE is that GABA-ergic agents such as benzodiazepines, barbiturates, and propofol work only early in the course of the prolonged seizures, and ketamine seems to work best later in the course. Naylor et al. (2005) elegantly showed in rats with SE induced with lithium-pilocarpine that synaptic inhibitory currents mediated by $GABA_A$ were reduced as the SE progressed. Also, special staining techniques were used that documented a reduction of cell surface $GABA_A$ receptors, which were relocalized intracellularly. The authors believed that excessive extracellular GABA levels caused this process. This combined with data showing up-regulation of NMDA receptors on the cell surface during SE could be a reason that, as SE progresses, GABA-ergic agents become less effective (as their receptors decline) and NMDA receptor blockers such as ketamine become more effective (as their receptors increase). This has become known as the *receptor trafficking hypothesis* of SE.

Stroke

Simon et al. (1984) made rat brains ischemic with carotid artery occlusion, thus mimicking human stroke. The occlusions lasted for 30 minutes and were followed by 2 hours of reperfusion, after which the animal was killed and the brain was sectioned for histological examination, focusing on the hippocampus, an area of the brain known to be sensitive to ischemic damage. One side of each rat's brain had been infused with the NMDA receptor blocking agent 2-amino-7-phosphonoheptanoic acid, an analogue of glutamate and a competitive blocker at the glutamate receptor. The brain areas infused with this drug ended up with much less brain damage than the untreated sides. This report appears to be the first showing a neuroprotective effect of an NMDA receptor blocker (albeit not ketamine). It also buttressed the then-new notion of excitatory amino acid excess (excitotoxicity) as a cause of brain damage from stroke. This set the stage for the eventual proposal that ketamine or other receptor blockers could be clinically useful for stroke syndromes.

The theory is that loss of oxygen and glucose from the stroke leads to a breakdown in ionic transcellular gradients, which causes release of excessive calcium intracellularly, which is known to lead to cell death. Recall that stimulation of NMDA receptors causes calcium ions to flow into the cell— thus, blockade of these receptors may be protective in situations of excessive intracellular calcium. Many studies of various compounds thought to block aspects of NMDA receptor function have failed in such trials, however. Why would this be the case, especially considering that these drugs are so good at providing neuroprotection in rodent models?

Ikonomidou and Turski (2002) commented on this clinical disappointment and dissonance between animal and human data. These authors postulated that glutamate is necessary for cell survival after a neuro-insult such as stroke or traumatic brain injury and that blocking it is deleterious. They believe that glutamate excess, and thus excitotoxicity, occurs immediately after the insult and only for a short time and that thereafter, glutamate levels return to normal and undertake usual functions. The authors speculated that when it comes to blocking NMDA receptors in these settings, isoform-specific blockade (e.g., GluN2B versus GluN2A subunit) or blockade of extrasynaptic receptors (those on the periphery of the postsynaptic membrane versus the postsynaptic density receptors) may be helpful. Of note, ketamine is not specific to subunits or NMDA receptor locations in its blockade.

The thrust of a very good paper by Lai et al. (2014) is that the reason previous NMDA receptor blockers failed is lack of specificity of subunit or synaptic location blockade. There is also the issue of timing of administration of the putative neuroprotectant drug: there is probably a frustratingly short window after stroke onset in which NMDA receptor modulators may be neuroprotective (and it may be before the patient reaches the hospital). The authors provide an erudite description of the possible cascade of molecular actions, starting with cellular receptor activity and ending with gene transcription intracellularly, in which interventions may be neuroprotective. Whether ketamine fills the bill remains to be seen, if only it can be tested in humans someday.

A Cochrane database study (Muir and Lees 2003) summarized 36 trials involving 11,209 patients with acute stroke in which amino acid antagonists (either glutamate release inhibitors or NMDA receptor antagonists) were tested for neuroprotective action. There was no evidence that any of the compounds (which did not include ketamine) provided any benefit.

In summary, as far as a role for ketamine in stroke neuroprotection goes, after decades of speculation, there still has not been a good human clinical trial. It would be fairly easy. Patients who present to an emergency department with an acute ischemic stroke could be randomized to a dose of ketamine versus saline placebo, in addition to care as usual. Outcome measures would be mortality, neurological function, cognition, neuroradiologic findings, and mental health, all easy to obtain. Such a study should not be terribly expensive, and given the enormous financial burden of stroke in the population, any benefit of ketamine would be quite welcome. The field awaits.

Traumatic Brain Injury

Traumatic brain injury (TBI) is common, often devastating, and expensive. The initial brain damage from the injury is permanent, but continued neuronal events in the subsequent days and weeks (the secondary injury) may extend this damage, and this is the target of neuroprotection. As with other acute neurological events, the literature in rodents for neuroprotection is much more compelling than that for humans.

Shapira et al. (1992) induced head trauma in rats, with ketamine-treated and non–ketamine-treated subgroups. They were behaviorally tested at serial intervals for 2 days, and then the brains were sectioned for histology. Behavioral abnormalities were less intense and infarct sizes smaller in the ketamine-treated group. This appears to be the first study documenting a neuroprotective effect of ketamine in TBI, albeit in rodents.

Chang et al. (2013) summarized the state of neuroprotection with ketamine for traumatic brain injury. The proposed mechanisms of ketamine-induced neuroprotection for this setting are similar to other settings and include reduction of excitotoxicity, anti-inflammatory actions, maintenance of hemodynamic stability (i.e., cerebral perfusion pressure), and reduction of cortical spreading depolarizations. They cited several studies showing hemodynamic safety of ketamine for anesthesia induction in traumatic brain injury but lamented that so far nothing had been done showing neuroprotection (e.g., follow-up cognitive testing).

Zanza et al. (2022) provided a nice review of ketamine in acute brain injury, specifically sedation in brain-injured patients. Outcomes in the 11 studies reviewed focused on intracranial pressure, cerebral perfusion, cortical spreading depolarizations, mortality, and neurological function. There were no studies in which ketamine was added strictly for presumed neuroprotection. The main findings were that intracranial pressure does not rise with ketamine, cerebral perfusion pressure increases, and spreading depolarizations are suppressed, which may have implications for neuroprotection. In other reviews, Jeffcote et al. (2023) and Gregers et al. (2020) reached similar conclusions.

Bebarta et al. (2020) studied Afghanistan war soldiers who suffered brain injuries in combat. Forty-six were treated presurgically with ketamine, 45 with another analgesic, and 69 with no analgesic. There were similar outcomes acutely in terms of gross functionality, but no neuropsychological testing was done. In another military sample, Grathwohl et al. (2008) compared ketamine to volatile anesthetics for combat-related head injury surgery (nonrandomized). An analysis of the ketamine anesthesia group found no differences in mortality or functional outcomes.

Maheswari et al. (2023) randomized 25 head-injury patients to anesthesia with ketamine/propofol (ketofol) versus 25 to propofol. There were no differences in functional outcomes at 30 and 90 days after surgery. There was less intra-operative vasopressor use with ketofol. On postoperative day 3, levels of glial fibrillary acid protein (a marker of brain injury) were lower in the ketofol group. Brain relaxation assessed intraoperatively (subjectively) by the neurosurgeon based on observations of tightness and swelling did not differ between the two groups. This is so far the closest study to a neuroprotection outcome assessment in head-injury patients receiving ketamine versus something else, and there were no functional differences at 3 months. To document a neuroprotective effect (if indeed it exists) for ketamine in traumatic brain injury, it may need to be given at some other time point or in some other dosage format, or the outcome needs to be something more subtle than a gross functional assessment (e.g., neuropsychological testing).

Subarachnoid Hemorrhage

Subarachnoid hemorrhage (SAH) constitutes a potentially catastrophic acute neurologic event often causing death or permanent neurological disability. SAH is usually caused by bursting of arterial aneurysms. When diagnosed, neurosurgery to clip the aneurysm is often performed.

In what appears to be the first-ever report of use of ketamine in subarachnoid hemorrhage patients, Langelaar et al. (1996) indicated that in patients after clipping of aneurysms that had caused subarachnoid hemorrhage, 66 received intravenous nimodipine (a calcium channel blocker commonly used for vascular stabilization in this setting), and 49 received nimodipine plus ketamine and lignocaine. These regimens were used for several days while the patients were in the neuro-intensive care unit. No differences in functional outcome emerged between the two groups.

Von der Brelie et al. (2017) pointed out that in subarachnoid hemorrhage, delayed cerebral ischemia is common and can cause new infarcts (this would be an example of secondary brain injury, which may be amenable to a neuroprotective agent). The mechanisms of delayed cerebral ischemia include vasospasm, inflammation, microthrombosis, and cortical spreading depolarizations. This was a retrospective study comparing outcomes of subarachnoid hemorrhage patients treated with ketamine versus without ketamine as a sedative in the neuro-intensive care unit. Ketamine was added if midazolam and fentanyl were ineffective and was given at a maximum dose of 500 mg/hour, which gives the reader an idea of how much ketamine is used for intensive care sedation. Scales of agitation as well as evidence of delayed infarcts were the outcomes of interest. Forty-one patients received ketamine; 23 did not. The incidence of delayed cerebral infarcts was 7.3% when ketamine was used versus 25% when it was not, indicating a possible neuroprotective effect of ketamine. Use of vasopressors to keep blood pressure from falling was less frequent when ketamine was used, which is very important since drops in blood pressure in the acute neurological event setting can cause further secondary brain injury. Extended Glasgow Outcome Scale (an 8-point scale with 1 being death and 8 being excellent functional recovery) scores did not differ between the two groups (i.e., ketamine versus not ketamine). Finally, ketamine resulted in lower intracranial pressure in 93.1% of patients given it.

The authors attributed the lower incidence of delayed infarctions with ketamine to three possible mechanisms: 1) ketamine reduced cortical spreading depolarizations; 2) ketamine's NMDA receptor blockade reduced intracellular calcium influx and therefore resulted in less excitotoxic cell injury; or 3) ketamine's cerebral hemodynamic effect caused increased cerebral perfusion pressure, which is good for the recently injured brain.

Santos et al. (2019) described 66 patients after subarachnoid hemorrhage, 33 of whom were treated in the neuro-intensive care unit with esketamine as part of their sedative regimen (midazolam was concurrently used). Intracranial pressure increased with esketamine, but the authors did not think it was a significant rise. Extended Glasgow Outcome Scale scores were lower with the esketamine-treated patients, which the authors attributed to their being the sickest patients to begin with (the choice of using esketamine was not random). Overall rate of medical complications was similar between the two groups as well.

Bhardwaj et al. (2020) randomized aneurysm-related subarachnoid hemorrhage patients undergoing aneurysm clipping to ketofol versus propofol alone for anesthesia. Only short-term outcomes were reported, and no differences emerged in intracranial pressure or neurosurgeon-rated brain relaxation. There was less intraoperative decrease in blood pressure with ketofol. Longer-term functional outcomes were not reported.

In summary, the clinical data on a neuroprotective effect of ketamine in subarachnoid hemorrhage are scarce. A prospective randomized study of ketamine for either anesthesia induction/maintenance or neuro-intensive care sedation would be quite welcome.

What About Neurodegenerative Disorders, Excitotoxicity, and Ketamine?

The original excitotoxicity literature focused on mechanisms of brain damage in acute neurological events such as those discussed in this chapter. However, Olney also theorized that excitotoxicity may be at play in chronic, insidious neurodegenerative disorders such as Huntington disease (Olney and de Gubareff 1978). In fact, one medication approved by the FDA for treatment of Alzheimer disease, memantine, is an NMDA receptor blocker, albeit weakly so. There is one rather esoteric paper (Foster et al. 1991) showing that a ketamine dose seemed to elicit temporary memory improvements in Alzheimer disease patients. However, one could hardly conceptualize ketamine as a pragmatic option for such patients: can we really imagine giving Alzheimer patients multiple, daily ketamine doses in an ongoing manner? Surely not. However, if ongoing excitotoxicity is really happening with these neurodegenerative diseases, perhaps ketamine in the lab or in very brief clinical studies may help shed some light in the search for suitable clinically usable compounds.

Epilogue

And on that somewhat esoteric note, the book ends. But of course, the story of ketamine will reach no such end. Papers on ketamine keep coming out at a furious pace—the National Library of Medicine listed more than 1,800 citations for ketamine for the year 2023 alone. Where will the ketamine story go next? In what avenue, heretofore untraveled, will ketamine pop up? After all these decades of fascination with ketamine, despite intensive searching, an alternative for its various uses has not been found. To paraphrase the famous line in *Risky Business* ("Porsche. There is no substitute"), perhaps ketamine simply has no substitute.

References

Aalto S, Hirvonen J, Kajander J, et al: Ketamine does not decrease striatal dopamine D2 receptor binding in man. Psychopharmacology (Berl) 164(4):401–406, 2002 12457270

Abdallah CG, De Feyter HM, Averill LA, et al: The effects of ketamine on prefrontal glutamate neurotransmission in healthy and depressed subjects. Neuropsychopharmacology 43(10):2154–2160, 2018 29977074

Abdallah CG, Roache JD, Averill LA, et al; Consortium to Alleviate PTSD: Repeated ketamine infusions for antidepressant-resistant PTSD: methods of a multicenter, randomized, placebo-controlled clinical trial. Contemp Clin Trials 81:11–18, 2019 30999057

Abdallah CG, Averill LA, Gueorguieva R, et al: Modulation of the antidepressant effects of ketamine by the mTORC1 inhibitor rapamycin. Neuropsychopharmacology 45(6):990–997, 2020 32092760

Abdallah CG, Roache JD, Gueorguieva R, et al: Dose-related effects of ketamine for antidepressant-resistant symptoms of posttraumatic stress disorder in veterans and active duty military: a double-blind, randomized, placebo-controlled multi-center clinical trial. Neuropsychopharmacology 47(8):1574–1581, 2022 35046508

Abel KM, Allin MPG, Kucharska-Pietura K, et al: Ketamine alters neural processing of facial emotion recognition in healthy men: an fMRI study. NeuroReport 14(3):387–391, 2003a 12634489

Abel KM, Allin MPG, Hemsley DR, Geyer MA: Low dose ketamine increases prepulse inhibition in healthy men. Neuropharmacology 44(6):729–737, 2003b 12681371

Abuhelwa AY, Somogyi AA, Loo CK, et al: Population pharmacokinetics and pharmacodynamics of the therapeutic and adverse effects of ketamine in patients with treatment-refractory depression. Clin Pharmacol Ther 112(3):720–729, 2022 35560226

Ahn K-H, Youn T, Cho SS, et al: N-methyl-D-aspartate receptor in working memory impairments in schizophrenia: event-related potential study of late stage of working memory process. Prog Neuropsychopharmacol Biol Psychiatry 27(6):993–999, 2003 14499316

Aiyer R, Mehta N, Gungor S, Gulati A: A systematic review of NMDA receptor antagonists for treatment of neuropathic pain in clinical practice. Clin J Pain 34(5):450–467, 2018 28877137

Albott CS, Lim KO, Forbes MK, et al: Efficacy, safety, and durability of repeated ketamine infusions for comorbid posttraumatic stress disorder and treatment-resistant depression. J Clin Psychiatry 79(3):e1–e8, 2018 29727073

Allen AC, Robles J, Dovenski W, Calderon S: PCP: a review of synthetic methods for forensic clandestine investigation. Forensic Sci Int 61(2–3):85–100, 1993 8307527

American Psychiatric Association: Diagnostic and Statistical Manual of Mental Disorders, Third Edition. Washington, DC, American Psychiatric Association, 1980

American Psychiatric Association: Diagnostic and Statistical Manual of Mental Disorders, Fifth Edition—Text Revision. Washington, DC, American Psychiatric Association, 2023

Amr YM: Multi-day low dose ketamine infusion as adjuvant to oral gabapentin in spinal cord injury related chronic pain: a prospective, randomized, double blind trial. Pain Physician 13(3):245–249, 2010 20495588

Anand A, Charney DS, Oren DA, et al: Attenuation of the neuropsychiatric effects of ketamine with lamotrigine: support for hyperglutamatergic effects of N-methyl-D-aspartate receptor antagonists. Arch Gen Psychiatry 57(3):270–276, 2000 10711913

Anand A, Mathew SJ, Sanacora G, et al: Ketamine versus ECT for nonpsychotic treatment-resistant major depression. N Engl J Med 388(25):2315–2325, 2023 37224232

Andreasen NC: Negative symptoms in schizophrenia. Definition and reliability. Arch Gen Psychiatry 39(7):784–788, 1982 7165477

Andreasen NC, Arndt S, Miller D, et al: Correlational studies of the Scale for the Assessment of Negative Symptoms and the Scale for the Assessment of Positive Symptoms: an overview and update. Psychopathology 28(1):7–17, 1995 7871123

Aniline O, Allen RE, Pitts FN Jr, et al: The urban epidemic of phencyclidine use: laboratory evidence from a public psychiatric hospital inpatient service. Biol Psychiatry 15(5):813–817, 1980 7417634

Anis NA, Berry SC, Burton NR, Lodge D: The dissociative anaesthetics, ketamine and phencyclidine, selectively reduce excitation of central mammalian neurones by N-methyl-aspartate. Br J Pharmacol 79(2):565–575, 1983 6317114

Anonymous: The perils of PCP. Drug Enforcement 1(3):8–9, 1974

Anticevic A, Corlett PR, Cole MW, et al: N-methyl-D-aspartate receptor antagonist effects on prefrontal cortical connectivity better model early than chronic schizophrenia. Biol Psychiatry 77(6):569–580, 2015 25281999

Araújo-de-Freitas L, Santos-Lima C, Mendonca-Filho E, et al: Neurocognitive aspects of ketamine and esketamine on subjects with treatment-resistant depression: a comparative, randomized and double-blind study. Psychiatry Res 303:114058, 2021

Avila MT, Weiler MA, Lahti AC, et al: Effects of ketamine on leading saccades during smooth-pursuit eye movements may implicate cerebellar dysfunction in schizophrenia. Am J Psychiatry 159(9):1490–1496, 2002 12202268

Azari P, Lindsay DR, Briones D, et al: Efficacy and safety of ketamine in patients with complex regional pain syndrome: a systematic review. CNS Drugs 26(3):215–228, 2012 22136149

Azhari N, Hu H, O'Malley KY, et al: Ketamine-facilitated behavioral treatment for cannabis use disorder: a proof of concept study. Am J Drug Alcohol Abuse 47(1):92–97, 2021 33175580

Backonja M, Arndt G, Gombar KA, et al: Response of chronic neuropathic pain syndromes to ketamine: a preliminary study. Pain 56(1):51–57, 1994 8159441

Bahji A, Vazquez GH, Zarate CA Jr: Comparative efficacy of racemic ketamine and esketamine for depression: a systematic review and meta-analysis. J Affect Disord 278:542–555, 2021 33022440

Bakker CB, Amini FB: Observations on the psychotomimetic effects of Sernyl. Compr Psychiatry 2:269–280, 1961 13864199

Ban TA, Lohrenz JJ, Lehmann HE: Observations on the action of Sernyl-a new psychotropic drug. Can Psychiatr Assoc J 6(3):150–157, 1961 13686510

Barany E: Applanation tonometry and ophthalmoscopy of the vervet monkey (cercopithecus ethiops) in phencyclidine catalepsia. Invest Ophthalmol 2(4):322–324, 1963 14092157

Bebarta VS, Mora AG, Bebarta EK, et al: Prehospital use of ketamine in the combat setting: a sub-analysis of patients with head injuries evaluated in the prospective Life Saving Intervention study. Mil Med 185(Suppl 1):136–142, 2020 32074369

Beck K, Hindley G, Borgan F, et al: Association of ketamine with psychiatric symptoms and implications for its therapeutic use and for understanding schizophrenia: a systematic review and meta-analysis. JAMA Netw Open 3(5):e204693, 2020 32437573

Becker B, Steffens M, Zhao Z, et al: General and emotion-specific neural effects of ketamine during emotional memory formation. Neuroimage 150:308–317, 2017 28232170

Beech HR, Davies BM, Morgenstern FS: Preliminary investigations of the effects of Sernyl upon cognitive and sensory processes. J Ment Sci 107:509–513, 1961 13688613

Bell JD: In vogue: ketamine for neuroprotection in acute neurologic injury. Anesth Analg 124(4):1237–1243, 2017 28079589

Bentley S, Artin H, Mehaffey E, et al: Response to intravenous racemic ketamine after switch from intranasal (S)-ketamine on symptoms of treatment-resistant depression and post-traumatic stress disorder in veterans: a retrospective case series. Pharmacotherapy 42(3):272–279, 2022 35122282

Berman RM, Cappiello A, Anand A, et al: Antidepressant effects of ketamine in depressed patients. Biol Psychiatry 47(4):351–354, 2000 10686270

Betzler F, Ernst F, Helbig J, et al: Substance use and prevention programs in Berlin's party scene: results of the SuPrA-study. Eur Addict Res 25(6):283–292, 2019 31302656

Bhardwaj A, Panda N, Chauhan R, et al: Comparison of ketofol (combination of ketamine and propofol) and propofol anesthesia in aneurysmal clipping surgery: a prospective randomized control trial. Asian J Neurosurg 15(3):608–613, 2020 33145214

Bhutta A-T, Schmitz ML, Swearingen C, et al: Ketamine as a neuroprotective and anti-inflammatory agent in children undergoing surgery on cardiopulmonary bypass: a pilot randomized, double-blind, placebo-controlled trial. Pediatr Crit Care Med 13(3):328–337, 2012 21926656

Blagrove M, Morgan CJA, Curran HV, et al: The incidence of unpleasant dreams after sub-anaesthetic ketamine. Psychopharmacology (Berl) 203(1):109–120, 2009 18949459

Bloch MH, Wasylink S, Landeros-Weisenberger A, et al: Effects of ketamine in treatment-refractory obsessive-compulsive disorder. Biol Psychiatry 72(11):964–970, 2012 22784486

Blonk MI, Koder BG, van den Bemt PM, Huygen FJ: Use of oral ketamine in chronic pain management: a review. Eur J Pain 14(5):466–472, 2010 19879174

Bodi T, Share I, Levy H, Moyer JH: Clinical trial of phencyclidíne (sernyl) in patients with psychoneurosis. Antibiotic Med Clin Ther 6(2):79–84, 1959 13628032

Boeijinga PH, Soufflet L, Santoro F, Luthringer R: Ketamine effects on CNS responses assessed with MEG/EEG in a passive auditory sensory-gating paradigm: an attempt for modelling some symptoms of psychosis in man. J Psychopharmacol 21(3):321–337, 2007 17591659

Bojesen KB, Andersen KA, Rasmussen SN, et al: Glutamate levels and resting cerebral blood flow in anterior cingulate cortex are associated at rest and immediately following infusion of S-ketamine in healthy volunteers. Front Psychiatry 9:22, 2018 29467681

Bonanno FG: Ketamine in war/tropical surgery (a final tribute to the racemic mixture). Injury 33(4):323–327, 2002 12091028

Bonaventura J, Gomez JL, Carlton ML, et al: Target deconvolution studies of (2R,6R)-hydroxynorketamine: an elusive search. Mol Psychiatry 27(10):4144–4156, 2022 35768639

Bottemanne H, Arnould A: Ketamine augmentation of exposure response prevention therapy for obsessive-compulsive disorder. Innov Clin Neurosci 18(10–12):9–11, 2021 35096475

Bottemanne H, Baldacci A, Muller C, et al: Ketamine Augmented Psychotherapy (KAP) in mood disorder: user guide [in French]. Encephale 48(3):304–312, 2022 34876279

Bourgoin A, Albanèse J, Wereszczynski N, et al: Safety of sedation with ketamine in severe head injury patients: comparison with sufentanil. Crit Care Med 31(3):711–717, 2003 12626974

Brambrink AM, Evers AS, Avidan MS, et al: Ketamine-induced neuroapoptosis in the fetal and neonatal rhesus macaque brain. Anesthesiology 116(2):372–384, 2012 22222480

Breier A, Malhotra AK, Pinals DA, et al: Association of ketamine-induced psychosis with focal activation of the prefrontal cortex in healthy volunteers. Am J Psychiatry 154(6):805–811, 1997 9167508

Breier A, Adler CM, Weisenfeld N, et al: Effects of NMDA antagonism on striatal dopamine release in healthy subjects: application of a novel PET approach. Synapse 29(2):142–147, 1998 9593104

Bremner JD, Krystal JH, Putnam FW, et al: Measurement of dissociative states with the Clinician-Administered Dissociative States Scale. J Trauma Stress 11(1):125–136, 1998 9479681

Brinck ECV, Tiippana E, Heesen M, et al: Perioperative intravenous ketamine for acute postoperative pain in adults. Cochrane Database Syst Rev 12(12):CD012033, 2018 30570761

Bryant JE, Frölich M, Tran S, et al: Ketamine induced changes in regional cerebral blood flow, interregional connectivity patterns, and glutamate metabolism. J Psychiatr Res 117:108–115, 2019 31376621

Burns RS, Lerner SE, Corrado R, et al: Phencyclidine—states of acute intoxication and fatalities. West J Med 123(5):345–349, 1975 1210329

Calabrese L: Titrated serial ketamine infusions stop outpatient suicidality and avert ER visits and hospitalizations. Int J Psychiatr Res 2(6):1–12, 2019

Calle P, Maudens K, Lemoyne S, et al: Lessons to be learned from toxicological analyses in intoxicated patients and seized materials at an electronic music dance festival. Forensic Sci Int 299:174–179, 2019 31039545

Canuso CM, Singh JB, Fedgchin M, et al: Efficacy and safety of intranasal esketamine for the rapid reduction of symptoms of depression and suicidality in patients at imminent risk for suicide: results of a double-blind, randomized, placebo-controlled study. Am J Psychiatry 175(7):620–630, 2018 29656663

Carlson AP, Abbas M, Alunday RL, et al: Spreading depolarization in acute brain injury inhibited by ketamine: a prospective, randomized, multiple crossover trial. J Neurosurg 130:1–7, 2018 29799344

Carpenter WT Jr: The schizophrenia ketamine challenge study debate. Biol Psychiatry 46(8):1081–1091, 1999 10536744

Carr DB, Goudas LC, Denman WT, et al: Safety and efficacy of intranasal ketamine for the treatment of breakthrough pain in patients with chronic pain: a randomized, double-blind, placebo-controlled, crossover study. Pain 108(1–2):17–27, 2004 15109503

Chan KWS, Lee TMC, Siu AM, et al: Effects of chronic ketamine use on frontal and medial temporal cognition. Addict Behav 38(5):2128–2132, 2013 23435274

Chan WM, Xu J, Fan M, et al: Downregulation in the human and mice cerebella after ketamine versus ketamine plus ethanol treatment. Microsc Res Tech 75(3):258–264, 2012 21809417

Chang C-M, Wu TL, Ting T-T, et al: Mis-anaesthetized society: expectancies and recreational use of ketamine in Taiwan. BMC Public Health 19(1):1307, 2019 31623586

Chang LC, Raty SR, Ortiz J, et al: The emerging use of ketamine for anesthesia and sedation in traumatic brain injuries. CNS Neurosci Ther 19(6):390–395, 2013 23480625

Chen G: Evaluation of phencyclidine-type cataleptic activity. Arch Int Pharmacodyn Ther 157(1):193–201, 1965 5894555

Chen G: The neuropharmacology of phencyclidine, in PCP (Phencyclidine): Historical and Current Perspectives. Edited by Domino EF. Ann Arbor, MI, NPP Books, 1981, pp 9–16

Chen GM, Weston JK: The analgesic and anesthetic effect of 1-(1-phenylcyclo-hexyl) piperidine HCl on the monkey. Anesth Analg 39(2):132–137, 1960 13809588

Chen G, Ensor CR, Russell D, Bohner B: The pharmacology of 1-(1-phenylcyclo-hexyl) piperidine-HCl. J Pharmacol Exp Ther 127:241–250, 1959 13809587

Chen G, Ensor CR, Bohner B: The neuropharmacology of 2-(omicron-chlorophe-nyl)-2-methylaminocyclohexanone hydrochloride. J Pharmacol Exp Ther 152(2):332–339, 1966 4380271

Chen M-H, Li C-T, Lin WC, et al: Cognitive function of patients with treatment-resistant depression after a single low dose of ketamine infusion. J Affect Disord 241:1–7, 2018 30081380

Cheng W-C, Dao K-L: The occurrence of alcohol/drugs by toxicological examination of selected drivers in Hong Kong. Forensic Sci Int 275:242–253, 2017 28412576

Cheng W-C, Dao K-L: Prevalence of drugs of abuse found in testing of illicit drug seizures and urinalysis of selected population in Hong Kong. Forensic Sci Int 299:6–16, 2019 30954006

Cheng W-J, Chen C-H, Chen C-K, et al: Similar psychotic and cognitive profile between ketamine dependence with persistent psychosis and schizophrenia. Schizophr Res 199:313–318, 2018 29510925

Chong C, Schug SA, Page-Sharp M, et al: Development of a sublingual/oral for-mulation of ketamine for use in neuropathic pain: preliminary findings from a three-way randomized, crossover study. Clin Drug Investig 29(5):317–324, 2009 19366273

Chu PSK, Kwok SC, Lam KM, et al: 'Street ketamine'-associated bladder dysfunc-tion: a report of ten cases. Hong Kong Med J 13(4):311–313, 2007 17592176

Clements JA, Nimmo WS, Grant IS: Bioavailability, pharmacokinetics, and analge-sic activity of ketamine in humans. J Pharm Sci 71(5):539–542, 1982 7097501

Cohen BD, Luby ED, Rosenbaum G, Gottlieb JS: Combined sernyl and sensory deprivation. Compr Psychiatry 1:345–348, 1960 13694346

Cohen BD, Rosenbaum G, Luby ED, Gottlieb JS: Comparison of phencyclidine hydrochloride (Sernyl) with other drugs. Simulation of schizophrenic perfor-mance with phencyclidine hydrochloride (Sernyl), lysergic acid diethylamide (LSD-25), and amobarbital (Amytal) sodium; II. Symbolic and sequential think-ing. Arch Gen Psychiatry 6:395–401, 1962 13880223

Cohen S: Angel dust. JAMA 238(6):515–516, 1977 577581

Cohen SP, Bhatia A, Buvanendran A, et al: Consensus guidelines on the use of in-travenous ketamine infusions for chronic pain from the American Society of Re-gional Anesthesia and Pain Medicine, the American Academy of Pain Medicine, and the American Society of Anesthesiologists. Reg Anesth Pain Med 43(5):521–546, 2018 29870458

Collier BB: Ketamine and the conscious mind. Anaesthesia 27(2):120–134, 1972 5021517

Connolly SB, Prager JP, Harden RN: A systematic review of ketamine for complex regional pain syndrome. Pain Med 16(5):943–969, 2015 25586192

Coppel DL, Bovill JG, Dundee JW: The taming of ketamine. Anaesthesia 28(3):293–296, 1973 4713950

Corazza O, Schifano F: Near-death states reported in a sample of 50 misusers. Subst Use Misuse 45(6):916–924, 2010 20397876

Corazza O, Assi S, Schifano F: From "Special K" to "Special M": the evolution of the recreational use of ketamine and methoxetamine. CNS Neurosci Ther 19(6):454–460, 2013 23421859

Corlett PR, Honey GD, Aitken MRF, et al: Frontal responses during learning predict vulnerability to the psychotogenic effects of ketamine: linking cognition, brain activity, and psychosis. Arch Gen Psychiatry 63(6):611–621, 2006 16754834

Correia-Melo FS, Leal GC, Vieira F, et al: Efficacy and safety of adjunctive therapy using esketamine or racemic ketamine for adult treatment-resistant depression: a randomized, double-blind, non-inferiority study. J Affect Disord 264:527–534, 2020 31786030

Correll GE, Maleki J, Gracely EJ, et al: Subanesthetic ketamine infusion therapy: a retrospective analysis of a novel therapeutic approach to complex regional pain syndrome. Pain Med 5(3):263–275, 2004 15367304

Corssen G: Clinical use of CI-581. Acta Anaesthesiol Scand Suppl 25:416–418, 1966 6003314

Corssen G, Domino EF: Dissociative anesthesia: further pharmacologic studies and first clinical experience with the phencyclidine derivative CI-581. Anesth Analg 45(1):29–40, 1966 5325977

Corssen G, Miyasaka M, Domino EF: Changing concepts in pain control during surgery: dissociative anesthesia with CI-581. A progress report. Anesth Analg 47(6):746–759, 1968 5749338

Cristea IA, Naudet F: US Food and Drug Administration approval of esketamine and brexanolone. Lancet Psychiatry 6(12):975–977, 2019 31680013

Crumb MW, Bryant C, Atkinson TJ: Emerging trends in pain medication management: back to the future: a focus on ketamine. Am J Med 131(8):883–886, 2018 29730359

Curic S, Leicht G, Thiebes S, et al: Reduced auditory evoked gamma-band response and schizophrenia-like clinical symptoms under subanesthetic ketamine. Neuropsychopharmacology 44(7):1239–1246, 2019 30758327

Curran HV, Monaghan L: In and out of the K-hole: a comparison of the acute and residual effects of ketamine in frequent and infrequent ketamine users. Addiction 96(5):749–760, 2001 11331033

Curran HV, Morgan C: Cognitive, dissociative and psychotogenic effects of ketamine in recreational users on the night of drug use and 3 days later. Addiction 95(4):575–590, 2000 10829333

Dadabayev AR, Joshi SA, Reda MH, et al: Low dose ketamine infusion for comorbid posttraumatic stress disorder and chronic pain: a randomized double-blind clinical trial. Chronic Stress (Thousand Oaks) 4:2470547020981670, 2020 33426410

Dahan A, Olofsen E, Sigtermans M, et al: Population pharmacokinetic-pharmaco-dynamic modeling of ketamine-induced pain relief of chronic pain. Eur J Pain 15(3):258–267, 2011 20638877

Dakwar E, Levin F, Foltin RW, et al: The effects of subanesthetic ketamine infu-sions on motivation to quit and cue-induced craving in cocaine-dependent re-search volunteers. Biol Psychiatry 76(1):40–46, 2014a 24035344

Dakwar E, Anerella C, Hart CL, et al: Therapeutic infusions of ketamine: do the psy-choactive effects matter? Drug Alcohol Depend 136:153–157, 2014b 24480515

Dakwar E, Hart CL, Levin FR, et al: Cocaine self-administration disrupted by the N-methyl-D-aspartate receptor antagonist ketamine: a randomized, crossover trial. Mol Psychiatry 22(1):76–81, 2017 27090301

Dakwar E, Nunes EV, Hart CL, et al: A sub-set of psychoactive effects may be crit-ical to the behavioral impact of ketamine on cocaine use disorder: results from a randomized, controlled laboratory study. Neuropharmacology 142:270–276, 2018 29309770

Dakwar E, Nunes EV, Hart CL, et al: A single ketamine infusion combined with mindfulness-based behavioral modification to treat cocaine dependence: a ran-domized clinical trial. Am J Psychiatry 176(11):923–930, 2019 31230464

Dakwar E, Levin F, Hart CL, et al: A single ketamine infusion combined with mo-tivational enhancement therapy for alcohol use disorder: a randomized midaz-olam-controlled pilot trial. Am J Psychiatry 177(2):125–133, 2020 31786934

Dalgarno PJ, Shewan D: Illicit use of ketamine in Scotland. J Psychoactive Drugs 28(2):191–199, 1996 8811587

Daly EJ, Singh JB, Fedgchin M, et al: Efficacy and safety of intranasal esketamine adjunctive to oral antidepressant therapy in treatment-resistant depression: a randomized clinical trial. JAMA Psychiatry 75(2):139–148, 2018 29282469

Daly EJ, Trivedi MH, Janik A, et al: Efficacy of esketamine nasal spray plus oral antidepressant treatment for relapse prevention in patients with treatment-resistant depression: a randomized clinical trial. JAMA Psychiatry 76(9):893–903, 2019 31166571

Dames S, Kryskow P, Watler C: A cohort-based case report: the impact of ket-amine-assisted therapy embedded in a community of practice framework for healthcare providers with PTSD and depression. Front Psychiatry 12:803279, 2022 35095617

Dandash O, Harrison BJ, Adapa R, et al: Selective augmentation of striatal func-tional connectivity following NMDA receptor antagonism: implications for psy-chosis. Neuropsychopharmacology 40(3):622–631, 2015 25141922

Das RK, Gale G, Walsh K, et al: Ketamine can reduce harmful drinking by phar-macologically rewriting drinking memories. Nat Commun 10(1):5187, 2019 31772157

Daumann J, Heekeren K, Neukirch A, et al: Pharmacological modulation of the neural basis underlying inhibition of return (IOR) in the human 5-HT2A ago-nist and NMDA antagonist model of psychosis. Psychopharmacology (Berl) 200(4):573–583, 2008 18649072

Daumann J, Wagner D, Heekeren K, et al: Neuronal correlates of visual and auditory alertness in the DMT and ketamine model of psychosis. J Psychopharmacol 24(10):1515–1524, 2010 19304859

Davies BM: A preliminary report on the use of sernyl in psychiatric illness. J Ment Sci 106:1073–1079, 1960 13720083

Davies BM: Oral Sernyl in obsessive states. J Ment Sci 107:109–114, 1961 13720084

Davies BM, Beech HR: The effect of 1-arylcylohexylamine (sernyl) on twelve normal volunteers. J Ment Sci 106:912–924, 1960 13720081

Deakin JFW, Lees J, McKie S, et al: Glutamate and the neural basis of the subjective effects of ketamine: a pharmaco-magnetic resonance imaging study. Arch Gen Psychiatry 65(2):154–164, 2008 18250253

de la Salle S, Choueiry J, Shah D, et al: Effects of ketamine on resting-state EEG activity and their relationship to perceptual/dissociative symptoms in healthy humans. Front Pharmacol 7:348, 2016 27729865

De Luca MT, Meringolo M, Spagnolo PA, Badiani A: The role of setting for ketamine abuse: clinical and preclinical evidence. Rev Neurosci 23(5–6):769–780, 2012 23159868

deRoux SJ, Sgarlato A, Marker E: Phencyclidine: a 5-year retrospective review from the New York City Medical Examiner's Office. J Forensic Sci 56(3):656–659, 2011 21291469

De Simoni S, Schwarz AJ, O'Daly OG, et al: Test-retest reliability of the BOLD pharmacological MRI response to ketamine in healthy volunteers. Neuroimage 64:75–90, 2013 23009959

Diamond PR, Farmery AD, Atkinson S, et al: Ketamine infusions for treatment resistant depression: a series of 28 patients treated weekly or twice weekly in an ECT clinic. J Psychopharmacol 28(6):536–544, 2014 24699062

Diazgranados N, Ibrahim L, Brutsche NE, et al: A randomized add-on trial of an N-methyl-D-aspartate antagonist in treatment-resistant bipolar depression. Arch Gen Psychiatry 67(8):793–802, 2010 20679587

Dillon P, Copeland J, Jansen K: Patterns of use and harms associated with nonmedical ketamine use. Drug Alcohol Depend 69(1):23–28, 2003 12536063

Di Vincenzo JD, Siegel A, Lipsitz O, et al: The effectiveness, safety and tolerability of ketamine for depression in adolescents and older adults: a systematic review. J Psychiatr Res 137:232–241, 2021 33706168

Dogoloff LI: Federal response to the PCP problem 1979. J Psychedelic Drugs 12(3–4):185–190, 1980 7431412

Domany Y, Shelton RC, McCullumsmith CB: Ketamine for acute suicidal ideation. An emergency department intervention: a randomized, double-blind, placebo-controlled, proof-of-concept trial. Depress Anxiety 37(3):224–233, 2020 31733088

Dominici P, Kopec K, Manur R, et al: Phencyclidine intoxication case series study. J Med Toxicol 11(3):321–325, 2015 25502414

Domino EF: History and pharmacology of PCP and PCP-related analogs. J Psychedelic Drugs 12(3–4):223–227, 1980 7431418

Domino EF: Taming the ketamine tiger. 1965. Anesthesiology 113(3):678–684, 2010 20693870

Domino EF, Luby ED: Phencyclidine/schizophrenia: one view toward the past, the other to the future. Schizophr Bull 38(5):914–919, 2012 22390879

Domino EF, Chodoff F, Corssen G: Human pharmacology of CI-581, and new intravenous agent chemically related to phencyclidine (abstract number 771). FASEB J 24:268, 1965

Douglas SR, Shenoda BB, Qureshi RA, et al: Analgesic response to intravenous ketamine is linked to a circulating microRNA signature in female patients with complex regional pain syndrome. J Pain 16(9):814–824, 2015 26072390

Doyle OM, De Simoni S, Schwarz AJ, et al: Quantifying the attenuation of the ketamine pharmacological magnetic resonance imaging response in humans: a validation using antipsychotic and glutamatergic agents. J Pharmacol Exp Ther 345(1):151–160, 2013 23370794

Driesen NR, McCarthy G, Bhagwagar Z, et al: Relationship of resting brain hyperconnectivity and schizophrenia-like symptoms produced by the NMDA receptor antagonist ketamine in humans. Mol Psychiatry 18(11):1199–1204, 2013a 23337947

Driesen NR, McCarthy G, Bhagwagar Z, et al: The impact of NMDA receptor blockade on human working memory-related prefrontal function and connectivity. Neuropsychopharmacology 38(13):2613–2622, 2013b 23856634

D'Souza DC, Berman RM, Krystal JH, Charney DS: Symptom provocation studies in psychiatric disorders: scientific value, risks, and future. Biol Psychiatry 46:1060–1080, 1999

D'Souza DC, Singh N, Elander J, et al: Glycine transporter inhibitor attenuates the psychotomimetic effects of ketamine in healthy males: preliminary evidence. Neuropsychopharmacology 37(4):1036–1046, 2012a 22113087

D'Souza DC, Ahn K, Bhakta S, et al: Nicotine fails to attenuate ketamine-induced cognitive deficits and negative and positive symptoms in humans: implications for schizophrenia. Biol Psychiatry 72(9):785–794, 2012b 22717030

D'Souza DC, Carson RE, Driesen N, et al; Yale GlyT1 Study Group: Dose-related target occupancy and effects on circuitry, behavior, and neuroplasticity of the glycine transporter-1 inhibitor PF-03463275 in healthy and schizophrenia subjects. Biol Psychiatry 84(6):413–421, 2018 29499855

Dualé C, Sibaud F, Guastella V, et al: Perioperative ketamine does not prevent chronic pain after thoracotomy. Eur J Pain 13(5):497–505, 2009 18783971

Duek O, Levy I, Yutong L, et al: PTSD augmented psychotherapy with ketamine (KPE) – First results (abstract). Biol Psychiatry 85:s122, 2019

Duncan EJ, Madonick SH, Parwani A, et al: Clinical and sensorimotor gating effects of ketamine in normals. Neuropsychopharmacology 25(1):72–83, 2001 11377920

Eichenberger U, Neff F, Sveticic G, et al: Chronic phantom limb pain: the effects of calcitonin, ketamine, and their combination on pain and sensory thresholds. Anesth Analg 106(4):1265–1273, 2008 18349204

Eide PK, Jørum E, Stubhaug A, et al: Relief of post-herpetic neuralgia with the N-methyl-D-aspartic acid receptor antagonist ketamine: a double-blind, cross-over comparison with morphine and placebo. Pain 58(3):347–354, 1994 7838584

Eide PK, Stubhaug A, Øye I, Breivik H: Continuous subcutaneous administration of the N-methyl-D-aspartic acid (NMDA) receptor antagonist ketamine in the treatment of post-herpetic neuralgia. Pain 61(2):221–228, 1995a 7659432

Eide PK, Stubhaug A, Stenehjem AE: Central dysesthesia pain after traumatic spinal cord injury is dependent on N-methyl-D-aspartate receptor activation. Neurosurgery 37(6):1080–1087, 1995b 8584148

Ekstrand J, Fattah C, Persson M, et al: Racemic ketamine as an alternative to electroconvulsive therapy for unipolar depression: a randomized, open-label, noninferiority trial (KetECT). Int J Neuropsychopharmacol 25(5):339–349, 2022 35020871

Evans J, Rosen M, Weeks RD, Wise C: Ketamine in neurosurgical procedures (letter). Lancet 1(7688):40–41, 1971 4099342

Falls HF, Hoy JE, Corssen G: CI-581: an intravenous or intramuscular anesthetic for office ophthalmic surgery. Am J Ophthalmol 61(5 Pt 2):1093–1095, 1966 5937988

Fan N, Xu K, Ning Y, et al: Profiling the psychotic, depressive and anxiety symptoms in chronic ketamine users. Psychiatry Res 237:311–315, 2016 26805565

Farmer CA, Gilbert JR, Moaddel R, et al: Ketamine metabolites, clinical response, and gamma power in a randomized, placebo-controlled, crossover trial for treatment-resistant major depression. Neuropsychopharmacology 45(8):1398–1404, 2020 32252062

Fauman MA, Fauman BJ: Violence associated with phencyclidine abuse. Am J Psychiatry 136(12):1584–1586, 1979 507211

Fauman MA, Fauman BJ: Chronic phencyclidine (PCP) abuse: a psychiatric perspective. J Psychedelic Drugs 12(3–4):307–315, 1980a 7431430

Fauman MA, Fauman BJ: Chronic phencyclidine (PCP) abuse: a psychiatric perspective—Part I: General aspects and violence [proceedings]. Psychopharmacol Bull 16(4):70–72, 1980b 7454944

Fava M, Freeman MP, Flynn M, et al: Double-blind, placebo-controlled, dose-ranging trial of intravenous ketamine as adjunctive therapy in treatment-resistant depression (TRD). Mol Psychiatry 25(7):1592–1603, 2020 30283029

Feder A, Parides MK, Murrough JW, et al: Efficacy of intravenous ketamine for treatment of chronic posttraumatic stress disorder: a randomized clinical trial. JAMA Psychiatry 71(6):681–688, 2014 24740528

Feder A, Costi S, Rutter SB, et al: A randomized controlled trial of repeated ketamine administration for chronic posttraumatic stress disorder. Am J Psychiatry 178(2):193–202, 2021 33397139

Fedgchin M, Trivedi M, Daly EJ, et al: Efficacy and safety of fixed-dose esketamine nasal spray combined with a new oral antidepressant in treatment-resistant depression: results of a randomized, double-blind, active-controlled study (TRANSFORM-1). Int J Neuropsychopharmacol 22(10):616–630, 2019 31290965

Feldman HW, Waldorf D: Angel Dust in Four American Cities: An Ethnographic Study of PCP Users. NIDA Services Research Report. US Department of Health and Human Services. Public Health Service. Alcohol, Drug Abuse, and Mental Health Administration. DHHS publ. no. (ADM) 81-1039, 1980

Fernández-Calderón F, Cleland CM, Palamar JJ: Polysubstance use profiles among electronic dance music party attendees in New York City and their relation to use of new psychoactive substances. Addict Behav 78:85–93, 2018 29128711

Finch PM, Knudsen L, Drummond PD: Reduction of allodynia in patients with complex regional pain syndrome: a double-blind placebo-controlled trial of topical ketamine. Pain 146(1–2):18–25, 2009 19703730

Fine J, Finestone SC: Sensory disturbances following ketamine anesthesia: recurrent hallucinations. Anesth Analg 52(3):428–430, 1973 4735997

Fleming LM, Javitt DC, Carter CS, et al: A multicenter study of ketamine effects on functional connectivity: large scale network relationships, hubs and symptom mechanisms. Neuroimage Clin 22:101739, 2019 30852397

Fond G, Bourbon A, Auquier P, et al: Venus and Mars on the benches of the faculty: influence of gender on mental health and behavior of medical students. Results from the BOURBON national study. J Affect Disord 239:146–151, 2018 30005328

Fontana AE, Loschi JA: Antidepressive therapy with CI 581 [in Spanish]. Acta Psiquiatr Psicol Am Lat 20(1):32–39, 1974 4455018

Food and Drug Administration: Ketamine abuse. FDA Drug Bull 9(4):24, 1979 488583

Foster NL, Giordani B, Mellow A, et al: Memory effects of low-dose ketamine in Alzheimer's disease [Abstract]. Neurology 41(Suppl 1):214, 1991

Francois J, Grimm O, Schwarz AJ, et al: Ketamine suppresses the ventral striatal response to reward anticipation: a cross-species translational neuroimaging study. Neuropsychopharmacology 41(5):1386–1394, 2016 26388147

Freeman TP, Morgan CJA, Klaassen E, et al: Superstitious conditioning as a model of delusion formation following chronic but not acute ketamine in humans. Psychopharmacology (Berl) 206(4):563–573, 2009 19436994

Fu CHY, Abel KM, Allin MPG, et al: Effects of ketamine on prefrontal and striatal regions in an overt verbal fluency task: a functional magnetic resonance imaging study. Psychopharmacology (Berl) 183(1):92–102, 2005 16228196

Gałuszko-Węgielnik M, Chmielewska Z, Jakuszkowiak-Wojten K, et al: Ketamine as add-on treatment in psychotic treatment-resistant depression. Brain Sci 13(1):142, 2023 DOI: 10.3390/brainsci13010142 36672123

Gardner AE, Olson BE, Lichtiger M: Cerebrospinal-fluid pressure during dissociative anesthesia with ketamine. Anesthesiology 35(2):226–228, 1971 5568142

Gardner AE, Dannemiller FJ, Dean D: Intracranial cerebrospinal fluid pressure in man during ketamine anesthesia. Anesth Analg 51(5):741–745, 1972 4672167

Gattaz WF, Gasser T, Beckmann H: Multidimensional analysis of the concentrations of 17 substances in the CSF of schizophrenics and controls. Biol Psychiatry 20(4):360–366, 1985 2858227

Ghasemi M, Kazemi MH, Yoosefi A, et al: Rapid antidepressant effects of repeated doses of ketamine compared with electroconvulsive therapy in hospitalized patients with major depressive disorder. Psychiatry Res 215(2):355–361, 2014 24374115

Gill H, Gill B, Rodrigues NB, et al: The effects of ketamine on cognition in treatment-resistant depression: a systematic review and priority avenues for future research. Neurosci Biobehav Rev 120:78–85, 2021 33242561

Giuliano K, Etchill E, Velez AK, et al: Ketamine mitigates neurobehavioral deficits in a canine model of hypothermic circulatory arrest. Semin Thorac Cardiovasc Surg 35(2):251–258, 2023 34995752

Glavonic E, Mitic M, Adzic M: Hallucinogenic drugs and their potential for treating fear-related disorders: through the lens of fear extinction. J Neurosci Res 100(4):947–969, 2022 35165930

Glue P, Medlicott NJ, Harland S, et al: Ketamine's dose-related effects on anxiety symptoms in patients with treatment refractory anxiety disorders. J Psychopharmacol 31(10):1302–1305, 2017 28441895

Glue P, Neehoff SM, Medlicott NJ, et al: Safety and efficacy of maintenance ketamine treatment in patients with treatment-refractory generalised anxiety and social anxiety disorders. J Psychopharmacol 32(6):663–667, 2018 29561204

Glue P, Neehoff S, Sabadel A, et al: Effects of ketamine in patients with treatment-refractory generalized anxiety and social anxiety disorders: exploratory double-blind psychoactive-controlled replication study. J Psychopharmacol 34(3):267–272, 2020 31526207

Goebel A, Jayaseelan S, Sachane K, et al: Racemic ketamine 4.5-day infusion treatment of long-standing complex regional pain syndrome—a prospective service evaluation in five patients (letter). Br J Anaesth 115(1):146–147, 2015 26089467

Goldberg ME, Domsky R, Scaringe D, et al: Multi-day low dose ketamine infusion for the treatment of complex regional pain syndrome. Pain Physician 8(2):175–179, 2005 16850072

Goldberg ME, Torjman MC, Schwartzman RJ, et al: Pharmacodynamic profiles of ketamine (R)- and (S)- with 5-day inpatient infusion for the treatment of complex regional pain syndrome. Pain Physician 13(4):379–387, 2010 20648207

Goldberg ME, Torjman MC, Schwartzman RJ, et al: Enantioselective pharmacokinetics of (R)- and (S)-ketamine after a 5-day infusion in patients with complex regional pain syndrome. Chirality 23(2):138–143, 2011 20803495

Good P, Tullio F, Jackson K, et al: Prospective audit of short-term concurrent ketamine, opioid and anti-inflammatory ('triple-agent') therapy for episodes of acute on chronic pain. Intern Med J 35(1):39–44, 2005 15667467

Gool RY, Clarke HL: Anaesthesia for under-doctored areas. A trial of phencyclidine in Nigeria. Anaesthesia 19(2):265–270, 1964 14150681

Gorelova NA, Koroleva VI, Amemori T, et al: Ketamine blockade of cortical spreading depression in rats. Electroencephalogr Clin Neurophysiol 66(4):440–447, 1987 2435524

Gottrup H, Bach FW, Juhl G, Jensen TS: Differential effect of ketamine and lidocaine on spontaneous and mechanical evoked pain in patients with nerve injury
pain. Anesthesiology 104(3):527–536, 2006 16508401

Gouzoulis-Mayfrank E, Heekeren K, Neukirch A, et al: Inhibition of return in the
human 5HT2A agonist and NMDA antagonist model of psychosis. Neuropsychopharmacology 31(2):431–441, 2006 16123739

Grabski M, McAndrew A, Lawn W, et al: Adjunctive ketamine with relapse preven-
tion-based psychological therapy in the treatment of alcohol use disorder. Am J
Psychiatry 179(2):152–162, 2022 35012326

Granata L, Niebergall H, Langner R, et al: Ketamine i.v. for the treatment of cluster
headaches: an observational study [in German]. Schmerz 30:286–288, 2016
27067225

Grathwohl KW, Black IH, Spinella PC, et al: Total intravenous anesthesia including ketamine versus volatile gas anesthesia for combat-related operative traumatic brain injury. Anesthesiology 109(1):44–53, 2008 18580171

Graven-Nielsen T, Kendall SA, Henriksson KG, et al: Ketamine reduces muscle
pain, temporal summation, and referred pain in fibromyalgia patients. Pain
85(3):483–491, 2000 10781923

Green SM, Roback MG, Kennedy RM, Krauss B: Clinical practice guideline for
emergency department ketamine dissociative sedation: 2011 update. Ann Emerg
Med 57(5):449–461, 2011 21256625

Gregers MCT, Mikkelsen S, Lindvig KP, Brøchner AC: Ketamine as an anesthetic
for patients with acute brain injury: a systematic review. Neurocrit Care
33(1):273–282, 2020 32328972

Grégoire M-C, MacLellan DL, Finley GA: A pediatric case of ketamine-associated
cystitis (letter). Urology 71(6):1232–1233, 2008 18455768

Greifenstein FE, Devault M, Yoshitake J, Gajewski JE: A study of a 1-aryl cyclo
hexyl amine for anesthesia. Anesth Analg 37(5):283–294, 1958 13583607

Grent-'t-Jong T, Rivolta D, Gross J, et al: Acute ketamine dysregulates task-related
gamma-band oscillations in thalamo-cortical circuits in schizophrenia. Brain
141(8):2511–2526, 2018 30020423

Greyson B: The near-death experience scale. Construction, reliability, and validity.
J Nerv Ment Dis 171(6):369–375, 1983 6854303

Grimm O, Gass N, Weber-Fahr W, et al: Acute ketamine challenge increases resting state prefrontal-hippocampal connectivity in both humans and rats. Psychopharmacology (Berl) 232(21–22):4231–4241, 2015 26184011

Grunebaum MF, Ellis SP, Keilp JG, et al: Ketamine versus midazolam in bipolar
depression with suicidal thoughts: a pilot midazolam-controlled randomized
clinical trial. Bipolar Disord 19(3):176–183, 2017 28452409

Grunebaum MF, Galfalvy HC, Choo T-H, et al: Ketamine for rapid reduction of
suicidal thoughts in major depression: a midazolam-controlled randomized clinical trial. Am J Psychiatry 175(4):327–335, 2018 29202655

Grunebaum MF, Galfalvy HC, Choo T-H, et al: Ketamine metabolite pilot study
in a suicidal depression trial. J Psychiatr Res 117:129–134, 2019 31415914

Guedj E, Cammilleri S, Colavolpe C, et al: Follow-up of pain processing recovery after ketamine in hyperalgesic fibromyalgia patients using brain perfusion ECD-SPECT. Eur J Nucl Med Mol Imaging 34(12):2115–2119, 2007 18278530

Guerra GG, Robertson CMT, Alton GY, et al; Western Canadian Complex Pediatric Therapies Follow-up Group: Neurodevelopmental outcome following exposure to sedative and analgesic drugs for complex cardiac surgery in infancy. Paediatr Anaesth 21(9):932–941, 2011 21507125

Gunduz-Bruce H, Reinhart RMG, Roach BJ, et al: Glutamatergic modulation of auditory information processing in the human brain. Biol Psychiatry 71(11):969–977, 2012 22036036

Guo L, Li P, Pan S, et al: Associations of childhood maltreatment with subsequent illicit drug use among Chinese adolescents: the moderating role of the child's sex. Psychiatry Res 269:361–368, 2018 30173042

Hallak JEC, Dursun SM, Bosi DC, et al: The interplay of cannabinoid and NMDA glutamate receptor systems in humans: preliminary evidence of cannabidiol and ketamine in healthy human subjects. Prog Neuropsychopharmacol Biol Psychiatry 35:198–202, 2011 21062637

Halstead M, Reed S, Krause R, Williams MT: Ketamine-assisted psychotherapy for PTSD related to racial discrimination. Clin Case Stud 20(4):310–330, 2021

Hamilton HK, D'Souza DC, Ford JM, et al: Interactive effects of an N-methyl-d-aspartate receptor antagonist and a nicotinic acetylcholine receptor agonist on mismatch negativity: implications for schizophrenia. Schizophr Res 191:87–94, 2018 28711472

Hartberg J, Garrett-Walcott S, De Gioannis A: Impact of oral ketamine augmentation on hospital admissions in treatment-resistant depression and PTSD: a retrospective study. Psychopharmacology (Berl) 235(2):393–398, 2018 29151192

Hart JB, McChesney JD, Greif M, Schulz G: Composition of illicit drugs and the use of drug analysis in abuse abatement. J Psychedelic Drugs 5(1):83–88, 1972

Hashimoto K: The R-stereoisomeer of ketamine as an alternative for ketamine for treatment-resistant major depression. Clin Psychopharmacol Neurosci 12(1):72–73, 2014 24851126

Hashimoto K: The NMDA Receptors. Humana Press, Cham, Switzerland, 2017

Heekeren K, Neukirch A, Daumann J, et al: Prepulse inhibition of the startle reflex and its attentional modulation in the human S-ketamine and N,N-dimethyltryptamine (DMT) models of psychosis. J Psychopharmacol 21(3):312–320, 2007 17591658

Heekeren K, Daumann J, Neukirch A, et al: Mismatch negativity generation in the human 5HT2A agonist and NMDA antagonist model of psychosis. Psychopharmacology (Berl) 199(1):77–88, 2008 18488201

Helbok R, Hartings JA, Schiefecker A, et al: What should a clinician do when spreading depolarizations are observed in a patient? Neurocrit Care 32(1):306–310, 2020 31338747

Hernández-Cáceres J, Macias-González R, Brozek G, Bures J: Systemic ketamine blocks cortical spreading depression but does not delay the onset of terminal anoxic depolarization in rats. Brain Res 437(2):360–364, 1987 3435842

Hertle DN, Dreier JP, Woitzik J, et al; Cooperative Study of Brain Injury Depolarizations (COSBID): Effect of analgesics and sedatives on the occurrence of spreading depolarizations accompanying acute brain injury. Brain 135(Pt 8):2390–2398, 2012 22719001

Hijazi Y, Boulieu R: Contribution of CYP3A4, CYP2B6, and CYP2C9 isoforms to N-demethylation of ketamine in human liver microsomes. Drug Metab Dispos 30(7):853–858, 2002 12065445

Hoegberg LCG, Christiansen C, Soe J, et al: Recreational drug use at a major music festival: trend analysis of anonymised pooled urine. Clin Toxicol (Phila) 56(4):245–255, 2018 28814125

Hoffmann V, Coppejans H, Vercauteren M, Adriaensen H: Successful treatment of postherpetic neuralgia with oral ketamine. Clin J Pain 10(3):240–242, 1994 7833583

Höflich A, Hahn A, Küblböck M, et al: Ketamine-induced modulation of the thalamo-cortical network in healthy volunteers as a model for schizophrenia. Int J Neuropsychopharmacol 18(9):1–11, 2015 25896256

Holcomb HH, Lahti AC, Medoff DR, et al: Sequential regional cerebral blood flow brain scans using PET with H2(15)O demonstrate ketamine actions in CNS dynamically. Neuropsychopharmacology 25(2):165–172, 2001 11425500

Holcomb HH, Lahti AC, Medoff DR, et al: Effects of noncompetitive NMDA receptor blockade on anterior cingulate cerebral blood flow in volunteers with schizophrenia. Neuropsychopharmacology 30(12):2275–2282, 2005 16034443

Honey GD, Honey RAE, O'Loughlin C, et al: Ketamine disrupts frontal and hippocampal contribution to encoding and retrieval of episodic memory: an fMRI study. Cereb Cortex 15(6):749–759, 2005 15537676

Honey GD, Corlett PR, Absalom AR, et al: Individual differences in psychotic effects of ketamine are predicted by brain function measured under placebo. J Neurosci 28(25):6295–6303, 2008 18562599

Hong LE, Summerfelt A, Buchanan RW, et al: Gamma and delta neural oscillations and association with clinical symptoms under subanesthetic ketamine. Neuropsychopharmacology 35(3):632–640, 2010 19890262

Hong YL, Yee CH, Tam YH, et al: Management of complications of ketamine abuse: 10 years' experience in Hong Kong. Hong Kong Med J 24(2):175–181, 2018 29632275

Hood RW: The construction and preliminary validation of a measure of reported mystical experience. J Sci Study Relig 14:29–41, 1975

Horacek J, Brunovsky M, Novak T, et al: Subanesthetic dose of ketamine decreases prefrontal theta cordance in healthy volunteers: implications for antidepressant effect. Psychol Med 40(9):1443–1451, 2010 19995475

Horowitz MA, Moncrieff J: Are we repeating mistakes of the past? A review of the evidence for esketamine. Br J Psychiatry 219(5):614–617, 2021 32456714

Hudetz JA, Pagel PS: Neuroprotection by ketamine: a review of the experimental and clinical evidence. J Cardiothorac Vasc Anesth 24(1):131–142, 2010 19640746

Hudetz JA, Iqbal Z, Gandhi SD, et al: Ketamine attenuates post-operative cognitive dysfunction after cardiac surgery. Acta Anaesthesiol Scand 53(7):864–872, 2009a 19422355

Hudetz JA, Patterson KM, Iqbal Z, et al: Ketamine attenuates delirium after cardiac surgery with cardiopulmonary bypass. J Cardiothorac Vasc Anesth 23(5):651–657, 2009b 19231245

Huge V, Lauchart M, Magerl W, et al: Effects of low-dose intranasal (S)-ketamine in patients with neuropathic pain. Eur J Pain 14(4):387–394, 2010 19733106

Ikonomidou C, Turski L: Why did NMDA receptor antagonists fail clinical trials for stroke and traumatic brain injury? Lancet Neurol 1(6):383–386, 2002 12849400

Ikonomidou C, Bosch F, Miksa M, et al: Blockade of NMDA receptors and apoptotic neurodegeneration in the developing brain. Science 283(5398):70–74, 1999 9872743

Ionescu DF, Bentley KH, Eikermann M, et al: Repeat-dose ketamine augmentation for treatment-resistant depression with chronic suicidal ideation: a randomized, double blind, placebo controlled trial. J Affect Disord 243:516–524, 2019 30286416

Ishihara H, Kudo H, Murakawa T, et al: Uneventful total intravenous anaesthesia with ketamine for schizophrenic surgical patients. Eur J Anaesthesiol 14(1):47–51, 1997 9049558

Itil T, Keskiner A, Kiremitci N, Holden JM: Effect of phencyclidine in chronic schizophrenics. Can Psychiatr Assoc J 12(2):209–212, 1967 6040448

Iwatsuki K, Aoba Y, Sato K, Iwatsuki N: Clinical study on CI-581, a phencyclidine derivative. Tohoku J Exp Med 93(1):39–48, 1967 5586563

Jansen K: Near death experience and the NMDA receptor (letter). BMJ 298(6689):1708, 1989 2547469

Jansen KLR: Ketamine—can chronic use impair memory? Int J Addict 25(2):133–139, 1990 2228329

Jansen KLR: The ketamine model of the near-death experience: a central role for the N-methyl-d-aspartate receptor. J Near Death Stud 16(1):5–26, 1997

Jansen K: Ketamine: Dreams and Realities. Boca Raton, FL, Multidisciplinary Association for Psychedelic Studies, 2001

Javitt DC: Negative schizophrenic symptomatology and the PCP (phencyclidine) model of schizophrenia. Hillside J Clin Psychiatry 9(1):12–35, 1987 2820854

Javitt DC, Zukin SR: Recent advances in the phencyclidine model of schizophrenia. Am J Psychiatry 148(10):1301–1308, 1991 1654746

Javitt DC, Carter CS, Krystal JH, et al: Utility of imaging-based biomarkers for glutamate-targeted drug development in psychotic disorders: a randomized clinical trial. JAMA Psychiatry 75(1):11–19, 2018 29167877

Jeevakumar V, Driskill C, Paine A, et al: Ketamine administration during the second postnatal week induces enduring schizophrenia-like behavioral symptoms and reduces parvalbumin expression in the medial prefrontal cortex of adult mice. Behav Brain Res 282:165–175, 2015 25591475

Jeffcote T, Weir T, Anstey J, et al: The impact of sedative choice on intracranial and systemic physiology in moderate to severe traumatic brain injury: a scoping review. J Neurosurg Anesthesiol 35(3):265–273, 2023 35142704

Jeffrey F, Lilly JC: John Lilly, So Far.... Los Angeles, CA, Jeremy P. Tarcher, 1990

Jia Z, Liu Z, Chu P, et al: Tracking the evolution of drug abuse in China, 2003–10: a retrospective, self-controlled study. Addiction 110(Suppl 1):4–10, 2015 25533859

Joe Laidler KA: The rise of club drugs in a heroin society: the case of Hong Kong. Subst Use Misuse 40(9–10):1257–1278, 2005 16048816

Joe-Laidler K, Hunt G: Sit down to float: the cultural meaning of ketamine use in Hong Kong. Addict Res Theory 16(3):259–271, 2008 19759834

Johnson BD: Psychosis and ketamine (letter). BMJ 4(5784):428–429, 1971 5124451

Johnstone M: The use of Sernyl in clinical anaesthesia [in German]. Anaesthetist 9:114–115, 1960

Johnstone M, Evans V, Baigel S: Sernyl (CI-395) in clinical anaesthesia. Br J Anaesth 31:433–439, 1959 14407580

Jørum E, Warncke T, Stubhaug A: Cold allodynia and hyperalgesia in neuropathic pain: the effect of N-methyl-D-aspartate (NMDA) receptor antagonist ketamine—a double-blind, cross-over comparison with alfentanil and placebo. Pain 101(3):229–235, 2003 12583865

Joules R, Doyle OM, Schwarz AJ, et al: Ketamine induces a robust whole-brain connectivity pattern that can be differentially modulated by drugs of different mechanism and clinical profile. Psychopharmacology (Berl) 232(21–22):4205–4218, 2015 25980482

Jovaisa T, Laurinenas G, Vosylius S, et al: Effects of ketamine on precipitated opiate withdrawal. Medicina (Kaunas) 42(8):625–634, 2006 16963828

Kalopita K, Armakolas A, Philippou A, et al: Ketamine-induced neurotoxicity in neurodevelopment: a synopsis of main pathways based on recent in vivo experimental findings. J Anaesthesiol Clin Pharmacol 37(1):37–42, 2021 34103820

Kang MJY, Hawken E, Vazquez GH: The mechanisms behind rapid antidepressant effects of ketamine: a systematic review with a focus on molecular neuroplasticity. Front Psychiatry 13:860882, 2022 35546951

Kapural L, Kapural M, Bensitel T, Sessler DI: Opioid-sparing effect of intravenous outpatient ketamine infusions appears short-lived in chronic-pain patients with high opioid requirements. Pain Physician 13(4):389–394, 2010 20648208

Kay SR, Fiszbein A, Opler LA: The positive and negative syndrome scale (PANSS) for schizophrenia. Schizophr Bull 13(2):261–276, 1987 3616518

Ke X, Ding Y, Xu K, et al: The profile of cognitive impairments in chronic ketamine users. Psychiatry Res 266:124–131, 2018 29864611

Kegeles LS, Abi-Dargham A, Zea-Ponce Y, et al: Modulation of amphetamine-induced striatal dopamine release by ketamine in humans: implications for schizophrenia. Biol Psychiatry 48(7):627–640, 2000 11032974

Kegeles LS, Martinez D, Kochan LD, et al: NMDA antagonist effects on striatal dopamine release: positron emission tomography studies in humans. Synapse 43(1):19–29, 2002 11746730

Keizer BM, Roache JD, Jones JR, et al: Continuous ketamine infusion for pain as an opportunity for psychotherapy for PTSD: a case series of ketamine-enhanced psychotherapy for PTSD and pain (KEP-P2) (letter). Psychother Psychosom 89(5):326–329, 2020 32248200

Kheirabadi D, Kheirabadi GR, Mirlohi Z, et al: Comparison of rapid antidepressant and antisuicidal effects of intramuscular ketamine, oral ketamine, and electroconvulsive therapy in patients with major depressive disorder: a pilot study. J Clin Psychopharmacol 40(6):588–593, 2020 33060432

Kheirabadi G, Vafaie M, Kheirabadi D, et al: Comparative effect of intravenous ketamine and electroconvulsive therapy in major depression: a randomized controlled trial. Adv Biomed Res 8:25, 2019 31123668

Khlestova E, Johnson JW, Krystal JH, Lisman J: The role of GluN2C-containing NMDA receptors in ketamine's psychotogenic action and in schizophrenia models. J Neurosci 36(44):11151–11157, 2016 27807157

Khorramzadeh E, Lotfy AO: The use of ketamine in psychiatry. Psychosomatics 14(6):344–346, 1973 4800188

Kiefer RT, Rohr P, Ploppa A, et al: Efficacy of ketamine in anesthetic dosage for the treatment of refractory complex regional pain syndrome: an open-label phase II study. Pain Med 9(8):1173–1201, 2008a 18266808

Kiefer R-T, Rohr P, Ploppa A, et al: A pilot open-label study of the efficacy of subanesthetic isomeric S(+)-ketamine in refractory CRPS patients. Pain Med 9(1):44–54, 2008b 18254766

Kim JS, Kornhuber HH, Holzmüller B, et al: Reduction of cerebrospinal fluid glutamic acid in Huntington's chorea and in schizophrenic patients. Arch Psychiatr Nervenkr 228(1):7–10, 1980a 6104477

Kim JS, Kornhuber HH, Schmid-Burgk W, Holzmüller B: Low cerebrospinal fluid glutamate in schizophrenic patients and a new hypothesis on schizophrenia. Neurosci Lett 20(3):379–382, 1980b 6108541

Kim M, Cho S, Lee J-H: The effects of long-term ketamine treatment on cognitive function in complex regional pain syndrome: a preliminary study. Pain Med 17(8):1447–1451, 2016 26921891

Kim YH, Lee PB, Oh TK: Is magnesium sulfate effective for pain in chronic postherpetic neuralgia patients comparing with ketamine infusion therapy? J Clin Anesth 27(4):296–300, 2015 25792176

Klass A, Sánchez-Porras R, Santos E: Systematic review of the pharmacological agents that have been tested against spreading depolarizations. J Cereb Blood Flow Metab 38(7):1149–1179, 2018

Kleinloog D, Rombouts S, Zoethout R, et al: Subjective effects of ethanol, morphine, ?(9)-tetrahydrocannabinol, and ketamine following a pharmacological challenge are related to functional brain connectivity. Brain Connect 5(10):641–648, 2015a 26390148

Kleinloog D, Uit den Boogaard A, Dahan A, et al: Optimizing the glutamatergic challenge model for psychosis, using S+ -ketamine to induce psychomimetic symptoms in healthy volunteers. J Psychopharmacol 29(4):401–413, 2015b 25693889

Klepstad P, Borchgrevink PC: Four years' treatment with ketamine and a trial of dextromethorphan in a patient with severe post-herpetic neuralgia. Acta Anaesthesiol Scand 41(3):422–426, 1997 9113190

Knott V, McIntosh J, Millar A, et al: Nicotine and smoker status moderate brain electric and mood activation induced by ketamine, an N-methyl-D-aspartate (NMDA) receptor antagonist. Pharmacol Biochem Behav 85(1):228–242, 2006 17023037

Knott VJ, Millar AM, McIntosh JF, et al: Separate and combined effects of low dose ketamine and nicotine on behavioural and neural correlates of sustained attention. Biol Psychol 88(1):83–93, 2011 21742012

Koffler SP, Hampstead BM, Irani F, et al: The neurocognitive effects of 5 day anesthetic ketamine for the treatment of refractory complex regional pain syndrome. Arch Clin Neuropsychol 22(6):719–729, 2007 17611073

Kofke WA, Bloom MJ, Van Cott A, Brenner RP: Electrographic tachyphylaxis to etomidate and ketamine used for refractory status epilepticus controlled with isoflurane. J Neurosurg Anesthesiol 9(3):269–272, 1997 9239591

Kolenda H, Gremmelt A, Rading S, et al: Ketamine for analgosedative therapy in intensive care treatment of head-injured patients. Acta Neurochir (Wien) 138(10):1193–1199, 1996 8955439

Kolp E, Friedman HL, Young MS, Krupitsky E: Ketamine enhanced psychotherapy: preliminary clinical observations on its effectiveness in treating alcoholism. Humanist Psychol 34(4):399–422, 2006

Kolp E, Young MS, Friedman H, et al: Ketamine-enhanced psychotherapy: preliminary clinical observations on its effects in treating death anxiety. Int J Transpers Stud 26(1):1–17, 2007

Kolp E, Krupitsky E, Friedman H, Young MS: Entheogen-enhanced transpersonal psychotherapy of addictions: focus on clinical applications of ketamine for treating alcoholism, in The Praeger International Collection on Addictions. Edited by Browne-Miller A. Westport, CT, Praeger, 2009, pp 403–417

Kolp E, Friedman HL, Krupitsky E, et al: Ketamine psychedelic psychotherapy: focus on its pharmacology, phenomenology, and clinical applications. Int J Transpers Stud 33(2):84–140, 2014

Kong D: Debatable Forms of Consent. Boston Globe. November 16:A1, 1998a

Kong D: Rights Bill for Mental Patients Advances. House Expected to OK Amended Measure. Boston Globe. November 17:B,1:5, 1998b

Kong D: Panel Urges Review of Patient Studies. Boston Globe. November 18:A1, 1998c

Kong D: Drug Studies Are Questioned. Boston Globe. December 31:A1, 1998d

Kong D: Mental Health Body Will Review Tests: Decision Follows a Series of Reports. Boston Globe. January 22:A20, 1999a

Kong D: US Agency Curbs Psychosis Tests, Reviews Funding. Boston Globe. February 6:A1, 1999b

Korpi ER, Kaufmann CA, Marnela K-M, Weinberger DR: Cerebrospinal fluid amino acid concentrations in chronic schizophrenia. Psychiatry Res 20(4):337–345, 1987 2885877

Kort NS, Ford JM, Roach BJ, et al: Role of N-methyl-d-aspartate receptors in action-based predictive coding deficits in schizophrenia. Biol Psychiatry 81(6):514–524, 2017 27647218

Koychev I, William Deakin JF, El-Deredy W, Haenschel C: Effects of acute ketamine infusion on visual working memory: event-related potentials. Biol Psychiatry Cogn Neurosci Neuroimaging 2(3):253–262, 2017 29528296

Kraguljac NV, Frölich MA, Tran S, et al: Ketamine modulates hippocampal neurochemistry and functional connectivity: a combined magnetic resonance spectroscopy and resting-state fMRI study in healthy volunteers. Mol Psychiatry 22(4):562–569, 2017 27480494

Krediet E, Bostoen T, Breeksema J, et al: Reviewing the potential of psychedelics for the treatment of PTSD. Int J Neuropsychopharmacol 23(6):385–400, 2020 32170326

Kreitschmann-Andermahr I, Rosburg T, Demme U, et al: Effect of ketamine on the neuromagnetic mismatch field in healthy humans. Brain Res Cogn Brain Res 12(1):109–116, 2001 11489614

Kroll WR: Experience with sernylan in zoo animals. Int Zoo Yearb 4:131–141, 1962

Krupitsky EM: Ketamine psychedelic therapy (KPT) of alcoholism and neurosis. Multidisciplinary Association for Psychedelic Studies Newsletter 3(4):24–28, 1992

Krupitsky EM, Grinenko AY: Ketamine psychedelic therapy (KPT): a review of the results of ten years of research. J Psychoactive Drugs 29(2):165–183, 1997 9250944

Krupitsky EM, Grinenko AY, Karandashova GF, et al: Metabolism of biogenic amines induced by alcoholism narcopsychotherapy with ketamine administration. Biog Amines 7(6):577–582, 1990

Krupitsky EM, Grinenko AY, Berkaliev TN, et al: The combination of psychedelic and aversive approaches in alcoholism treatment: the affective contra-attribution method. Alcohol Treat Q 9(1):99–105, 1992

Krupitsky EM, Burakov AM, Romanova TN, et al: Attenuation of ketamine effects by nimodipine pretreatment in recovering ethanol dependent men: psychopharmacologic implications of the interaction of NMDA and L-type calcium channel antagonists. Neuropsychopharmacology 25(6):936–947, 2001 11750186

Krupitsky E, Burakov A, Romanova T, et al: Ketamine psychotherapy for heroin addiction: immediate effects and two-year follow-up. J Subst Abuse Treat 23(4):273–283, 2002 12495789

Krupitsky EM, Burakov AM, Dunaevsky IV, et al: Single versus repeated sessions of ketamine-assisted psychotherapy for people with heroin dependence. J Psychoactive Drugs 39(1):13–19, 2007 17523581

Krystal JH, Karper LP, Seibyl JP, et al: Subanesthetic effects of the noncompetitive NMDA antagonist, ketamine, in humans. Psychotomimetic, perceptual, cognitive, and neuroendocrine responses. Arch Gen Psychiatry 51(3):199–214, 1994 8122957

Krystal JH, Karper LP, Bennett A, et al: Interactive effects of subanesthetic ketamine and subhypnotic lorazepam in humans. Psychopharmacology (Berl) 135(3):213–229, 1998 9498724

Krystal JH, D'Souza DC, Karper LP, et al: Interactive effects of subanesthetic ketamine and haloperidol in healthy humans. Psychopharmacology (Berl)
145(2):193–204, 1999 10463321

Krystal JH, Abi-Saab W, Perry E, et al: Preliminary evidence of attenuation of the
disruptive effects of the NMDA glutamate receptor antagonist, ketamine, on
working memory by pretreatment with the group II metabotropic glutamate receptor agonist, LY354740, in healthy human subjects. Psychopharmacology
(Berl) 179(1):303–309, 2005a 15309376

Krystal JH, Perry EB Jr, Gueorguieva R, et al: Comparative and interactive human
psychopharmacologic effects of ketamine and amphetamine: implications for
glutamatergic and dopaminergic model psychoses and cognitive function. Arch
Gen Psychiatry 62(9):985–994, 2005b 16143730

Krystal JH, Madonick S, Perry E, et al: Potentiation of low dose ketamine effects
by naltrexone: potential implications for the pharmacotherapy of alcoholism.
Neuropsychopharmacology 31(8):1793–1800, 2006 16395307

Kurtzke JF: The use of cyclohexylamines in thalamic pain. Neurology 11:390–394,
1961 13755336

Kushwaha SKS, Keshari RK, Rai AK: Advances in nasal trans-mucosal drug delivery. J Appl Pharm Sci 1(7):21–28, 2011

Kvarnström A, Karlsten R, Quiding H, et al: The effectiveness of intravenous ketamine and lidocaine on peripheral neuropathic pain. Acta Anaesthesiol Scand
47(7):868–877, 2003 12859309

Kvarnström A, Karlsten R, Quiding H, Gordh T: The analgesic effect of intravenous ketamine and lidocaine on pain after spinal cord injury. Acta Anaesthesiol
Scand 48(4):498–506, 2004 15025615

Labruyere J, Fuller TA, Olney JW, et al: Phencyclidine and ketamine protect
against kainic acid-induced seizures and seizure-related brain damage. Abstr Soc
Neurosci 12:344, 1986

Lahti AC, Koffel B, LaPorte D, Tamminga CA: Subanesthetic doses of ketamine
stimulate psychosis in schizophrenia. Neuropsychopharmacology 13(1):9–19,
1995a 8526975

Lahti AC, Holcomb HH, Medoff DR, Tamminga CA: Ketamine activates psychosis
and alters limbic blood flow in schizophrenia. NeuroReport 6(6):869–872,
1995b 7612873

Lahti AC, Weiler MA, Parwani A, et al: Blockade of ketamine-induced psychosis
with olanzapine (abstract). Schizophr Res 36:310, 1999

Lahti AC, Weiler MA, Tamara Michaelidis BA, et al: Effects of ketamine in normal
and schizophrenic volunteers. Neuropsychopharmacology 25(4):455–467,
2001a 11557159

Lahti AC, Warfel D, Michaelidis T, et al: Long-term outcome of patients who receive ketamine during research. Biol Psychiatry 49(10):869–875, 2001b
11343683

Lai TW, Zhang S, Wang YT: Excitotoxicity and stroke: identifying novel targets
for neuroprotection. Prog Neurobiol 115:157–188, 2014 24361499

Langelaar G, Leeuwenkamp OR, Sterkman LGW, et al: The effect of nimodipine monotherapy and combined treatment with ketamine and lignocaine in aneurysmal subarachnoid haemorrhage. J Int Med Res 24(5):425–432, 1996 8895046

Langrehr D, Alai P, Andjelkovic J, Kluge I: On anesthesia using ketamine (CI-581): report of 1st experience in 500 cases [in German]. Anaesthesist 16(10):308–318, 1967 5590495

Lankenau SE, Clatts MC: Ketamine injection among high risk youth: preliminary findings from New York City. J Drug Issues 32(3):893–905, 2002 17440604

Lankenau SE, Clatts MC: Drug injection practices among high-risk youths: the first shot of ketamine. J Urban Health 81(2):232–248, 2004 15136657

LaPorte DJ, Lahti AC, Koffel B, Tamminga CA: Absence of ketamine effects on memory and other cognitive functions in schizophrenia patients. J Psychiatr Res 30(5):321–330, 1996 8923336

Lara DR, Bisol LW, Munari LR: Antidepressant, mood stabilizing and procognitive effects of very low dose sublingual ketamine in refractory unipolar and bipolar depression. Int J Neuropsychopharmacol 16(9):2111–2117, 2013 23683309

Le TT, Di Vincenzo JD, Teopiz KM, et al: Ketamine for psychotic depression: an overview of the glutamatergic system and ketamine's mechanisms associated with antidepressant and psychotomimetic effects. Psychiatr Res 306:114231, 2021

Le TT, Cordero IP, Jawad MY, et al: The abuse liability of ketamine: a scoping review of preclinical and clinical studies. J Psychiatr Res 151:476–496, 2022 35623124

Leal GC, Bandeira ID, Correia-Melo FS, et al: Intravenous arketamine for treatment-resistant depression: open-label pilot study. Eur Arch Psychiatry Clin Neurosci 271(3):577–582, 2021 32078034

Leal GC, Souza-Marques B, Mello RP, et al: Arketamine as adjunctive therapy for treatment-resistant depression: a placebo-controlled pilot study. J Affect Disord 330:7–15, 2023 36871913

Lee HH, Chen SC, Lee JF, et al: Simultaneous drug identification in urine of sexual assault victims by using liquid chromatography tandem mass spectrometry. Forensic Sci Int 282:35–40, 2018 29149685

Lemming D, Sörensen J, Graven-Nielsen T, et al: The responses to pharmacological challenges and experimental pain in patients with chronic whiplash-associated pain. Clin J Pain 21(5):412–421, 2005 16093747

Lenze EJ, Farber NB, Kharasch E, et al: Ninety-six hour ketamine infusion with co-administered clonidine for treatment-resistant depression: a pilot randomised controlled trial. World J Biol Psychiatry 17(3):230–238, 2016 26919405

Leung A, Wallace MS, Ridgeway B, Yaksh T: Concentration-effect relationship of intravenous alfentanil and ketamine on peripheral neurosensory thresholds, allodynia and hyperalgesia of neuropathic pain. Pain 91(1–2):177–187, 2001 11240090

Leung KW, Wong ZCF, Ho JYM, et al: Determination of hair ketamine cut-off value from Hong Kong ketamine users by LC-MS/MS analysis. Forensic Sci Int 259:53–58, 2016 26750989

Leung KW, Wong ZCF, Ho JYM, et al: Surveillance of drug abuse in Hong Kong by hair analysis using LC-MS/MS. Drug Test Anal 10(6):977–983, 2018 29205946

Levy L, Cameron DE, Aitken RCB: Observation on two psychotomimetic drugs of piperidine derivation—CI 395 (sernyl) and CI 400. Am J Psychiatry 116:843–844, 1960 14416411

Li C-T, Chen M-H, Lin W-C, et al: The effects of low-dose ketamine on the prefrontal cortex and amygdala in treatment-resistant depression: a randomized controlled study. Hum Brain Mapp 37(3):1080–1090, 2016 26821769

Li F, Liu J, Yip PSF, et al: Mortalities of methamphetamine, opioid, and ketamine abusers in Shanghai and Wuhan, China. Forensic Sci Int 306:110093, 2020 31816483

Li N, Lee B, Liu R-J, et al: mTOR-dependent synapse formation underlies the rapid antidepressant effects of NMDA antagonists. Science 329(5994):959–964, 2010 20724638

Liang HJ, Tang KL, Chan F, et al: Ketamine users have high rates of psychosis and/or depression. J Addict Nurs 26(1):8–13, 2015 25761158

Liao Y, Tang J, Ma M, et al: Frontal white matter abnormalities following chronic ketamine use: a diffusion tensor imaging study. Brain 133(Pt 7):2115–2122, 2010 20519326

Liao Y, Tang J, Corlett PR, et al: Reduced dorsal prefrontal gray matter after chronic ketamine use. Biol Psychiatry 69(1):42–48, 2011 21035788

Liao Y, Tang J, Fornito A, et al: Alterations in regional homogeneity of resting-state brain activity in ketamine addicts. Neurosci Lett 522(1):36–40, 2012 22698584

Liao Y, Tang YL, Hao W: Ketamine and international regulations. Am J Drug Alcohol Abuse 43(5):495–504, 2017 28635347

Lilly JC: The Scientist: A Novel Autobiography. New York, Lippincott, 1978

Lin EP, Lee J-R, Lee CS, et al: Do anesthetics harm the developing human brain? An integrative analysis of animal and human studies. Neurotoxicol Teratol 60:117–128, 2017 27793659

Lipschitz DS, D'Souza DC, White JA, et al: Clozapine blockade of ketamine effects in healthy subjects (abstract). Biol Psychiatry 41:23S, 1997

Liu SYW, Ng SKK, Tam YH, et al: Clinical pattern and prevalence of upper gastrointestinal toxicity in patients abusing ketamine. J Dig Dis 18(9):504–510, 2017 28749602

Liu W, Zhou Y, Zheng W, et al: Repeated intravenous infusions of ketamine: neurocognition in patients with anxious and nonanxious treatment-resistant depression. J Affect Disord 259:1–6, 2019 31430662

Liu Y, Lin D, Wu B, Zhou W: Ketamine abuse potential and use disorder. Brain Res Bull 126(Pt 1):68–73, 2016 27261367

Lo RSC, Krishnamoorthy R, Freeman JG, Austin AS: Cholestasis and biliary dilatation associated with chronic ketamine abuse: a case series. Singapore Med J 52(3):e52, 2011

Lodge D: The history of the pharmacology and cloning of ionotropic glutamate receptors and the development of idiosyncratic nomenclature. Neuropharmacology 56(1):6–21, 2009 18765242

Lodge D, Berry SC: Psychotomimetic effects of sigma opiates may be mediated by block of central excitatory synapses utilising receptors for aspartate-like amino acids. Neurol Neurobiol (Tallinn) 12:503–518, 1984

Lodge D, Mercier MS: Ketamine and phencyclidine: the good, the bad and the unexpected. Br J Pharmacol 172(17):4254–4276, 2015 26075331

Longnecker DE, Mackey SC, Newman MF, et al (eds): Anesthesiology (3rd Edition). New York, McGraw-Hill, 2018.

Loo C, Glozier N, Barton D, et al: Efficacy and safety of a 4-week course of repeated subcutaneous ketamine injections for treatment-resistant depression (KADS study): randomised double-blind active controlled trial. Br J Psychiatry 1–9, 2023

Luby ED: Phencyclidine revisited [proceedings]. Psychopharmacol Bull 16(4):85–86, 1980 7454950

Luby ED, Cohen BD, Rosenbaum G, et al: Study of a new schizophrenomimetic drug; sernyl. AMA Arch Neurol Psychiatry 81(3):363–369, 1959 13626287

Lugg W: The parable of the Therapeutic Goods Administration approval of esketamine (Spravato) in Australia. Australas Psychiatry 31(2):186–189, 2023 36802863

Luisada PV: The phencyclidine psychosis: phenomenology and treatment, in Phencyclidine (PCP) Use: An Appraisal. Edited by Petersen RC, Stillman RC. National Institute on Drug Abuse, DHEW publ. no. (ADM) 79-728. Washington, DC, Supt. of Docs., US Govt. Printing Office, 1978

Lynch ME, Clark AJ, Sawynok J, Sullivan MJL: Topical 2% amitriptyline and 1% ketamine in neuropathic pain syndromes: a randomized, double-blind, placebo-controlled trial. Anesthesiology 103(1):140–146, 2005 15983466

Macciardi F, Lucca A, Catalano M, et al: Amino acid patterns in schizophrenia: some new findings. Psychiatry Res 32(1):63–70, 1990 2161549

Maddox VH: The historical development of phencyclidine, in PCP (Phencyclidine): Historical and Current Perspectives. Edited by Domino EF. Ann Arbor, MI, NPP Books, 1981, pp 1–8

Madonick SH, D'Souza DC, Brush L, et al: Assessment of glutamate-opiate interactions: a contribution to the pathophysiology of schizophrenia? (abstract). Schizophr Res 36:310–311, 1999

Maheswari N, Panda NB, Mahajan S, et al: Ketofol as an anesthetic agent in patients with isolated moderate to severe traumatic brain injury: a prospective, randomized double-blind controlled study. J Neurosurg Anesthesiol 35(1):49–55, 2023 36745167

Mahoney JM, Vardaxis V, Moore JL, et al: Topical ketamine cream in the treatment of painful diabetic neuropathy: a randomized, placebo-controlled, double-blind initial study. J Am Podiatr Med Assoc 102(3):178–183, 2012 22659759

Majić T, Schmidt TT, Gallinat J: Peak experiences and the afterglow phenomenon: when and how do therapeutic effects of hallucinogens depend on psychedelic experiences? J Psychopharmacol 29(3):241–253, 2015 25670401

Malhotra AK, Pinals DA, Adler CM, et al: Ketamine-induced exacerbation of psychotic symptoms and cognitive impairment in neuroleptic-free schizophrenics. Neuropsychopharmacology 17(3):141–150, 1997a 9272481

Malhotra AK, Adler CM, Kennison SD, et al: Clozapine blunts N-methyl-D-aspartate antagonist-induced psychosis: a study with ketamine. Biol Psychiatry 42(8):664–668, 1997b 9325559

Malhotra AK, Breier A, Goldman D, et al: The apolipoprotein E epsilon 4 allele is associated with blunting of ketamine-induced psychosis in schizophrenia. A preliminary report. Neuropsychopharmacology 19(5):445–448, 1998 9778666

Mankowitz E, Brock-Utne JG, Cosnett JE, Green-Thompson R: Epidural ketamine. A preliminary report. S Afr Med J 61(12):441–442, 1982 7064021

Marks J: The Search for the "Manchurian Candidate." New York, WW Norton and Co., 1991

Mathai DS, Meyer MJ, Storch EA, Kosten TR: The relationship between subjective effects induced by a single dose of ketamine and treatment response in patients with major depressive disorder: a systematic review. J Affect Disord 264:123–129, 2020 32056741

Mathai DS, Mora V, Garcia-Romeu A: Toward synergies of ketamine and psychotherapy. Front Psychol 13:868103, 2022 35401323

Mathalon DH, Ahn K-H, Perry EB Jr, et al: Effects of nicotine on the neurophysiological and behavioral effects of ketamine in humans. Front Psychiatry 5:3, 2014 24478731

Mathisen LC, Skjelbred P, Skoglund LA, Øye I: Effect of ketamine, an NMDA receptor inhibitor, in acute and chronic orofacial pain. Pain 61(2):215–220, 1995 7659431

Matusch A, Hurlemann R, Rota Kops E, et al: Acute S-ketamine application does not alter cerebral [18F]altanserin binding: a pilot PET study in humans. J Neural Transm (Vienna) 114(11):1433–1442, 2007 17541696

Max MB, Byas-Smith MG, Gracely RH, Bennett GJ: Intravenous infusion of the NMDA antagonist, ketamine, in chronic posttraumatic pain with allodynia: a double-blind comparison to alfentanil and placebo. Clin Neuropharmacol 18(4):360–368, 1995 8665549

Mayberg TS, Lam AM, Matta BF, et al: Ketamine does not increase cerebral blood flow velocity or intracranial pressure during isoflurane/nitrous oxide anesthesia in patients undergoing craniotomy. Anesth Analg 81(1):84–89, 1995 7598288

McCarthy DA: History of the development of cataleptoid anesthetics of the phencyclidine type, in PCP (Phencyclidine): Historical and Current Perspectives. Edited by Domino EF. Ann Arbor, MI, NPP Books, 1981, pp 17–23

McCarthy DA, Chen G, Kaump DH, Ensor C: General anesthetic and other pharmacological properties of 2-(O-chlorophenyl)-2-methylamino cyclohexanone HCl (CI-58L). J New Drugs 5(1):21–33, 1965 14283065

McGhee LL, Maani CV, Garza TH, et al: The correlation between ketamine and posttraumatic stress disorder in burned service members. J Trauma 64(2)(Suppl):S195–S198, Discussion S197–S198, 2008 18376165

McGhee LL, Maani CV, Garza TH, et al: The intraoperative administration of ketamine to burned U.S. service members does not increase the incidence of posttraumatic stress disorder. Mil Med 179(8)(Suppl):41–46, 2014 25102548

McGirr A, Berlim MT, Bond DJ, et al: A systematic review and meta-analysis of randomized, double-blind, placebo-controlled trials of ketamine in the rapid treatment of major depressive episodes. Psychol Med 45(4):693–704, 2015 25010396

McIntyre RS, Rosenblat JD, Rodrigues NB, et al: The effect of intravenous ketamine on cognitive functions in adults with treatment-resistant major depressive or bipolar disorders: results from the Canadian rapid treatment center of excellence (CRTCE). Psychiatry Res 302:113993, 2021 34034067

McMullen EP, Lee Y, Lipsitz O, et al: Strategies to prolong ketamine's efficacy in adults with treatment-resistant depression. Adv Ther 38(6):2795–2820, 2021 33929660

Medoff DR, Holcomb HH, Lahti AC, Tamminga CA: Probing the human hippocampus using rCBF: contrasts in schizophrenia. Hippocampus 11(5):543–550, 2001 11732707

Mendola C, Cammarota G, Netto R, et al: S(+)-ketamine for control of perioperative pain and prevention of post thoracotomy pain syndrome: a randomized, double-blind study. Minerva Anestesiol 78(7):757–766, 2012 22441361

Meyers FH, Rose AJ, Smith DE: Incidents involving the Haight-Ashbury population and some uncommonly used drugs. J Psychedelic Drugs 1(2):139–146, 1967

Michelet D, Brasher C, Horlin A-L, et al: Ketamine for chronic non-cancer pain: a meta-analysis and trial sequential analysis of randomized controlled trials. Eur J Pain 22(4):632–646, 2018 29178663

Milak MS, Rashid R, Dong Z, et al: Assessment of relationship of ketamine dose with magnetic resonance spectoscopy of Glx and GABA responses in adults with major depression: a randomized clinical trial. JAMA Netw Open 3(8):e2013211, 2020 32785636

Mills IH, Park GR, Manara AR, Merriman RJ: Treatment of compulsive behaviour in eating disorders with intermittent ketamine infusions. QJM 91(7):493–503, 1998 9797933

Mion G, Villevieille T: Ketamine pharmacology: an update (pharmacodynamics and molecular aspects, recent findings). CNS Neurosci Ther 19(6):370–380, 2013 23575437

Mion G, Le Masson J, Granier C, Hoffman C: A retrospective study of ketamine administration and the development of acute or post-traumatic stress disorder in 274 war-wounded soldiers. Anaesthesia 72:1476–1483, 2017

Mitchell AC: An unusual case of chronic neuropathic pain responds to an optimum frequency of intravenous ketamine infusions. J Pain Symptom Manage 21(5):443–446, 2001 11369165

Mitchell AC, Fallon MT: A single infusion of intravenous ketamine improves pain relief in patients with critical limb ischaemia: results of a double blind randomised controlled trial. Pain 97(3):275–281, 2002 12044624

Mollaahmetoglu OM, Keeler J, Ashbullby KJ, et al: "This is something that changed my life": a qualitative study of patients' experiences in a clinical trial of ketamine treatment for alcohol use disorders. Front Psychiatry 12:695335, 2021 34483991

Moody RA: Life After Life. New York, Mockingbird Books, 1975

Moore M, Alltounian H: Journeys Into the Bright World. Rockport, MA, Para Research, 1978

Morgan CJA, Curran HV: Acute and chronic effects of ketamine upon human memory: a review. Psychopharmacology (Berl) 188(4):408–424, 2006 17006715

Morgan CJA, Mofeez A, Brandner B, et al: Ketamine impairs response inhibition and is positively reinforcing in healthy volunteers: a dose-response study. Psychopharmacology (Berl) 172(3):298–308, 2004a 14727004

Morgan CJA, Mofeez A, Brandner B, et al: Acute effects of ketamine on memory systems and psychotic symptoms in healthy volunteers. Neuropsychopharmacology 29(1):208–218, 2004b 14603267

Morgan CJA, Monaghan L, Curran HV: Beyond the K-hole: a 3-year longitudinal investigation of the cognitive and subjective effects of ketamine in recreational users who have substantially reduced their use of the drug. Addiction 99(11):1450–1461, 2004c 15500598

Morgan CJA, Riccelli M, Maitland CH, Curran HV: Long-term effects of ketamine: evidence for a persisting impairment of source memory in recreational users. Drug Alcohol Depend 75(3):301–308, 2004d 15283951

Morgan CJA, Rossell SL, Pepper F, et al: Semantic priming after ketamine acutely in healthy volunteers and following chronic self-administration in substance users. Biol Psychiatry 59(3):265–272, 2006a 16140283

Morgan CJA, Perry EB, Cho H-S, et al: Greater vulnerability to the amnestic effects of ketamine in males. Psychopharmacology (Berl) 187(4):405–414, 2006b 16896964

Morgan CJA, Rees H, Curran HV: Attentional bias to incentive stimuli in frequent ketamine users. Psychol Med 38(9):1331–1340, 2008 18177527

Morgan CJA, Huddy V, Lipton M, et al: Is persistent ketamine use a valid model of the cognitive and oculomotor deficits in schizophrenia? Biol Psychiatry 65(12):1099–1102, 2009 19111280

Morgan CJA, Muetzelfeldt L, Curran HV: Consequences of chronic ketamine self-administration upon neurocognitive function and psychological wellbeing: a 1-year longitudinal study. Addiction 105(1):121–133, 2010 19919593

Morgan CJA, Curran HV; Independent Scientific Committee on Drugs: Ketamine use: a review. Addiction 107(1):27–38, 2012 21777321

Morgan CJA, Dodds CM, Furby H, et al: Long-term heavy ketamine use is associated with spatial memory impairment and altered hippocampal activation. Front Psychiatry 5:149, 2014 25538631

Morgan HL, Turner DC, Corlett PR, et al: Exploring the impact of ketamine on the experience of illusory body ownership. Biol Psychiatry 69(1):35–41, 2011 20947068

Morgan JP, Kagan D: The dusting of America: the image of phencyclidine (PCP) in the popular media. J Psychedelic Drugs 12(3–4):195–204, 1980 7431414

Morris PJ, Burke RD, Sharma AK, et al: A comparison of the pharmacokinetics and NMDAR antagonism-associated neurotoxicity of ketamine, (2R,6R)-hydroxynorketamine and MK-801. Neurotoxicol Teratol 87:106993, 2021 33945878

Mueller F, Musso F, London M, et al: Pharmacological fMRI: effects of subanesthetic ketamine on resting-state functional connectivity in the default mode network, salience network, dorsal attention network and executive control network. Neuroimage Clin 19:745–757, 2018 30003027

Muetzelfeldt L, Kamboj SK, Rees H, et al: Journey through the K-hole: phenomenological aspects of ketamine use. Drug Alcohol Depend 95(3):219–229, 2008 18355990

Muir BJ, Evans V, Mulcahy JJ: Sernyl analgesia for children's burn dressings. A preliminary communication. Br J Anaesth 33:51–53, 1961 13773625

Muir KW, Lees KR: Excitatory amino acid antagonists for acute stroke. Cochrane Database Syst Rev 2003(3):CD001244, 2003 12917902

Murck H, Spitznagel H, Ploch M, et al: Hypericum extract reverses S-ketamine-induced changes in auditory evoked potentials in humans—possible implications for the treatment of schizophrenia. Biol Psychiatry 59(5):440–445, 2006 16165104

Murrough JW, Iosifescu DV, Chang LC, et al: Antidepressant efficacy of ketamine in treatment-resistant major depression: a two-site randomized controlled trial. Am J Psychiatry 170(10):1134–1142, 2013a 23982301

Murrough JW, Perez AM, Pillemer S, et al: Rapid and longer-term antidepressant effects of repeated ketamine infusions in treatment-resistant major depression. Biol Psychiatry 74(4):250–256, 2013b 22840761

Murrough JW, Burdick KE, Levitch CF, et al: Neurocognitive effects of ketamine and association with antidepressant response in individuals with treatment-resistant depression: a randomized controlled trial. Neuropsychopharmacology 40(5):1084–1090, 2015 25374095

Musso F, Brinkmeyer J, Ecker D, et al: Ketamine effects on brain function—simultaneous fMRI/EEG during a visual oddball task. Neuroimage 58(2):508–525, 2011 21723949

Nagels A, Kirner-Veselinovic A, Krach S, Kircher T: Neural correlates of S-ketamine induced psychosis during overt continuous verbal fluency. Neuroimage 54(2):1307–1314, 2011 20727411

Nagels A, Kirner-Veselinovic A, Wiese R, et al: Effects of ketamine-induced psychopathological symptoms on continuous overt rhyme fluency. Eur Arch Psychiatry Clin Neurosci 262(5):403–414, 2012 22189657

Nagels A, Cabanis M, Oppel A, et al: S-ketamine-induced NMDA receptor blockade during natural speech production and its implications for formal thought disorder in schizophrenia: a pharmaco-fMRI study. Neuropsychopharmacology 43(6):1324–1333, 2018 29105665

Nagels W, Demeyere R, Van Hemelrijck J, et al: Evaluation of the neuroprotective effects of S(+)-ketamine during open-heart surgery. Anesth Analg 98(6):1595–1603, 2004 15155311

Narendran R, Frankle WG, Keefe R, et al: Altered prefrontal dopaminergic function in chronic recreational ketamine users. Am J Psychiatry 162(12):2352–2359, 2005 16330601

National Institute on Drug Abuse. Trends in Annual Prevalence of Use of Various Drugs in Grades 8, 10, and 12. National Institute on Drug Abuse, 2023. Available at: https://monitoringthefuture.org/wp-content/uploads/2022/12/mtf2022table02.pdf. Accessed December 5, 2023.

Naylor DE, Liu H, Wasterlain CG: Trafficking of GABA(A) receptors, loss of inhibition, and a mechanism for pharmacoresistance in status epilepticus. J Neurosci 25(34):7724–7733, 2005 16120773

Newcomer JW, Farber NB, Selke G, et al: Guanabenz prevention of NMDA-antagonist-induced mental symptoms in healthy humans (abstract). Schizophr Res 36:311–312, 1999

Niciu MJ, Grunschel BD, Corlett PR, et al: Two cases of delayed-onset suicidal ideation, dysphoria and anxiety after ketamine infusion in patients with obsessive-compulsive disorder and a history of major depressive disorder. J Psychopharmacol 27(7):651–654, 2013a 23676198

Niciu MJ, Luckenbaugh DA, Ionescu DF, et al: Subanesthetic dose ketamine does not induce an affective switch in three independent samples of treatment-resistant maor depression [Letter]. Biol Psychiatry 74:e23–e24, 2013b

Niciu MJ, Luckenbaugh DA, Ionescu DF, et al: Clinical predictors of ketamine response in treatment-resistant major depression. J Clin Psychiatry 75(5):e417–e423, 2014 24922494

Nicolodi M, Sicuteri F: Exploration of NMDA receptors in migraine: therapeutic and theoretic implications. Int J Clin Pharmacol Res 15(5–6):181–189, 1995 8835616

Niesters M, Martini C, Dahan A: Ketamine for chronic pain: risks and benefits. Br J Clin Pharmacol 77(2):357–367, 2014 23432384

Nikolajsen L, Hansen CL, Nielsen J, et al: The effect of ketamine on phantom pain: a central neuropathic disorder maintained by peripheral input. Pain 67(1):69–77, 1996 8895233

Nogo D, Nazal H, Song Y, et al: A review of potential neuropathological changes associated with ketamine. Expert Opin Drug Saf 21(6):813–831, 2022 35502632

Noppers I, Niesters M, Swartjes M, et al: Absence of long-term analgesic effect from a short-term S-ketamine infusion on fibromyalgia pain: a randomized, prospective, double blind, active placebo-controlled trial. Eur J Pain 15(9):942–949, 2011 21482474

Northoff G, Richter A, Bermpohl F, et al: NMDA hypofunction in the posterior cingulate as a model for schizophrenia: an exploratory ketamine administration study in fMRI. Schizophr Res 72(2–3):235–248, 2005 15560968

Nutt D, King LA, Saulsbury W, Blakemore C: Development of a rational scale to assess the harm of drugs of potential misuse. Lancet 369(9566):1047–1053, 2007 17382831

Ochs-Ross R, Daly EJ, Zhang Y, et al: Efficacy and safety of esketamine nasal spray plus an oral antidepressant in elderly patients with treatment-resistant depression— TRANSFORM-3. Am J Geriatr Psychiatry 28(2):121–141, 2020 31734084

O'Connell NE, Wand BM, McAuley J, et al: Interventions for treating pain and disability in adults with complex regional pain syndrome (Review). Cochrane Database Syst Rev 2013(4):CD009416, 2013 23633371

Olney JW: Toxic effects of glutamate and related amino acids on the developing central nervous system, in Heritable Disorders of Amino Acid Metabolism: Patterns of Clinical Expression and Genetic Variation. Edited by Nyhan WL. New York, Wiley and Sons, 1974, pp 501–512

Olney JW: Excitatory transmitters and neuropsychiatric disorders, in Neurobiology of Amino Acids, Peptides, and Trophic Factors. Edited by Ferrendelli JA, Collins RC, Johnson EM. New York, Kluwer Academic, 1988, pp 51–61

Olney JW: Excitatory amino acids and neuropsychiatric disorders. Biol Psychiatry 26(5):505–525, 1989 2571362

Olney JW: Excitotoxicity: an overview. Can Dis Wkly Rep 16(Suppl 1E):47–57, discussion 57–58, 1990 1966279

Olney JW, de Gubareff T: Glutamate neurotoxicity and Huntington's chorea. Nature 271(5645):557–559, 1978 146165

Olney JW, Farber NB: Efficacy of clozapine compared with other antipsychotics in preventing NMDA-antagonist neurotoxicity. J Clin Psychiatry 55(9)(Suppl B):43–46, 1994 7961572

Olney JW, Farber NB: NMDA antagonists as neurotherapeutic drugs, psychotogens, neurotoxins, and research tools for studying schizophrenia. Neuropsychopharmacology 13(4):335–345, 1995a 8747758

Olney JW, Farber NB: Glutamate receptor dysfunction and schizophrenia. Arch Gen Psychiatry 52(12):998–1007, 1995b 7492260

Olney JW, Labruyere J, Price MT: Pathological changes induced in cerebrocortical neurons by phencyclidine and related drugs. Science 244(4910):1360–1362, 1989 2660263

Olney JW, Newcomer JW, Farber NB: NMDA receptor hypofunction model of schizophrenia. J Psychiatr Res 33(6):523–533, 1999 10628529

Oranje B, van Berckel BNM, Kemner C, et al: The effects of a sub-anaesthetic dose of ketamine on human selective attention. Neuropsychopharmacology 22(3):293–302, 2000 10693157

Oranje B, Gispen-de Wied CC, Verbaten MN, Kahn RS: Modulating sensory gating in healthy volunteers: the effects of ketamine and haloperidol. Biol Psychiatry 52(9):887–895, 2002 12399142

Oranje B, Gispen-de Wied CC, Westenberg HGM, et al: Haloperidol counteracts the ketamine-induced disruption of processing negativity, but not that of the P300 amplitude. Int J Neuropsychopharmacol 12(6):823–832, 2009 19154656

Ornowska M, Wormsbecker A, Andolfatto G, et al: The use of ketamine as a neuroprotective agent following cardiac arrest: a scoping review of current literature. CNS Neurosci Ther 29(1):104–110, 2023 36184822

Ortega JJZ, Otter JIL: Phencyclidine for capture of stray dogs. J Am Vet Med Assoc 150(7):772–776, 1967 6068409

Overall JE, Gorham DR: The brief psychiatric rating scale. Psychol Rep 10:799–812, 1962

Øye I, Paulsen O, Maurset A: Effects of ketamine on sensory perception: evidence for a role of N-methyl-D-aspartate receptors. J Pharmacol Exp Ther 260(3):1209–1213, 1992 1312163

Øye I, Rabben T, Fagerlund TH: Analgesic effect of ketamine in a patient with neuropathic pain [in Norwegian]. Tidsskr Nor Laegeforen 116(26):3130–3131, 1996 8999575

Palamar JJ: What's in a name? Correlates of ecstasy users knowing or agreeing that Molly is ecstasy/MDMA. J Psychoactive Drugs 50(1):88–93, 2018 28937933

Pannacciulli E, Sordi L, Trazzi R: L'Allucinogeno CI 581 nel su impiego anestesiologico. G Ital Mal Torace 20(6):61–67, 1966

Parikh T, Walkup JT: The future of ketamine in the treatment of teen depression (editorial). Am J Psychiatry 178(4):288–289, 2021 33789452

Parkin MC, Turfus SC, Smith NW, et al: Detection of ketamine and its metabolites in urine by ultra high pressure liquid chromatography-tandem mass spectrometry. J Chromatogr B Analyt Technol Biomed Life Sci 876(1):137–142, 2008 18976970

Parwani A, Duncan EJ, Bartlett E, et al: Impaired prepulse inhibition of acoustic startle in schizophrenia. Biol Psychiatry 47(7):662–669, 2000 10745060

Passie T, Karst M, Borsutzky M, et al: Effects of different subanaesthetic doses of (S)-ketamine on psychopathology and binocular depth inversion in man. J Psychopharmacol 17(1):51–56, 2003 12680739

Patil S, Anitescu M: Efficacy of outpatient ketamine infusions in refractory chronic pain syndromes: a 5-year retrospective analysis. Pain Med 13(2):263–269, 2012 21939497

Paule MG, Li M, Allen RR, et al: Ketamine anesthesia during the first week of life can cause long-lasting cognitive deficits in rhesus monkeys. Neurotoxicol Teratol 33(2):220–230, 2011 21241795

Perception Neuroscience: Atai Life Sciences Announces Results from the Phase 1 IV-to-Subcutaneous Bridging Study of PCN-101 (R-Ketamine). Press Release, August 8, 2023. Available at: https://www.perceptionns.com/s/atai-Life-Sciences-Announces-Results-from-the-Phase-1-IV-to-Subcutaneous-Bridging-Study-of-PCN-101-R.pdf. Accessed February 21, 2024.

Perel A, Davidson JT: Recurrent hallucinations following ketamine. Anaesthesia 31(8):1081–1083, 1976 984361

Perez-Ruixo C, Rossenu S, Zannikos P, et al: Population pharmacokinetics of es-ketamine nasal spray and its metabolite noresketamine in healthy subjects and patients with treatment-resistant depression. Clin Pharmacokinet 60(4):501–516, 2021 33128208

Persson J, Hasselström J, Wiklund B, et al: The analgesic effect of racemic ketamine in patients with chronic ischemic pain due to lower extremity arteriosclerosis ob-literans. Acta Anaesthesiol Scand 42(7):750–758, 1998 9698948

Persson J, Hasselström J, Maurset A, et al: Pharmacokinetics and non-analgesic ef-fects of S- and R-ketamines in healthy volunteers with normal and reduced met-abolic capacity. Eur J Clin Pharmacol 57(12):869–875, 2002 11936706

Peters RJ Jr, Kelder SH, Meshack A, et al: Beliefs and social norms about cigarettes or marijuana sticks laced with embalming fluid and phencyclidine (PCP): why youth use "fry." Subst Use Misuse 40(4):563–571, 2005 15830737

Pfenninger EG, Durieux ME, Himmelseher S: Cognitive impairment after small-dose ketamine isomers in comparison to equianalgesic racemic ketamine in hu-man volunteers. Anesthesiology 96(2):357–366, 2002 11818769

Phillips JL, Norris S, Talbot J, et al: Single, repeated, and maintenance ketamine infusions for treatment-resistant depression: a randomized controlled trial. Am J Psychiatry 176(5):401–409, 2019 30922101

Pickering AE, McCabe CS: Prolonged ketamine infusion as a therapy for complex regional pain syndrome: synergism with antagonism? Br J Clin Pharmacol 77(2):233–238, 2014 23701138

Podlesh I, Zindler M: 1st experience with the phencyclidine derivative ketamine (CI-581), a new intravenous and intramuscular anesthetic. Anaesthetist 16(10):299–303, 1967

Pollak TA, De Simoni S, Barimani B, et al: Phenomenologically distinct psychoto-mimetic effects of ketamine are associated with cerebral blood flow changes in functionally relevant cerebral foci: a continuous arterial spin labelling study. Psychopharmacology (Berl) 232(24):4515–4524, 2015 26438425

Polomano RC, Buckenmaier CC 3rd, Kwon KH, et al: Effects of low-dose IV ket-amine on peripheral and central pain from major limb injuries sustained in com-bat. Pain Med 14(7):1088–1100, 2013 23590428

Pomeroy JL, Marmura MJ, Nahas SJ, Viscusi ER: Ketamine infusions for treatment refractory headache. Headache 57(2):276–282, 2017 28025837

Popova V, Daly EJ, Trivedi M, et al: Efficacy and safety of flexibly dosed esketamine nasal spray combined with a newly initiated oral antidepressant in treatment-resistant depression: a randomized double-blind active-controlled study. Am J Psychiatry 176(6):428–438, 2019 31109201

Portmann S, Kwan HY, Theurillat R, et al: Enantioselective capillary electropho-resis for identification and characterization of human cytochrome P450 enzymes which metabolize ketamine and norketamine in vitro. J Chromatogr A 1217(51):7942–7948, 2010 20609441

Poterucha TJ, Murphy SL, Rho RH, et al: Topical amitriptyline-ketamine for treat-ment of rectal, genital, and perineal pain and discomfort. Pain Physician 15(6):485–488, 2012 23159965

Pradhan B, Rossi G: Combining ketamine, brain stimulation (rTMS) and mindfulness therapy (TIMBER) for opioid addiction. Cureus 12(11):e11798, 2020 33409043

Pradhan B, Gray R, Parikh T, et al: Trauma interventions using mindfulness based extinction and reconsolidation (TIMBER©) as monotherapy for chronic PTSD: a pilot study. Adolesc Psychiatry (Hilversum) 5:125–131, 2015

Pradhan B, Wainer IW, Moaddel R, et al: Trauma interventions using mindfulness based extinction and reconsolidation (TIMBER) psychotherapy to prolong the therapeutic effects of single ketamine infusion on posttraumatic stress disorder and comorbed depression: a pilot randomized, placebo-controlled, crossover clinical trial. Asia Pacific Journal of Clinical Trials: Nervous System Diseases 2(3):80–90, 2017

Pradhan B, Mitrev L, Moaddell R, Wainer IW: d-Serine is a potential biomarker for clinical response in treatment of post-traumatic stress disorder using (R,S)-ketamine infusion and TIMBER psychotherapy: a pilot study. Biochim Biophys Acta Proteins Proteom 1866(7):831–839, 2018 29563072

Quinlan J: The use of a subanesthetic infusion of intravenous ketamine to allow withdrawal of medically prescribed opioids in people with chronic pain, opioid tolerance and hyperalgesia: outcome at 6 months (letter). Pain Med 13(11):1524–1525, 2012 22978408

Radant AD, Bowdle TA, Cowley DS, et al: Does ketamine-mediated N-methyl-D-aspartate receptor antagonism cause schizophrenia-like oculomotor abnormalities? Neuropsychopharmacology 19(5):434–444, 1998 9778665

Rainey JM Jr, Crowder MK: Prevalence of phencyclidine in street drug preparations (letter). N Engl J Med 290(8):466–467, 1974a 4811036

Rainey JM Jr, Crowder MK: Ketamine or phencyclidine (letter). JAMA 230(6):824, 1974b 4479446

Ramsay JG, Rappaport BA: SmartTots: a multidisciplinary effort to determine anesthetic safety in young children. Anesth Analg 113(5):963–964, 2011 22021790

Ranganathan M, DeMartinis N, Huguenel B, et al: Attenuation of ketamine-induced impairment in verbal learning and memory in healthy volunteers by the AMPA receptor potentiator PF-04958242. Mol Psychiatry 22(11):1633–1640, 2017 28242871

Rasmussen KG: Principles and Practice of Electroconvulsive Therapy. Washington, DC, American Psychiatric Association Publishing, 2019

Rasmussen KG, Lineberry TW, Galardy CW, et al: Serial infusions of low-dose ketamine for major depression. J Psychopharmacol 27(5):444–450, 2013 23428794

Reier CE: Ketamine—"dissociative agent" or hallucinogen? (letter). N Engl J Med 284(14):791–792, 1971 5548039

Reiff CM, Richman EE, Nemeroff CB, et al; the Work Group on Biomarkers and Novel Treatments, a Division of the American Psychiatric Association Council of Research: Psychedelics and psychedelic-assisted psychotherapy. Am J Psychiatry 177(5):391–410, 2020 32098487

Richeval C, Dumestre-Toulet V, Wiart J-F, et al: New psychoactive substances in oral fluid of drivers around a music festival in south-west France in 2017. Forensic Sci Int 297:265–269, 2019 30851602

Rivolta D, Heidegger T, Scheller B, et al: Ketamine dysregulates the amplitude and connectivity of high-frequency oscillations in cortical-subcortical networks in humans: evidence from resting-state magnetoencephalography recordings. Schizophr Bull 41(5):1105–1114, 2015 25987642

Roberts RE, Curran HV, Friston KJ, Morgan CJA: Abnormalities in white matter microstructure associated with chronic ketamine use. Neuropsychopharmacology 39(2):329–338, 2014 23929545

Robison R, Lafrance A, Brendle M, et al: A case series of group-based ketamine-assisted psychotherapy for patients in residential treatment for eating disorders with comorbid depression and anxiety disorders. J Eat Disord 10(1):65, 2022 35524316

Rodin EA, Luby ED, Meyer JS: Electroencephalographic findings associated with sernyl infusion. Electroencephalogr Clin Neurophysiol 11:796–798, 1959 14438167

Rodriguez CI, Kegeles LS, Levinson A, et al: Randomized controlled crossover trial of ketamine in obsessive-compulsive disorder: proof-of-concept. Neuropsychopharmacology 38(12):2475–2483, 2013 23783065

Rodriguez CI, Kegeles LS, Levinson A, et al: In vivo effects of ketamine on glutamate-glutamine and gamma-aminobutyric acid in obsessive-compulsive disorder: proof of concept. Psychiatry Res 233(2):141–147, 2015 26104826

Rodriguez CI, Levinson A, Zwerling J, et al: Open-label trial on the effects of memantine in adults with obsessive-compulsive disorder after a single ketamine infusion (letter). J Clin Psychiatry 77(5):688–689, 2016a 27249077

Rodriguez CI, Wheaton M, Zwerling J, et al: Can exposure-based CBT extend the effects of intravenous ketamine in obsessive-compulsive disorder? An open-label trial (letter). J Clin Psychiatry 77(3):408–409, 2016b 27046314

Rodriguez CI, Lapidus KAB, Zwerling J, et al: Challenges in testing intranasal ketamine in obsessive-compulsive disorder (letter). J Clin Psychiatry 78(4):466–467, 2017 28448699

Romeo B, Choucha W, Fossati P, Rotge J-Y: Meta-analysis of short- and mid-term efficacy of ketamine in unipolar and bipolar depression. Psychiatry Res 230(2):682–688, 2015 26548981

Rosati A, De Masi S, Guerrini R: Ketamine for refractory status epilepticus: a systematic review. CNS Drugs 32(11):997–1009, 2018 30232735

Rosch RE, Auksztulewicz R, Leung PD, et al: Selective prefrontal disinhibition in a roving auditory oddball paradigm under N-methyl-d-aspartate receptor blockade. Biol Psychiatry Cogn Neurosci Neuroimaging 4(2):140–150, 2019 30115499

Rosenbaum G, Cohen BD, Luby ED, et al: Comparison of sernyl with other drugs: simulation of schizophrenic performance with sernyl, LSD-25, and amobarbital (amytal) sodium; I. Attention, motor function, and proprioception. AMA Arch Gen Psychiatry 1:651–656, 1959 14438905

Roser P, Haussleiter IS, Chong H-J, et al: Inhibition of cerebral type 1 cannabinoid receptors is associated with impaired auditory mismatch negativity generation in the ketamine model of schizophrenia. Psychopharmacology (Berl) 218(4):611–620, 2011 21590281

Ross C, Jain R, Bonnett CJ, Wolfson P: High-dose ketamine infusion for the treatment of posttraumatic stress disorder in combat veterans. Ann Clin Psychiatry 31(4):271–279, 2019 31675388

Rothberg RL, Azhari N, Haug NA, Dakwar E: Mystical-type experiences occasioned by ketamine mediate its impact on at-risk drinking: results from a randomized, controlled trial. J Psychopharmacol 35(2):150–158, 2021 33307947

Rowland LM, Bustillo JR, Mullins PG, et al: Effects of ketamine on anterior cingulate glutamate metabolism in healthy humans: a 4-T proton MRS study. Am J Psychiatry 162(2):394–396, 2005 15677610

Rowland LM, Beason-Held L, Tamminga CA, Holcomb HH: The interactive effects of ketamine and nicotine on human cerebral blood flow. Psychopharmacology (Berl) 208(4):575–584, 2010 20066400

Rule A: A Rage to Kill and Other True Cases. New York, Pocket Star Books, 1999

Sadove MS, Shulman M, Hatano S, Fevold N: Analgesic effects of ketamine administered in subdissociative doses. Anesth Analg 50(3):452–457, 1971 5103784

Salas S, Frasca M, Planchet-Barraud B, et al: Ketamine analgesic effect by continuous intravenous infusion in refractory cancer pain: considerations about the clinical research in palliative care. J Palliat Med 15(3):287–293, 2012 22335487

Santos E, Olivares-Rivera A, Major S, et al: Lasting s-ketamine block of spreading depolarizations in subarachnoid hemorrhage: a retrospective cohort study. Crit Care 23(1):427, 2019 31888772

Sassano-Higgins S, Baron D, Juarez G, et al: A review of ketamine abuse and diversion. Depress Anxiety 33(8):718–727, 2016 27328618

Sator-Katzenschlager S, Deusch E, Maier P, et al: The long-term antinociceptive effect of intrathecal S(+)-ketamine in a patient with established morphine tolerance. Anesth Analg 93(4):1032–1034, 2001 11574378

Sawynok J: Topical and peripheral ketamine as an analgesic. Anesth Analg 119(1):170–178, 2014 24945127

Schatzberg AF: Some comments on psychedelic research (editorial). Am J Psychiatry 177(5):368–369, 2020 32354267

Schenberg EE: Psychedelic-assisted psychotherapy: a paradigm shift in psychiatric research and development. Front Pharmacol 9:733, 2018 30026698

Schiefecker AJ, Beer R, Pfausler B, et al: Clusters of cortical spreading depolarizations in a patient with intracerebral hemorrhage: a multimodal neuromonitoring study. Neurocrit Care 22(2):293–298, 2015 25142825

Schifano F, Corkery J, Oyefeso A, et al: Trapped in the "K-hole": overview of deaths associated with ketamine misuse in the UK (1993–2006) (letter). J Clin Psychopharmacol 28(1):114–116, 2008 18204359

Schmechtig A, Lees J, Perkins A, et al: The effects of ketamine and risperidone on eye movement control in healthy volunteers. Transl Psychiatry 3(12):e334, 2013 24326395

Schmidt A, Bachmann R, Kometer M, et al: Mismatch negativity encoding of prediction errors predicts S-ketamine-induced cognitive impairments. Neuropsychopharmacology 37(4):865–875, 2012 22030715

Schönenberg M, Reichwald U, Domes G, et al: Effects of peritraumatic ketamine medication on early and sustained posttraumatic stress symptoms in moderately injured accident victims. Psychopharmacology (Berl) 182(3):420–425, 2005 16012867

Schönenberg M, Reichwald U, Domes G, et al: Ketamine aggravates symptoms of acute stress disorder in a naturalistic sample of accident victims. J Psychopharmacol 22(5):493–497, 2008 18208917

Schwartz T, Trunko ME, Feifel D, et al: A longitudinal case series of IM ketamine for patients with severe and enduring eating disorders and comorbid treatment-resistant depression. Clin Case Rep 9(5):e03869, 2021 34026123

Schwartzman RJ, Alexander GM, Grothusen JR, et al: Outpatient intravenous ketamine for the treatment of complex regional pain syndrome: a double-blind placebo controlled study. Pain 147(1–3):107–115, 2009 19783371

Schwenk ES, Viscusi ER, Buvanendran A, et al: Consensus guidelines on the use of intravenous ketamine infusions for acute pain management from the American Society of Regional Anesthesia and Pain Medicine, the American Academy of Pain Medicine, and the American Society of Anesthesiologists. Reg Anesth Pain Med 43(5):456–466, 2018a 29870457

Schwenk ES, Dayan AC, Rangavajjula A, et al: Ketamine for refractory headache: a retrospective analysis. Reg Anesth Pain Med 43(8):875–879, 2018b 29923953

Shahani R, Streutker C, Dickson B, Stewart RJ: Ketamine-associated ulcerative cystitis: a new clinical entity. Urology 69(5):810–812, 2007 17482909

Shahzad K, Suec A, Al-Koussayer O, et al: Analgesic ketamine use leading to cystectomy: a case report. Br J Med Surg Urol 5:188–191, 2012

Shapira Y, Artru AA, Lam AM: Ketamine decreases cerebral infarct volume and improves neurological outcome following experimental head trauma in rats. J Neurosurg Anesthesiol 4(4):231–240, 1992 15815471

Sharma LP, Thamby A, Balachander S, et al: Clinical utility of repeated intravenous ketamine treatment for resistant obsessive-compulsive disorder. Asian J Psychiatr 52:102183, 2020 32554207

Shcherbinin S, Doyle O, Zelaya FO, et al: Modulatory effects of ketamine, risperidone and lamotrigine on resting brain perfusion in healthy human subjects. Psychopharmacology (Berl) 232(21–22):4191–4204, 2015 26223493

Sheehy KA, Muller EA, Lippold C, et al: Subanesthetic ketamine infusions for the treatment of children and adolescents with chronic pain: a longitudinal study. BMC Pediatr 15:198, 2015 26620833

Shiroma PR, Albott CS, Johns B, et al: Neurocognitive performance and serial intravenous subanesthetic ketamine in treatment-resistant depression. Int J Neuropsychopharmacol 17(11):1805–1813, 2014 24963561

Shiroma P, McManos E, Voller E, et al: Repeated subanesthetic ketamine to enhance prolonged exposure therapy in post-traumatic stress disorder: a proof-of-concept study [Abstract]. Biol Psychiatry 87:s217, 2020a

Shiroma PR, Thuras P, Wels J, et al: A randomized, double-blind, active placebo-controlled study of efficacy, safety, and durability of repeated vs single subanesthetic ketamine for treatment-resistant depression. Transl Psychiatry 10(1):206, 2020b 32591498

Shiroma PR, Velit-Salazar MR, Vorobyov Y: A systematic review of neurocognitive effects of subanesthetic doses of intravenous ketamine in major depressive disorder, post-traumatic stress disorder, and healthy population. Clin Drug Investig 42(7):549–566, 2022 35672558

Siegel JS, Palanca BJA, Ances BM, et al: Prolonged ketamine infusion modulates limbic connectivity and induces sustained remission of treatment-resistant depression. Psychopharmacology (Berl) 238(4):1157–1169, 2021 33483802

Siegel RK: Phencyclidine and ketamine intoxication: a study of four populations of recreational users. NIDA Res Monogr 21(21):119–147, 1978 101865

Sigtermans MJ, van Hilten JJ, Bauer MCR, et al: Ketamine produces effective and long-term pain relief in patients with Complex Regional Pain Syndrome Type 1. Pain 145(3):304–311, 2009 19604642

Simon RP, Swan JH, Griffiths T, Meldrum BS: Blockade of N-methyl-D-aspartate receptors may protect against ischemic damage in the brain. Science 226(4676):850–852, 1984 6093256

Singh JB, Fedgchin M, Daly EJ, et al: A double-blind, randomized, placebo-controlled, dose-frequency study of intravenous ketamine in patients with treatment-resistant depression. Am J Psychiatry 173(8):816–826, 2016a 27056608

Singh JB, Fedgchin M, Daly E, et al: Intravenous esketamine in adult treatment-resistant depression: a double-blind, double-randomization, placebo-controlled study. Biol Psychiatry 80(6):424–431, 2016b 26707087

Singh JB, Fedgchin M, Daly EJ, Drevets WC: Relapse prevention in treatment-resistant major depressive disorder with rapid-acting antidepressants, in Rapid Acting Antidepressants. Edited by Duman RS, Krystal JH. Cambridge, MA, Elsevier (Academic Press), 2020, pp 237–259

Skolnick P, Layer RT, Popik P, et al: Adaptation of N-methyl-D-aspartate (NMDA) receptors following antidepressant treatment: implications for the pharmacotherapy of depression. Pharmacopsychiatry 29(1):23–26, 1996 8852530

Slikker W Jr, Zou X, Hotchkiss CE, et al: Ketamine-induced neuronal cell death in the perinatal rhesus monkey. Toxicol Sci 98(1):145–158, 2007 17426105

Smith DE: A clinical approach to the treatment of phencyclidine (PCP) abuse [proceedings]. Psychopharmacol Bull 16(4):67–70, 1980 7454943

Smith DE, Wesson DR: PCP abuse: diagnostic and psychopharmacological treatment approaches. J Psychedelic Drugs 12(3–4):293–299, 1980 7431428

Smith GS, Schloesser R, Brodie JD, et al: Glutamate modulation of dopamine measured in vivo with positron emission tomography (PET) and 11C-raclopride in normal human subjects. Neuropsychopharmacology 18(1):18–25, 1998 9408915

Smith-Apeldoorn SY, Veraart JKE, Spijker J, et al: Maintenance ketamine treatment for depression: a systematic review of efficacy, safety, and tolerability. Lancet Psychiatry 9(11):907–921, 2022 36244360

Snyder SH: Phencyclidine. Nature 285(5764):355–356, 1980 7189825

Sofia RD, Harakal JJ: Evaluation of ketamine HCl for anti-depressant activity. Arch Int Pharmacodyn Ther 214(1):68–74, 1975 1156026

Sörensen J, Bengtsson A, Bäckman E, et al: Pain analysis in patients with fibromyalgia. Effects of intravenous morphine, lidocaine, and ketamine. Scand J Rheumatol 24(6):360–365, 1995 8610220

Souza-Marques B, Telles M, Leal GC, et al: Esketamine for unipolar major depression with psychotic features: a retrospective chart review and comparison with nonpsychotic depression. J Clin Psychopharmacol 42(4):408–412, 2022 35727083

Steffens M, Becker B, Neumann C, et al: Effects of ketamine on brain function during smooth pursuit eye movements. Hum Brain Mapp 37(11):4047–4060, 2016 27342447

Steffens M, Neumann C, Kasparbauer A-M, et al: Effects of ketamine on brain function during response inhibition. Psychopharmacology (Berl) 235(12):3559–3571, 2018 30357437

Stevens C: Amino ketones. Abstr Pap Am Chem Soc 61:5569, 1964

Stone J, Erlandsson K, Arstad E, et al: Ketamine displacement of the NMDA ion channel SPET ligand [123I]CNS-1261 in vivo (abstract). Schizophr Bull 32(2):446, 2005

Stone JM, Erlandsson K, Årstad E, et al: Ketamine displaces the novel NMDA receptor SPET probe [(123)I]CNS-1261 in humans in vivo. Nucl Med Biol 33(2):239–243, 2006 16546678

Stone JM, Erlandsson K, Arstad E, et al: Relationship between ketamine-induced psychotic symptoms and NMDA receptor occupancy: a [(123)I]CNS-1261 SPET study. Psychopharmacology (Berl) 197(3):401–408, 2008 18176855

Stone JM, Abel KM, Allin MPG, et al: Ketamine-induced disruption of verbal self-monitoring linked to superior temporal activation. Pharmacopsychiatry 44(1):33–48, 2011 21154218

Stone JM, Pepper F, Fam J, et al: Glutamate, N-acetyl aspartate and psychotic symptoms in chronic ketamine users. Psychopharmacology (Berl) 231(10):2107–2116, 2014 24264567

Stone J, Kotoula V, Dietrich C, et al: Perceptual distortions and delusional thinking following ketamine administration are related to increased pharmacological MRI signal changes in the parietal lobe. J Psychopharmacol 29(9):1025–1028, 2015 26152321

Storr TM, Quibell R: Can ketamine prescribed for pain cause damage to the urinary tract? Palliat Med 23(7):670–672, 2009 19648225

Strong AJ, Fabricius M, Boutelle MG, et al: Spreading and synchronous depressions of cortical activity in acutely injured human brain. Stroke 33(12):2738–2743, 2002 12468763

Su T-P, Chen M-H, Li C-T, et al: Dose-related effects of adjunctive ketamine in Taiwanese patients with treatment-resistant depression. Neuropsychopharmacology 42(13):2482–2492, 2017 28492279

Tam YH, Ng CF, Wong YS, et al: Population-based survey of the prevalence of lower urinary tract symptoms in adolescents with and without psychotropic substance abuse. Hong Kong Med J 22(5):454–463, 2016 27516568

Tang WK, Liang HJ, Lau CG, et al: Relationship between cognitive impairment and depressive symptoms in current ketamine users. J Stud Alcohol Drugs 74(3):460–468, 2013 23490576

Tang WK, Morgan CJA, Lau GC, et al: Psychiatric morbidity in ketamine users attending counselling and youth outreach services. Subst Abus 36(1):67–74, 2015 25023206

Tavernor WD: A study of the effect of phencyclidine in the pig. Vet Rec 75(50):1377–1383, 1963

Taylor JH, Landeros-Weisenberger A, Coughlin C, et al: Ketamine for social anxiety disorder: a randomized, placebo-controlled crossover trial. Neuropsychopharmacology 43(2):325–333, 2018 28849779

Telles JPM, Welling LC, Coelho ACSDS, et al: Cortical spreading depolarization and ketamine: a short systematic review. Neurophysiol Clin 51(2):145–151, 2021 33610431

Thiebes S, Leicht G, Curic S, et al: Glutamatergic deficit and schizophrenia-like negative symptoms: new evidence from ketamine-induced mismatch negativity alterations in healthy male humans. J Psychiatry Neurosci 42(4):273–283, 2017 28556775

Tishler CL, Gordon LB: Ethical parameters of challenge studies inducing psychosis with ketamine. Ethics Behav 9(3):211–217, 1999 11657272

Trullas R, Skolnick P: Functional antagonists at the NMDA receptor complex exhibit antidepressant actions. Eur J Pharmacol 185(1):1–10, 1990 2171955

Truppman Lattie D, Nehoff H, Neehoff S, et al: Anxiolytic effects of acute and maintenance ketamine, as assessed by the Fear Questionnaire subscales and the Spielberger State Anxiety Rating Scale. J Psychopharmacol 35(2):137–141, 2021 32900266

Tung CK, Yeung SW, Chiang TP, et al: Reliability and validity of the Severity of Dependence Scale in a Chinese sample of treatment-seeking ketamine users. East Asian Arch Psychiatry 24(4):156–164, 2014 25482835

Turfus SC, Parkin MC, Cowan DA, et al: Use of human microsomes and deuterated substrates: an alternative approach for the identification of novel metabolites of ketamine by mass spectrometry. Drug Metab Dispos 37(8):1769–1778, 2009 19448136

Turkoz I, Lopena O, Salvadore G, et al: Treatment response to esketamine nasal spray in patients with major depressive disorder and acute suicidal ideation or behavior without evidence of early response: a pooled post hoc analysis of ASPIRE. CNS Spectr 1–7, 2022 35904046

Turner DM: The Essential Psychedelic Guide. San Francisco, CA, Panther Press, 1994

Turner EH: Esketamine for treatment-resistant depression: seven concerns about efficacy and FDA approval. Lancet Psychiatry 6(12):977–979, 2019 31680014

Uhlhaas PJ, Millard I, Muetzelfeldt L, et al: Perceptual organization in ketamine users: preliminary evidence of deficits on night of drug use but not 3 days later. J Psychopharmacol 21(3):347–352, 2007 17591661

Umbricht D, Schmid L, Koller R, et al: Ketamine-induced deficits in auditory and visual context-dependent processing in healthy volunteers: implications for models of cognitive deficits in schizophrenia. Arch Gen Psychiatry 57(12):1139–1147, 2000 11115327

Umbricht D, Koller R, Vollenweider FX, Schmid L: Mismatch negativity predicts psychotic experiences induced by NMDA receptor antagonist in healthy volunteers. Biol Psychiatry 51(5):400–406, 2002 11904134

U.S. Food and Drug Administration: Ketalar prescribing information. Available at: https://www.accessdata.fda.gov/drugsatfda_docs/label/2018/016812s040lbl.pdf. Accessed January 12, 2024.

Van Harreveld A: Compounds in brain extracts causing spreading depression of cerebral cortical activity and contraction of crustacean muscle. J Neurochem 3(4):300–315, 1959 13642064

Veen C, Jacobs G, Philippens I, Vermetten E: Subanesthetic dose ketamine in posttraumatic stress disorder: a role for reconsolidation during trauma-focused psychotherapy? Curr Topics Behav Neurosci 38:137–162, 2018

Veraart JKE, Smith-Apeldoorn SY, Spijker J, et al: Ketamine treatment for depression in patients with a history of psychosis or current psychotic symptoms: a systematic review. J Clin Psychiatry 82(4):20r13459, 2021

Vernaleken I, Klomp M, Moeller O, et al: Vulnerability to psychotogenic effects of ketamine is associated with elevated D2/3-receptor availability. Int J Neuropsychopharmacol 16:745–754, 2013 22906553

Vincent JP, Kartalovski B, Geneste P, et al: Interaction of phencyclidine ("angel dust") with a specific receptor in rat brain membranes. Proc Natl Acad Sci USA 76(9):4678–4682, 1979 41247

Virtue RW, Alanis JM, Mori M, et al: An anesthetic agent: 2-orthochlorophenyl, 2-methylamino cyclohexanone HCl (CI-581). Anesthesiology 28(5):823–833, 1967 6035012

Vollenweider FX, Leenders KL, Scharfetter C, et al: Metabolic hyperfrontality and psychopathology in the ketamine model of psychosis using positron emission tomography (PET) and [18F]fluorodeoxyglucose (FDG). Eur Neuropsychopharmacol 7(1):9–24, 1997a 9088881

Vollenweider FX, Leenders KL, Øye I, et al: Differential psychopathology and patterns of cerebral glucose utilisation produced by (S)- and (R)-ketamine in healthy volunteers using positron emission tomography (PET). Eur Neuropsychopharmacol 7(1):25–38, 1997b 9088882

Vollenweider FX, Vontobel P, Øye I, et al: Effects of (S)-ketamine on striatal dopamine: a [11C]raclopride PET study of a model psychosis in humans. J Psychiatr Res 34(1):35–43, 2000 10696831

Von der Brelie C, Seifert M, Rot S, et al: Sedation of patients with acute aneurysmal subarachnoid hemorrhage with ketamine is safe and might influence the occurrence of cerebral infarctions associated with delayed cerebral ischemia. World Neurosurg 97:374–382, 2017 27742511

Vondruska JF: Phencyclidine anesthesia in baboons. J Am Vet Med Assoc 147(10):1073–1074, 1965 4956237

Wajs E, Aluisio L, Holder R, et al: Esketamine nasal spray plus oral antidepressant in patients with treatment-resistant depression: assessment of long-term safety in a phase 3, open-label study (SUSTAIN-2). J Clin Psychiatry 81(3):19m12891, 2020

Walker MC, Howard RS, Smith SJ, et al: Diagnosis and treatment of status epilepticus on a neurological intensive care unit. QJM 89(12):913–920, 1996 9015485

Wang C, Zheng D, Xu J, et al: Brain damages in ketamine addicts as revealed by magnetic resonance imaging. Front Neuroanat 7(23):23, 2013 23882190

Wang L-J, Chen C-K, Lin S-K, et al: Cognitive profile of ketamine-dependent patients compared with methamphetamine-dependent patients and healthy controls. Psychopharmacology (Berl) 235(7):2113–2121, 2018a 29713787

Wang L-J, Chen M-Y, Lin C-Y, et al: Difference in long-term relapse rates between youths with ketamine use and those with stimulants use. Subst Abuse Treat Prev Policy 13(1):50, 2018b 30577882

Warner DO, Zaccariello MJ, Katusic SK, et al: Neuropsychological and behavioral outcomes after exposure of young children to procedures requiring general anesthesia: the Mayo Anesthesia Safety in Kids (MASK) study. Anesthesiology 129(1):89–105, 2018 29672337

Warner DO, Chelonis JJ, Paule MG, et al: Performance on the Operant Test Battery in young children exposed to procedures requiring general anaesthesia: the MASK study. Br J Anaesth 122(4):470–479, 2019 30857603

Watson TD, Petrakis IL, Edgecombe J, et al: Modulation of the cortical processing of novel and target stimuli by drugs affecting glutamate and GABA neurotransmission. Int J Neuropsychopharmacol 12(3):357–370, 2009 18771605

Webster LR, Walker MJ: Safety and efficacy of prolonged outpatient ketamine infusions for neuropathic pain. Am J Ther 13(4):300–305, 2006 16858163

Wei Y, Chang L, Hashimoto K: Molecular mechanisms underlying the antidepressant actions of arketamine: beyond the NMDA receptor. Mol Psychiatry 27(1):559–573, 2022 33963284

Weiler MA, Thaker GK, Lahti AC, Tamminga CA: Ketamine effects on eye movements. Neuropsychopharmacology 23(6):645–653, 2000 11063920

Whitaker R, Kong D: Testing Takes Toll. Boston Globe. November 15:A1, 1998

White PF, Ham J, Way WL, Trevor AJ: Pharmacology of ketamine isomers in surgical patients. Anesthesiology 52(3):231–239, 1980 6989292

White PF, Schüttler J, Shafer A, et al: Comparative pharmacology of the ketamine isomers. Studies in volunteers. Br J Anaesth 57(2):197–203, 1985 3970799

Whittaker E, Dadabayev AR, Joshi SA, Glue P: Systematic review and meta-analysis of randomized controlled trials of ketamine in the treatment of refractory anxiety spectrum disorders. Ther Adv Psychopharmacol 11:20451253211056743, 2021 34925757

Widman AJ, McMahon LL: Effects of ketamine and other rapidly acting antidepressants on hippocampal excitatory and inhibitory transmission, in Rapid Acting Antidepressants. Edited by Duncan RS, Krystal JH. Boston, Elsevier (ScienceDirect), 2020, pp 3–41

Wilkins LK, Girard TA, Cheyne JA: Ketamine as a primary predictor of out-of-body experiences associated with multiple substance use. Conscious Cogn 20(3):943–950, 2011 21324714

Wilkinson ST, Farmer C, Ballard ED, et al: Impact of midazolam vs. saline on effect size estimates in controlled trials of ketamine as a rapid-acting antidepressant. Neuropsychopharmacology 44(7):1233–1238, 2019 30653192

Wilkinson ST, Rhee TG, Joormann J, et al: Cognitive behavioral therapy to sustain the antidepressant effects of ketamine in treatment-resistant depression: a randomized clinical trial. Psychother Psychosom 90(5):318–327, 2021 34186531

Williams NR, Heifets BD, Bentzley BS, et al: Attenuation of antidepressant and antisuicidal effects of ketamine by opioid receptor antagonism. Mol Psychiatry 24(12):1779–1786, 2019 31467392

Williamson DJ, Gogate JP, Kern Sliwa JK, et al: Longitudinal course of adverse events with esketamine nasal spray: a post hoc analysis of pooled data from phase 3 trials in patients with treatment-resistant depression. J Clin Psychiatry 83(6):21m14318, 2022

Wilson JA, Nimmo AF, Fleetwood-Walker SM, Colvin LA: A randomised double blind trial of the effect of pre-emptive epidural ketamine on persistent pain after lower limb amputation. Pain 135(1–2):108–118, 2008 17583431

Wink LK, Reisinger DL, Horn P, et al: Intranasal ketamine in adolescents and young adults with autism spectrum disorder—initial results of a randomized, controlled, crossover, pilot study. J Autism Dev Disord 51(4):1392–1399, 2021 32642957

Winter H, Irle E: Hippocampal volume in adult burn patients with and without posttraumatic stress disorder. Am J Psychiatry 161(12):2194–2200, 2004 15569889

Wolfson P, Hartelius G (eds): The Ketamine Papers: Science, Therapy, and Transformation. Santa Cruz, CA, Multidisciplinary Association for Psychedelic Studies, 2016

Wong GL-H, Tam Y-H, Ng C-F, et al: Liver injury is common among chronic abusers of ketamine. Clin Gastroenterol Hepatol 12(10):1759–62.e1, 2014 24534547

World Health Organization: Model List of Essential Medicines. World Health Organization, 2024. Available at: https://list.essentialmeds.org/. Accessed February 19, 2024.

Wu P, Wang Q, Huang Z, et al: Clinical staging of ketamine-associated urinary dysfunction: a strategy for assessment and treatment. World J Urol 34(9):1329–1336, 2016 26803767

Xu K, Krystal JH, Ning Y, et al: Preliminary analysis of positive and negative syndrome scale in ketamine-associated psychosis in comparison with schizophrenia. J Psychiatr Res 61:64–72, 2015 25560772

Xu Y, Hackett M, Carter G, et al: Effects of low-dose and very low-dose ketamine among patients with major depression: a systematic review and meta-analysis. Int J Neuropsychopharmacol 19(4):1–15, 2016 26578082

Yanagihara Y, Ohtani M, Kariya S, et al: Plasma concentration profiles of ketamine and norketamine after administration of various ketamine preparations to healthy Japanese volunteers. Biopharm Drug Dispos 24(1):37–43, 2003 12516077

Yang C, Shirayama Y, Zhang JC, et al: R-ketamine: a rapid-onset and sustained antidepressant without psychotomimetic side effects. Transl Psychiatry 5(9):e632, 2015 26327690

Yang C, Qu Y, Abe M, et al: (R)-Ketamine shows greater potency and longer lasting antidepressant effects than its metabolite (2R, 6R)-hydroxynorketamine. Biol Psychiatry 82(5):e43–e44, 2017 28104224

Yee C-H, Lai PT, Lee W-M, et al: Clinical outcome of a prospective case series of patients with ketamine cystitis who underwent standardized treatment protocol. Urology 86(2):236–243, 2015 26199162

Yoon G, Petrakis IL, Krystal JH: Association of combined naltrexone and ketamine with depressive symptoms in a case series of patients with depression and alcohol use disorder (letter). JAMA Psychiatry 76(3):337–338, 2019 30624551

Young FA: Refraction of the monkey eye under general anesthesia. Vision Res 61:331–339, 1963 14168300

Yu W-L, Cho CC-M, Lung PF-C, et al: Ketamine-related cholangiopathy: a retrospective study on clinical and imaging findings. Abdom Imaging 39(6):1241–1246, 2014 24934474

Yurgelun-Todd DA, Renshaw PF, Goldsmith P, et al: A randomized, placebo-controlled, phase 1 study to evaluate the effects of TAK-063 on ketamine-induced changes in fMRI BOLD signal in healthy subjects. Psychopharmacology (Berl) 237(2):317–328, 2020 31773211

Zanos P, Moaddel R, Morris PJ, et al: NMDAR inhibition-independent antidepressant actions of ketamine metabolites. Nature 533(7604):481–486, 2016 27144355

Zanos P, Moaddel R, Morris PJ, et al: Ketamine and ketamine metabolite pharmacology: insights into therapeutic mechanisms. Pharmacol Rev 70(3):621–660, 2018 29945898

Zanza C, Piccolella F, Racca F, et al: Ketamine in acute brain injury: current opinion following cerebral circulation and electrical activity. Healthcare (Basel) 10(3):566, 2022 35327044

Zarate CA Jr, Singh JB, Carlson PJ, et al: A randomized trial of an N-methyl-D-aspartate antagonist in treatment-resistant major depression. Arch Gen Psychiatry 63(8):856–864, 2006 16894061

Zarate CA Jr, Brutsche NE, Ibrahim L, et al: Replication of ketamine's antidepressant efficacy in bipolar depression: a randomized controlled add-on trial. Biol Psychiatry 71(11):939–946, 2012a 22297150

Zarate CA Jr, Brutsche N, Laje G, et al: Relationship of ketamine's plasma metabolites with response, diagnosis, and side effects in major depression. Biol Psychiatry 72(4):331–338, 2012b 22516044

Zeiler FA, West M: Ketamine for status epilepticus: Canadian physician views and time to push forward. Can J Neurol Sci 42(2):132–134, 2015 25736810

Zeiler FA, Teitelbaum J, Gillman LM, West M: NMDA antagonists for refractory seizures. Neurocrit Care 20(3):502–513, 2014 24519081

Zekry O, Gibson SB, Aggarwal A: Subanesthetic, subcutaneous ketamine infusion therapy in the treatment of chronic nonmalignant pain. J Pain Palliat Care Pharmacother 30(2):91–98, 2016 27092576

Zeng MC, Niciu MJ, Luckenbaugh DA, et al: Acute stress symptoms do not worsen in posttraumatic stress disorder and abuse with a single subanesthetic dose of ketamine (letter). Biol Psychiatry 73(12):e37–e38, 2013 23245747

Zhang C, Tang WK, Liang HJ, et al: Other drug use does not impact cognitive impairments in chronic ketamine users. Drug Alcohol Depend 186:1–8, 2018 29518690

Zhang JC, Li SX, Hashimoto K: R (-)-ketamine shows greater potency and longer lasting antidepressant effects than S (+)-ketamine. Pharmacol Biochem Behav 116:137–141, 2014a 24316345

Zhang JC, Yao W, Hashimoto K: Arketamine, a new rapid-acting antidepressant: a historical review and future directions. Neuropharmacology 218:109219, 2022 35977629

Zhang MWB, Ho RCM: Controversies on the effect of ketamine on cognition. Front Psychiatry 7:47, 2016 27065891

Zhang Y, Xu Z, Zhang S, et al: Profiles of psychiatric symptoms among amphetamine type stimulant and ketamine using inpatients in Wuhan, China. J Psychiatr Res 53:99–102, 2014b 24613031

Zhao J, Wang Y, Wang D: The effect of ketamine infusion in the treatment of complex regional pain syndrome: a systemic review and meta-analysis. Curr Pain Headache Rep 22(2):12, 2018 29404715

Zorumski CF, Izumi Y, Mennerick S: Ketamine: NMDA receptors and beyond. J Neurosci 36(44):11158–11164, 2016 27807158

Zukin SR, Zukin RS: Specific [3H]phencyclidine binding in rat central nervous system. Proc Natl Acad Sci USA 76(10):5372–5376, 1979 291953

Index

Page numbers printed in **boldface** type refer to figures and tables.